Attachment in Adults

Attachment in Adults

Clinical and Developmental Perspectives

Edited by

MICHAEL B. SPERLING
Fairleigh Dickinson University

WILLIAM H. BERMAN
Fordham University

Foreword by Robert S. Weiss

1994

THE GUILFORD PRESS
New York   London

Printed in the United States of America

This book is printed on acid-free paper.

Last digit is print number: 9 8 7 6 5 4 3 2 1

Library of Congress Cataloging-in-Publication Data
Attachment in adults: clinical and developmental perspectives /
edited by Michael B. Sperling, William H. Berman; foreword by
Robert S. Weiss.
        p.   cm.
Includes bibliographical references and index.
ISBN 0-89862-547-5
    1. Attachment behavior.   2. Adulthood—Psychological aspects.
I. Sperling, Michael B., 1957-   . II. Berman, William H., 1954-
[DNLM: 1. Object Attachment.   WM 460.6.02 A883 1994]
BF575.A86A79   1994
155.6—dc20
DNLM/DLC
for Library of Congress   94-2524
                                                                CIP

Contributors

Kenneth S. Adam, MD, FRCP(C), Department of Psychiatry, McMaster University, Hamilton, Ontario, Canada

Toni C. Antonucci, PhD, Institute for Social Research, University of Michigan, Ann Arbor, Michigan

Joanna Batgos, MS, Department of Psychology, Yale University, New Haven, Connecticut

Ellen Raynes Berman, PsyD, Wilkins Center for Eating Disorders, Stamford, Connecticut

William H. Berman, PhD, Department of Psychology, Fordham University, Bronx, New York; Department of Psychology (Psychiatry), New York Hospital–Cornell Medical Center, White Plains, New York

Sidney J. Blatt, PhD, Departments of Psychiatry and Psychology, Yale University, New Haven, Connecticut

Maria L. Boccia, PhD, Department of Psychiatry, University of Colorado Health Sciences Center, Denver, Colorado

Sherrilyn Coffman, DNS, Division of Nursing, Florida Atlantic University, Boca Raton, Florida

Diana Diamond, PhD, Doctoral Program in Clinical Psychology, City University of New York, New York, New York; Department of Psychology (Psychiatry), New York Hospital–Cornell Medical Center, White Plains, New York

Judith A. Feeney, PhD, Department of Psychology, University of Queensland, Brisbane, Queensland, Australia

Nathalie Guacci-Franco, MS, Department of Psychology, Florida International University, North Miami, Florida

Mary Hanrahan, Department of Psychology, University of Queensland, Brisbane, Queensland, Australia; present address: Griffith University, Brisbane, Queensland, Australia

Carl G. Hindy, PhD, Private Practice, Nashua, New Hampshire

Adrienne Keller, PhD, Department of Psychiatry, University of Virginia, Charlottesville, Virginia

Bonnie J. Leadbeater, PhD, Department of Psychology, Yale University, New Haven, Connecticut

Mary J. Levitt, PhD, Department of Psychology, Florida International University, North Miami, Florida

Stephen C. Loveless, PhD (Deceased), Department of Public Administration, Florida International University, North Miami, Florida

Lisa Sandow Lyons, Department of Psychology, Fairleigh Dickinson University, Teaneck, New Jersey

Lauren Marcus, MS, Department of Psychology, Fordham University, Bronx, New York

Patricia Noller, PhD, Department of Psychology, University of Queensland, Brisbane, Queensland, Australia

Gordon Parker, MD, PhD, FRANZCP, School of Psychiatry, University of New South Wales, Sydney, Australia

Martin Reite, MD, Department of Psychiatry, University of Colorado Health Sciences Center, Denver, Colorado

Julie C. Rothbard, Department of Psychology, State University of New York at Buffalo, Buffalo, New York

J. Conrad Schwarz, PhD, Department of Psychology, University of Connecticut, Storrs, Connecticut

Phillip R. Shaver, PhD, Department of Psychology, University of California at Davis, Davis, California

Michael B. Sperling, PhD, Department of Psychology, Fairleigh Dickinson University, Teaneck, New Jersey; Department of Psychology (Psychiatry) (Visiting), New York Hospital–Cornell Medical Center, White Plains, New York

Robert S. Weiss, PhD, Work and Family Research Unit, University of Massachusetts at Boston, Boston, Massachusetts

Malcolm West, PhD, Department of Psychiatry, University of Calgary, Calgary, Alberta, Canada

Acknowledgments

So many people in our professional and personal lives have contributed to our interest in attachment theory and research that it is difficult to remember and credit everyone sufficiently. Teachers and supervisors who have influenced our thinking in attachment theory include Sidney Blatt, Harold Raush, Jerome L. Singer, and Kenneth Talan. Numerous colleagues, many of whom are represented in this book, have influenced our formulations and methods regarding attachment theory and therapy; our thanks go to these colleagues and to all the authors for making this work possible. In addition, the Psychoanalytic Study Group at Yale University provided the foundation for critical thinking in psychoanalytic, object relations, and attachment theory for William H. Berman, as did contemporaries and faculty at the University of Massachusetts at Amherst for Michael B. Sperling. Nancy Busch deserves appreciation for administrative and financial support at Fordham University.

Our undergraduate and graduate students have provided many vital and thoughtful contributions—new ideas, fresh perspectives, and ample legwork. Those particularly deserving of mention include Alex Barsdorf, Glenn Fagen, Pamela Foelsch, Glenn Heiss, Lisa Lyons, Lauren Marcus, Nicholas Radcliffe, and Valerie White.

Our patients, too, have had an enormous influence on our understanding of attachment. Through both their engagement and their resistance, they have taught us as much about the experience of attachment as the research foundation we operate within.

Kitty Moore, our editor at The Guilford Press, also deserves much thanks for her enthusiasm and skillful help with this book. She kept us on track, and provided a keen psychological sensibility that helped to move the book to a successful completion.

Finally, one's family usually contributes in some measure to a project such as this. In this case, our families have unusual significance as being both supports for our work and also critical foundations in the development and understanding of our own adult attachments. To our parents, and especially to our wives (Priscilla Fishler Sperling and Ellen Raynes Berman) and our children (Katherine Sperling and Daniel Berman), we offer our ongoing appreciation and enduring attachment.

MICHAEL B. SPERLING
WILLIAM H. BERMAN

Foreword

John Bowlby's wife, Ursula, told me that in 1951, when her husband completed his report for the World Health Organization on the close connection between maternal care and children's mental health (Bowlby, 1951), she asked him to what subject he would now turn his attention. She said that he answered, in his quiet way, "I think this topic might do for my lifetime." And indeed, with absolutely unwavering focus, Bowlby did devote a lifetime of research from a base in the Tavistock Institute and Clinic in London to understanding the emotional and behavioral systems that link children to their parents: their nature; the ways in which they are expressed and governed; their functions for the children; and the consequences for the children of interruption or loss of parental relationships.

Bowlby incorporated in his work whatever might advance understanding: evolutionary thought, ethological findings, and the insights of psychoanalysis. Always, he tested his developing theories against the reports of patients whom he was treating, the observations made by his colleagues, and, to a lesser extent, his own observations, of parents and children. Toward the end of his career, Bowlby presented his findings and theories in a magisterial three-volume work, *Attachment and Loss* (Bowlby, 1969, 1973, 1980). Alan Sroufe, writing in 1986 for a review of the preceding three decades of research in child development, said of *Attachment and Loss*, "[It] may well be judged by historians to be the most significant psychological work to appear during this period" (p. 841).

The chapters of *Attachment in Adults* show how fruitful Bowlby's work has been. They show how much his ideas, as further developed by talented students and colleagues and by their students and colleagues, have produced extraordinary advances in our understanding of affective life in adulthood as well as childhood.

Bowlby's theory of attachment had at its core the belief that, as a consequence of evolutionary processes, children are equipped with emotional and behavioral systems that impel them to establish proximity with caretakers (ordinarily their parents) when the children feel threatened or disturbed, or when they are for any reason concerned about the accessibility of the caretakers. For Bowlby, parental accessibility is children's primary source of security, and parental responsiveness is children's primary guide to development. Bowlby argued that the children's internalized representations of their parents and of the children's own selves—their "internal working models"—become anticipations that guide their relationships with their parents and others. The ability of children to move into a world with confidence, and to display initiative and independence, is largely dependent on the children's having learned to value themselves as the deserving recipients of their parents' caring attentiveness.

It was the inspiration of Mary Ainsworth, a younger colleague of Bowlby's, to classify children by the quality of their internal working models as these were displayed in the children's attitude toward attachment figures (Ainsworth, Blehar, Waters, & Wall, 1978). Ainsworth arranged for children to be brought into a strange situation—a laboratory room, glassed on one side, toys in a corner—where they were exposed to a graded series of mild disturbances that culminated in the brief departure of the parents who had brought them. On the basis of observations of the children's reactions to the parents' return, Ainsworth developed a typology that has become fundamental to thinking about individual attachment styles. Most children, she reported, reacted in a way she and her students could characterize as "secure." Some, however, displayed persisting anxiety and seemed fearful of further parental departures; others, although just as upset, seemed to deny the need for their parents' presence. This categorizing of children's attachment styles provided a foundation for work on the way in which parental behavior affected children, and on the different implications of secure and insecure attachment styles for the children's further functioning.

Although his own work was focused mostly on children and their relationships to their parents, Bowlby believed that attachment theory is not only a theory of child development. On a number of occasions he insisted that attachment phenomena are lifelong. For some time, however, work on "adult attachment" was slow and scattered. In 1969, about 10 years after Ainsworth began her observations of mothers and children in what was now known as the "Strange Situation," Colin Parkes, working with Bowlby, showed that attachment strivings similar to those of children were displayed by grieving adults (Parkes, 1969). His may have been the first empirical study to suggest just how attachment phenomena might appear in the lives of adults. A few years later, I showed that attachment strivings could also explain the desperation of loneliness and the confusion of divorce (Weiss, 1974, 1975). A few investigators, influenced by Bowlby, had begun work on the later-life consequences of having lost a parent in childhood, and one or two others were studying attachment phenomena in ongoing adult relationships, particularly marriage. Notable among these early investigators of adult attachment were Kenneth Adam, Gordon Parker, and William Berman, all contributors to this volume. But for the most part, until the middle of the 1980s, attachment studies considered only small children's attachments to their parents.

A major impetus to work in the area of adult attachment was the development of methods and concepts for studying attachment styles in adults. Just as Ainsworth's identification of attachment styles in children made it possible for psychologists to study in a comparative fashion the determinants and consequences of children's internal working models, so Cindy Hazan and Phillip Shaver's (1987) self-rating instrument for categorizing adult attachment styles made possible similar research with adults. Also, at about the same time as Hazan and Shaver presented their self-rating instrument, Mary Main and her students (Main, Kaplan, & Cassidy, 1985) developed a method for assessing adult attachment styles from transcripts of interviews. Their approach was to treat the interview materials as samples of cognitive functioning in the area of attachment relationships. They showed that the scores parents received on this test corresponded closely to the attachment styles of their children. The startling and impressive nature of their findings may have done as much as their test procedure—which is difficult to administer and score—to foster research interest in the area of adult attachment.

As the chapters in this volume demonstrate, work on adult attachment is now proceeding actively in several areas. These areas include the study of the attachment relationships of adult life; the contribution of early and current attachment experience to psychopathology in adults; the application of research findings to therapeutic interventions; and the physiological substructure of attachment in adults as well as in children. A brief overview of findings in these areas may suggest how fruitful work in adult attachment has already proven to be.

A central issue in the study of the attachment relationships of adult life must certainly be people's courtship behavior and mating—the way in which people establish and maintain the primary emotional partnerships of adult life. Chapters in this volume report work demonstrating that attachment style affects not only anticipations of success in courtship, but also tendencies toward jealousy and tendencies toward romantic obsession. Also in this volume, Berman and his colleagues describe their work with established marital pairs, including use of a test situation modeled on the Strange Situation. In Berman's test situation, one marital partner briefly leaves the room and then after a brief absence returns to his or her seat. Berman reports that at that point the partner who has remained in the room, if avoidant, actually leans away from the returned partner. Presumably, an anxious/ambivalent partner would somehow seek reassurance from the returned partner.

Within the domain of adult psychopathology, two particular areas are illuminated by chapters in this volume: the area of suicidal ideation and impulse, and the area of ordinary depression. In the first, Adam describes his effort to identify the genesis of the suicidal impulse in adolescents and adults. His early work led him to question the rather simplisitc hypothesis that childhood loss in itself potentiates later suicidal impulse. He now reports that absent or rejecting attachment relationships of any sort (not just experiences of loss), augmented by a chaotic living situation, set the stage for later suicidal ideation and behavior. Now he and his colleagues are going forward to develop methods for identifying young people at risk of suicidal impulse. In equally systematic fashion, Parker has explored the linkage between attachment experience and depression. In his chapter he reports that there are at least two forms of depression: one linked to attachment experiences, and presumably psychogenic; the other independent of attachment experiences, and presumably genetic in origin. Certainly this research must prove valuable to those who must prescribe for the depressed.

The chapter by Sperling and Lyons describes applications of the concepts and findings of adult attachment research in psychotherapy. In particular, they have found that attention to attachment issues arising in a patient's ongoing life can prove useful, even when the patient may not tolerate examination of transference issues. It might be noted, although Sperling and Lyons do not make this explicit in their chapter, how much attachment ideas have illuminated the notion of "transference"—the tendency to introduce into current relationships (especially, but not only, therapeutic encounters) emotional themes developed in childhood experience. Now it is possible to recognize that the persisting anticipation of certain developments in attachment relationships is the agency of transference.

Both Bowlby and Ainsworth believed that attachment served physiological functions, at the least regulating those physiological systems associated with security and insecurity. Reite and his colleagues have reported, on the basis of their search for the physiological substructures of attachment, that the regulatory functions of attachment extend to circadian rhythms. Their research gives further content to an observation sometimes made—that adult partners who maintain a well-functioning relationship of attachment describe themselves as "in tune" with each other or "on the same wavelength." Perhaps such pairs are quite literally in tune, in ways we are just beginning to recognize.

If much has been accomplished, there is much more still to be done. Concepts must be further clarified; a good many empirical questions require further exploration; and it may well be that measures can profitably be further developed.

What may be the central concept of attachment theory—the internal working model—is patently a metaphor. Much more work is needed to specify just what it is that produces the persistence of attachment style. It may be that what is responsible is neither as cognitive nor as coherent as the term "internal working model" suggests; it may be, for example, that a cascade of feelings occurs when people enter situations that bear emotional likeness to earlier situations, and those feelings (of need, hurt, or fear) trigger behavior sequences (see the discussion in Bretherton, Ridgeway, & Cassidy, 1990). We need the kind of work on internal working models that is being done on the visual and auditory systems—work that will identify pathways and processes.

In addition, there is a great deal to be learned about the functioning of the attachment relationships of adult life. I look forward to reading, in a few years, reports from studies of partner choice as a function of attachment style, and of the particular marital difficulties that accompany particular pairings of attachment styles. I hope work will also be done on the processes through which adult attachments are relinquished; perhaps this research will be conducted by people involved in grief counseling. Work is needed on the ways in which parental functioning expresses the parents' own attachment experiences, and the processes by which this comes about. And it would be good if we could learn how to help parents be good parents, whatever the nature of their own developmental experiences.

In work on adult psychopathology, I anticipate that attachment experience will prove to be linked to other psychopathologies in addition to those of suicidal impulse and depression. I think that the pathologies of anxiety, such as panic states and phobias, will be especially likely to prove linked to attachment experience. But others of the psychoneuroses and character disorders may also prove easier to understand when recast as disorders of attachment relationships.

Although adult attachment theory is already of enormous value for our understanding of ourselves, I believe it to be still in an early stage of development. As one expression of this, all the authors in this volume write from active research enterprises, and many of the chapters are presented as progress reports rather than final statements. What we now know is surely only the beginning. And yet, how much we have already learned.

The field of psychology quite regularly witnesses the advent of a bright idea whose ultimate yield turns out to be a series of ingenious tests of trivial hypotheses. What we see in this volume is very different. We see here research on the fundamental experiences of human life, including courtship and marriage; the determinants of resilience and of depression; and the vulnerability of some among the unhappy to suicidal ideation and action. Every topic discussed has been illuminated by attachment theory, so that we come away from each discussion with a deeper and surer understanding. The fact that study of the attachment system and its expressions should lead to chapters of the richness and scope of those included here is testimony to the fundamental importance of the attachment system for human functioning. This book establishes that if we are to have a social psychology worthy of the name—one that deals adequately with the sources and consequences of social behavior—it must give a central place to the study of attachment.

I was not as close to John Bowlby as were many others, nor as I wish I had been. I was a member of his seminar for 6 months in 1971. When I came to take my leave of him, before I departed from the Tavistock, we sat and talked through the afternoon. Although I saw him several times afterwards, we were perhaps closest at that moment. He said, then, that sometimes people find each other only at a point of departure. He also said that he regretted being marginal—as he then, for a time, was—to the world of English psychoanalysis. "But," he went on, referring to the colleagues who had distanced themselves from him, "when people stake their careers, and how they have affected other people's lives, on a particular world view, they can hardly relinquish it only because better data have become available."

This book presents, among much else, still more of the "better data" that John Bowlby so valued. The book would have pleased him.

ROBERT S. WEISS

REFERENCES

Ainsworth, M. D. S., Blehar, M. C., Waters, E., & Wall, S. (1978). *Patterns of attachment: A psychological study of the Strange Situation.* Hillsdale, NJ: Erlbaum.

Bowlby, J. (1951). *Maternal care and mental health.* Geneva: World Health Organization.

Bowlby, J. (1969). *Attachment and loss: Vol. 1. Attachment.* New York: Basic Books.

Bowlby, J. (1973). *Attachment and loss: Vol. 2. Separation: Anxiety and anger.* New York: Basic Books.

Bowlby, J. (1980). *Attachment and loss: Vol. 3. Loss: Sadness and depression.* New York: Basic Books.

Bretherton, I., Ridgeway, D., & Cassidy, J. (1990). Assessing internal working models of the attachment relationship: An attachment story completion task for three-year-olds. In M. T. Greenberg, D. Cicchetti, & E. M. Cummings (Eds.), *Attachment in the preschool years: Theory, research, and intervention* (pp. 273–308). Chicago: University of Chicago Press.

Hazan, C., & Shaver, P. R. (1987). Romantic love conceptualized as an attachment process. *Journal of Personality and Social Psychology, 52,* 511-524.

Main, M., Kaplan, N., & Cassidy, J. (1985). Security in infancy, childhood, and adulthood: A move to the level of representation. In I. Bretherton & E. Waters (Eds.), *Growing points of attachment theory and research. Monographs of the Society for Research in Child Development, 50*(1–2, Serial No. 209), 66–104.

Parkes, C. M. (1969). Separation anxiety: An aspect of the search for a lost object. In M. H. Lader (Ed.), *Studies of anxiety* (*British Journal of Psychiatry* Special Publication No. 3; pp. 87–92). Ashford, Kent: Headley Bros.

Sroufe, L. A. (1986). Appraisal: Bowlby's contribution to psychoanalytic theory and developmental psychology: Attachment, separation, loss. *Journal of Child Psychology and Psychiatry, 27*(6), 841–849.

Weiss, R. S. (1974). *Loneliness: The experience of emotional and social isolation.* Cambridge, MA: MIT Press.

Weiss, R. S. (1975). *Marital separation.* New York: Basic Books.

Contents

xvii

PART I

Introduction

CHAPTER 1

The Structure and Function of Adult Attachment

WILLIAM H. BERMAN
MICHAEL B. SPERLING

The study of attachment began as research into the earliest developmental origins of childhood and adult psychopathology, with John Bowlby's (1960) work at the Tavistock Clinic. This model represented a break from traditional psychoanalytic conceptualizations and investigations, both in its emphasis on prospective study and in its attention to the link between parental separation/loss and later emotional disturbances (1969, 1982a). From the beginning, however, Bowlby's overall goal was to understand "the adverse influences on personality development of inadequate maternal care during early childhood . . . [when] young children . . . [are] separated from those they know and love" (Bowlby, 1988b, p. 21).

Mary Ainsworth's involvement in Bowlby's research group altered the course of study of attachment, bringing to it experimental research methodologies and a child development orientation (Ainsworth, 1973; Ainsworth, Blehar, Waters, & Wall, 1978). Her work at Johns Hopkins University and the University of Virginia resulted in a generation of researchers committed to studying attachment as a normal developmental process in infants and young children (see Erickson, Sroufe, & Egeland, 1985; Main, Kaplan, & Cassidy, 1985). The empirical basis of attachment was considered to lie in mother–infant interactions and in Ainsworth's explicit emphasis on observable, quantifiable childhood behavior. In particular, attachment was defined in terms of the behavior exhibited by children in the Strange Situation, a laboratory recreation of the separation–reunion process. As a result, attachment theory in the United States was explored largely as a theory of social–emotional development in children, rather than as an exploration of the etiology of adult emotional disorders. In addition, attachment theory was largely rejected by mainstream psychoanalysis as too simplistic, too deviant from Freudian drive theory, and insufficiently comprehensive to replace Kleinian object relations theory (Bowlby, 1969, 1982a, 1982b).

3

Currently, interest in the relationship between parent-infant attachment and adult relationships and psychopathology has "come of age" (Bowlby, 1988a). There are now at least three lines of empirical inquiry with regard to attachment and personality or psychopathology in adults. Developmental psychology has begun to examine attachment as a life-span concept (see Ainsworth, 1985; Kobak & Sceery, 1988; Kobak & Hazan, 1991; Main et al., 1985), through a rather strict adherence to the operationalizations and methods used by Ainsworth. Studies from this group consist largely of interview (Kobak & Hazan, 1991; Main et al., 1985) or Q-sort methods (Kobak & Sceery, 1988) that try to assess the same attachment patterns as the original experimental procedure.

In a second line of inquiry, social and personality psychologists such as Phillip Shaver (e.g., Shaver, Hazan, & Bradshaw, 1988), Patricia Noller and Judith Feeney (Feeney & Noller, 1990), and Kim Bartholomew (Bartholomew & Horowitz, 1991) have used Ainsworth's and Bowlby's ideas and formulations, and have applied social-psychological methods such as questionnaires and large-scale surveys to the study of normative adult attachment. They have used self-report measures designed to assess attachment style or attachment security, maximizing the reliability of the instruments and their convergent validity. These studies have typically involved large convenience samples such as college students, although some researchers have sought out other populations such as married couples.

Finally, clinical researchers such as Gordon Parker (Parker, Tupling, & Brown, 1979; Parker, 1979), Malcolm West and his colleagues (West & Sheldon, 1988; West, Sheldon, & Reiffer, 1987, 1989), Kenneth Adam and his colleagues (Adam, Bouckoms, & Streiner, 1982), and ourselves (Berman, 1988a; Berman & Sperling, 1991; Sperling, 1988; Sperling & Berman, 1991; Sperling, Berman, & Fagen, 1992) have applied attachment theory to a variety of clinical contexts involving both normative and pathological attachment processes in adults. The aim of this research has been to examine the relationship between attachment experiences and later psychopathology. Retrospective accounts of attachment experiences are obtained through interviews, self-reports, and psychotherapies, and are related to current symptoms, psychopathology, and treatment response.

This book offers perspectives on adult attachment from all of these lines of inquiry. The unifying thread of these chapters is the application of the construct of attachment, originally developed and formulated with regard to the mother-infant bond, to a conceptual and empirical understanding of human relatedness across the life span. In studying adult relationships, attachment theory has an intuitive appeal. Compared to object relations theory, it is relatively simple to understand and seems parsimoniously to capture much of the variation in adult interpersonal relatedness. It relies less on the internal fantasies of the individual, and largely rejects drive-based formulations of close relationships in favor of genetically based behavioral systems with survival value. Like psychoanalytic theory, attachment theory retains a fundamental belief that one's earliest experiences of relationships are formative in later life. Attachment theory also integrates concepts from cognitive theory with emotion and childhood experience; this is particularly apparent in recent attention to the representational basis of attachment processes. Yet adult attachment is a new field. As such, the domains of the theory as it relates to adults are still somewhat fluid and in the process of definition. In this spirit, the chapters in this book are likely to raise as many questions as they answer.

The purpose of this introductory chapter is to clarify the meaning of adult attachment, to articulate the characteristics of adult attachment, and to highlight issues or questions that will be raised throughout the book. Our specific goals are as follows:

- To provide an overview of the basics of attachment theory as described by Bowlby, Ainsworth, Main, and others, from which all the chapters draw.
- To provide and discuss a working definition of adult attachment.
- To identify the different conceptualizations of adult attachment in research on the topic.
- To highlight the dimensions of adult attachment that determine its manifestation in specific relationships, including the type of relationship and the intensity and security of the attachment.
- To identify significant issues or problems that are raised in this book but for which resolution is not yet complete, and to provide an overview of the individual chapters as they relate to these concerns.

THE BASICS OF ATTACHMENT THEORY

Based in the theories of ethology and evolution, John Bowlby's attachment theory (1969, 1973, 1980, 1982a) rests on the concept of an "attachment behavioral system"—a homeostatic process that regulates infant proximity-seeking and contact-maintaining behaviors with one or a few specific individuals who provide physical or psychological safety or security. According to Bowlby (1969, 1982a), the attachment system is an independent behavioral system, equivalent in function to other drive-behavioral systems such as feeding, mating, and exploration. Attachment behaviors are organized around specific attachment figures, with the goal of felt security during the second half of the first year of life. The survival value of an attachment drive–namely, its role in keeping the infant alive–ensures that it will be passed on through processes of natural selection (Ainsworth, 1989). The development of the attachment system at about the time of locomotion and object permanence makes evolutionary sense, in that it serves to deter the infant from straying or exploring too far from the caregiver, and activates exploratory behavior in the protective presence of the caregiver. This pattern of interaction between infant and parent is known as "exploration from a secure base" (Ainsworth, 1967).

The attachment system operates according to principles of cybernetic or control systems theory. This model assumes that the control system has a set of environmental features that will activate or turn on the system. Once activated, the system engages in specific actions that will serve to achieve a set goal. A difference from simpler systems, however, is that these behaviors will change as proximity to the set goal changes. Once the goal is reached, the control system is deactivated, except for the detectors that are vigilant for environmental system activators. In the case of attachment, attachment behaviors are initiated when the child realizes that he or she can no longer easily reach the attachment figure, or when the child feels threatened or fearful. The child then engages in any of several behaviors designed to re-establish proximity, including calling, seeking, crying, gazing, or touching. Which behavior will be used depends on specific environmental factors, such as distance from the attachment figure and severity of anxiety. Once proximity is achieved, the child alters his or her behaviors to those designed to maintain proximity, such as hugging, cooing, clinging, and smiling. Attachment is then deactivated, and the child can use other behavioral systems such as exploration or feeding.

It is a fundamental assumption of attachment theory that in order to activate and deactivate the attachment system effectively and efficiently, the child must develop "internal working models" of the attachment figure and of the self in interaction with the attachment figure (Bowlby, 1988a). Such models allow the child to be aware that the attachment figure is missing and to recognize the attachment figure on his or her return. An internal working model is in many ways comparable to other descriptions of the way in which experience is encoded in the mind, including the "internal object" or "object representation" of psychoanalytic theory; the "schema," "script," or "personal construct" of cognitive and developmental psychology; or the "representation of interaction that has been generalized" in Stern's (1985) integrative developmental–clinical theory.

These descriptions of attachment and mental representations assume that the behavioral system has developed and been refined in an adaptive environment–that is, an environment in which activation, reaction, and deactivation occur in a consistent fashion and in which the set goal is being regularly achieved. There are many children whose early experiences neither are consistent nor reflect regular achievement of the secure base. Ainsworth's program of research documented these individual differences in attachment behavior through the regular observation of mother–child interaction during the first year of a child's life, culminating in the laboratory observation technique dubbed the Strange Situation. She identified several distinct types of attachment bonds that were most notable on reunion with the mother following brief, experimentally controlled separations (Ainsworth et al., 1978). The most common was the "secure" style, in which the child showed signs of distress when the parent left him or her alone or with a stranger, sought out the mother upon her return, held her for a period of time, and then returned to exploration and play. In addition to this pattern (which was found in a majority of the children) were two other patterns, which Ainsworth considered to represent "insecure" attachments: the "avoidant" style and the "anxious/ambivalent" style (Ainsworth et al., 1978). In the context of the Strange Situation, the avoidant style was characterized by distress during separation and by a lack of acknowledgment or rejection of the attachment figure during reunion. The anxious/ambivalent style was characterized by a high level of distress during the separation and by mixed approach and rejection during the reunion period. These patterns have been found to show stable differences in the natural environment as well (Bowlby, 1988b). Secure children are more likely to interact well, explore their environment, and show emotional resiliency. The avoidant children tend to be more anxious and fearful at home and angry, or attention-seeking in school. The anxious/ambivalent children tend to be clinging, fearful of the environment, and emotionally labile.

Longitudinal research on attachment has begun to document stable patterns of behavior from 1 year of age to at least the 10th year. Children's behavior in school, in home, and in social situations can be predicted by their attachment style (Sroufe, Egeland, & Kreutzer, 1990), and a child's attachment style is consistent with parenting characteristics and parental attachment style (Main et al., 1985). Attachment theory in general is also useful in explaining both children's and adults' reactions to separations, including the various patterns of anger, withdrawal, and reintegration found in bereavement (Parkes, 1972) and divorce (Weiss, 1975). Moreover, research has supported Bowlby's early notion that the child's early experiences of the close bond to the mother (and father) have a significant long-term effect on development. Specifically, significant disruptions in the parent–child bond, as well as parenting characteristics that parallel separation (rejection, hostility, or inconsistent responding), have been shown to have a detrimental impact on subsequent development (Rutter, 1985).

DEFINING ADULT ATTACHMENT

A Working Definition

Our working definition of "adult attachment" is as follows: Adult attachment is the stable tendency of an individual to make substantial efforts to seek and maintain proximity to and contact with one or a few specific individuals who provide the subjective potential for physical and/or psychological safety and security. This stable tendency is regulated by internal working models of attachment, which are cognitive-affective-motivational schemata built from the individual's experience in his or her interpersonal world.

This definition needs clarification in several ways. First, attachment defines a behavioral system that may or may not be active either in the person's life or in a particular relationship at any given time. In other words, adult attachment provides the potential for relationship security, rather than relationship security per se. Consistent with this, attachment in adults does not invariably provide felt security (Ainsworth, 1985, 1989). Quite the contrary: Many people have attachment relationships that provoke significant anxiety and anger. However, these relationships are maintained because the persons believe that their attachment figures have the potential to provide felt security. Second, attachment is manifested in, but not defined by, a limited set of characteristics that arise when distance from or accessibility of the attachment figure exceeds some individually defined limit. These characteristics include overt behaviors, emotional reactions, and cognitive activity. Some of the characteristics are trans-situational, whereas others are specific to certain situations. Finally, an internal working model is a representation in the mind that includes aspects of the self, the attachment figure, situational invariants for attachment interactions, and the affects that connect the two figures. Internal working models are based on a prior history of attachment relationships plus current interactions between the self and the attachment figure when the attachment behavioral system is activated. In addition, internal working models define the rules by which two individuals interact, including behaviors, feelings, and thoughts. These rules allow each individual to anticipate and plan (correctly or incorrectly) what the other person will do given a preceding set of actions, and hence may elicit reactions and behaviors that are not accurate in terms of the current situation.

Adult Attachment as Attachment plus Caregiving

We have referred above to the caregiving capacities of the adult toward his or her children as attachment behaviors. Within the domain of adult attachment, we suggest that the theory should combine the attachment system (originally characterized by care-seeking or proximity-seeking behaviors) with a nurturance system characterized by caregiving behaviors. With this recommendation, we depart significantly from Bowlby (1969, 1982a) and others (Hinde, 1982), who have maintained that the two systems are separate. Bowlby's original theory clearly indicated that "attachment" refers to the child's bond to the mother, whereas the mother's (and father's) bond to the child is a separate behavioral system referred to as "caregiving" (Bowlby, 1969, 1982a). In contrast to the perspective that attachment and caregiving are independent but related behavioral systems, we believe that the caregiving system is an integral component and direct outgrowth of the attachment system. This is particularly true in the realm of adult attachment, although it may be applicable to attachment across the life span.[1]

We make this argument for three reasons. First, we are influenced by general systems theory (Von Bertalanffy, 1968), in which the concept of a behavioral system in one individual without reference to the other individuals in the larger system is pointless. It is obvious that the attachment system is irrelevant in the absence of a parenting figure (or figures). In fact, it is exactly the disturbances in the dyadic relationship that account for differences in attachment style, and hence in later emotional and behavioral adjustment. In addition, just as the attachment behavior of the infant is shaped by the responsiveness and availability of the parent, the caregiving behavior of the parent is shaped by the responsiveness and reactivity of the infant.

Second, there are virtually no relationships between adults that have the extremes of caregiving and attachment found in the parent–child relationship. Clearly, functioning adult marital or sexual relationships require reciprocity and easy interchange between the caregiving and attachment roles (Ainsworth, 1985). The same can be said of parent–child relationships when the children are grown. It is rare that parents do not accept help, support, or nurturance from an adult child, even while they remain an attachment figure to their child.

Third, our personal and clinical experiences suggest that the emotional experiences that are bound up in attachment are exactly those that are bound up in caregiving. The fear of danger or threat triggers caregiving responses, just as it triggers attachment responses. Caregiving in relationships that parallel attachment relationships is just as intense an emotional experience, just as tied to security and anxiety, just as involved with anger, just as enduring, and just as unresponsive to punishment and extinction as is attachment per se. Indeed, one of the primary adult manifestations of disturbed attachments is "compulsive caregiving" (Bowlby, 1980), which suggests that noncompulsive caregiving is a normal outgrowth of attachment. Although it is beyond the scope of this chapter or this book to exhaustively address the nature of caregiving and its relationship to attachment, we are proposing that caregiving is directly and inextricably tied to attachment in adult close relationships.

CONCEPTUALIZING ADULT ATTACHMENT

Research on adult attachment has addressed different aspects of Bowlby's overall theory, and the techniques of measurement and nature of conclusions depend on which aspect of the theory is being addressed. Three major conceptualizations of adult attachment are represented in this book: attachment as a state-based syndrome or set of distressing symptoms that emerge when the attachment figure is unavailable; attachment as a trait-based tendency to form particular types of attachment relationships and to respond to these relationships similarly; and attachment as an interactive process between two people in an ongoing relationship. In this section, we elaborate briefly on each of these perspectives and indicate how they contribute to the overall theory.

Attachment as State: Attachment Distress

Bowlby's earliest research on attachment in infants dealt with the common responses of infants to separation from their attachment figures. These reactions were summarized in the stages of "protest," "despair," and "detachment" (Bowlby, 1973). In the earliest phase, efforts to re-establish contact with the attachment figure, including calling, crying, seeking, and making physical contact, were commonly seen behaviors. In despair, the child exhibited lethargy, tearfulness, passivity, and withdrawal. The earliest research in adult attachment also examined the common reaction of adults to disruption of the attachment bond. Most of this work assumed that adults form attachment bonds to other adults, typically in the context of marriage, and examined people's response to loss of their attachment figures. It was predicted that virtually all people would experience symptoms of loss equivalent to those found in a child at the loss of a parent. To summarize, adults do exhibit a consistent pattern of reactions to marital separation (Weiss, 1975) and death of a spouse (Parkes, 1972;

Glick, Weiss, & Parkes, 1974). These reactions are comparable to those seen in infants separated from their attachment figures and include stages of protest, despair, and detachment/reintegration. The behaviors are thought to be the normative reaction of an individual to the "intolerable inaccessibility of the attachment figure" (Weiss, 1975, p. 131).

In addition to studies of loss through traumatic events, several researchers have studied attachment distress through normative separation experiences, such as the transition from high school to college (Berman & Sperling, 1991; Kenny, 1987). Measures of attachment included a focus on cognitive activity through spontaneous thoughts about parents, and questionnaires assessing the quality of the parent-child relationship. Results from both studies suggested that college students in general maintain a continued attachment to their parents, and that this attachment may influence their adjustment and emotional distress during the college years.

Other research on normative changes in attachment has also shown a continued attachment of children to their parents. Levitt (Levitt, Weber, & Clark, 1986; Levitt, Coffman, Guacci-Franco, & Loveless, Chapter 9, this volume) and Antonucci (1976; Kahn & Antonucci, 1980; and Antonucci, Chapter 10, this volume) have also emphasized changes and continuities across the life cycle. One finding in these studies is that a loving and caring attachment to parents, spouses, and friends promotes adjustment and healthy adaptation despite numerous life stresses.

Attachment as Trait: The Internal Working Model

The most common conceptualization of adult attachment in recent research involves stable individual differences in attachment style. "Attachment styles" refer to particular internal working models of attachment that determine people's behavioral responses to real or imagined separation and reunion from their attachment figures. These internal working models are thought to be consistent across time and across relationships, and for most theorists they are direct outgrowths of initial attachment experience(s). The key difference between the trait or style and the state conceptualizations of attachment is the emphasis on stable individual differences in emotional experience versus a universal emotional reaction to separations and losses.

Attachment style is determined by the way in which the accessibility and responsiveness of the attachment figure, and complementary aspects of the self, are encoded in the internal working model of attachment (Bowlby, 1988a). These styles in children were initially identified by Ainsworth in her well-known Strange Situation research (Ainsworth et al., 1978) and have been supported in numerous subsequent studies. Research with children has supported the temporal stability of attachment style (Main et al., 1985; Sroufe et al., 1990), but there are significant variations in style across attachment figures (Ainsworth, 1989; Main et al., 1985). Maternal and paternal attachment styles are essentially uncorrelated, and may both contribute to a child's internal working model and subsequent adjustment (Bloom-Feshbach, 1987).

The relationship of children's internal working models of attachment to those of adults is not yet understood. There is a general consensus that adults exhibit stable characteristics in their intimate relationships, although these styles may have changed from the childhood experience and may show more stability during adulthood (Shaver et al., 1988). In addition, the relationship of different childhood attachments to the development of adult attachment as a single trait has not been clarified. For example, when a child has an attachment relationship with both mother and father, does only one, both, or a synthesis of both determine the type of attachment relationship one forms with adult intimate relationships?

The number of attachment styles among adults also remains unclear. In general, most theorists maintain that there is only one secure style (our own research in this regard is a notable exception) and numerous insecure styles. Some researchers have proposed two insecure attachment styles, others three, and still others four. Ainsworth's original tripartite model of "secure," "avoidant," and "anxious/ambivalent" was adopted by Shaver and his colleagues (Hazan & Shaver, 1987; Shaver et al., 1988) in several studies of heterosexual love as an attachment process. Main and her colleagues also adopted a tripartite model, which they later expanded to include four categories of adult attachment: "autonomous," "dismissing," "preoccupied," and "unresolved" (Main et al., 1985). In her childhood attachment research, Ainsworth also referred to a fourth, "punitive" style (Ainsworth, 1985), which may be related to Main et al.'s (1985) "disorganized/disoriented" style.

Sperling (1988; Sperling & Berman, 1991) has proposed a modification of this model, which emphasizes four attachment styles formed from dependent and aggressive interpersonal drives, plus an oblique dimension of security-insecurity. The resulting four categories are "dependent," "avoidant," "resistant/ambivalent," and "hostile" styles, each of which can contain different levels of security. Bartholomew and Horowitz (1991) have also proposed a four-category model, which emphasizes the individual's internal representation of self and other in determining the individual's experience of close relationships. In addition to the "secure" and "preoccupied" styles, their model identifies two subtypes of the avoidant style—one that is counterdependent (labeled "dismissing"), and one that conveys significant fear of closeness (labeled "fearful"). Bowlby (1980) himself initially proposed a number of adult variations of insecure infant attachment styles, including the "compulsive caregiving," "compulsive care-seeking," "compulsive self-reliant," and "angry withdrawn" styles. These four insecure styles, plus the implicit secure style, were adopted by West and his colleagues in their efforts to develop methods of assessing clinical manifestations of adult attachment (West & Sheldon, 1988).

A variation of this approach has been to examine the dimensions of attachment that underlie these styles. Parker (1983; Parker et al., 1979; see also Parker, Chapter 12, this volume) first explored attachment as it related to adult psychopathology by developing the Parental Bonding Instrument (PBI), which measures the dimensions of warmth/affection and protection/control. He viewed these as the two critical dimensions implicit in individuals' retrospective experience of their parental attachment relationships. With regard to current intimate relationships, the factor-analytically derived dimensions of closeness, dependency, and anxiety have been proposed to underlie Hazan and Shaver's tripartite model (Collins & Read, 1990). Research using these dimensions has provided some support for their utility in studying adult intimate relations.

Attachment as Interaction: Love and Marriage

There is little research that compares adult interactions with current attachment figures to parent–infant interactions. Although the above-described conceptualizations help clarify attachment from an individual perspective, neither approach incorporates the aspects of Bowlby's theory in which reciprocal interaction patterns and goal-corrected feedback mechanisms are emphasized. Recent research, however, has begun to examine attachment as it relates to momentary interactions within adult intimate relations.

Kobak and Hazan (1991) examined the relationship of adult attachment styles to specific interactions in married couples. Their data suggest that there are significant correlations between attachment security on the one hand, and marital interaction and marital quality on the other. One's own attachment security affects one's tendency to be rejecting of the partner. Cohn, Silver, Cowan, Cowan, and Pearson (1992) found that husbands with secure attachments had more positive interactions and fewer conflicts with their wives than husbands with insecure attachments. Interestingly, no differences in spousal interactions were found for wives with secure versus insecure attachments. Both Kobak and Hazan (1991) and Cohn et al. (1992) found some relationship between level of security and marital quality, but measured these in ways that did not allow comparability. Finally, Berman and his colleagues (see Berman, Marcus, & Berman, Chapter 8, this volume) have begun to examine the relationship of attachment to marital adjustment and interaction on the basis of behavior following a brief, potentially distressing separation, rather than behavior in standard conflict resolution or intimacy-seeking interactions. These data suggest that secure–secure marital dyads exhibit less proximity-seeking behavior following a distressing separation and are more satisfied in their marriages than insecure–secure dyads.

In summary, the different conceptualizations of attachment address different aspects of adult close relationships. The state model helps clarify the ubiquitous reaction to loss and separation among adults. The trait model sheds light on how people think about close relationships, and explains why people react to threat or loss in different yet stable ways. The interactional model may be most useful in exploring how attachment is manifested in specific close relationships, and why individuals respond differentially depending on characteristics of their partners. Future research should examine the relationship between attachment style and interactional behavior, or attachment style and attachment distress, in a variety of situations and in relationships with different histories. Attention should be given to particular attachment behaviors and to a clear distinction between attachment relationships and close relationships in general, in order to clarify the unique contribution of a hypothesized attachment behavioral system.

THE DIMENSIONS OF ADULT ATTACHMENT

Attachment theory is simple in principle, particularly in comparison to object relations theory. For example, the development of internal working models in attachment theory stems primarily from the interaction patterns between parent and child (Bowlby, 1969), whereas mental representations in object relations theory involve the complex interplay of external reality and internal fantasy (see Kernberg, 1976; see also Diamond & Blatt, Chapter 3, this volume). The details of the psychology of attachment, however, are quite complex. The qualities of attachment are multifaceted and intricate. Attachments exist over time and across relationships. Within a given relationship, attachment is comprised of a genetically determined behavioral system, a mental representation of attachment relationships, a particular relationship history, and a specific environmental context. As a result, one could say that although two different close relationships may both reflect attachment bonds, the nature of these relationships may be dramatically different.

Given this complexity, it becomes important to identify the characteristics of adult attachment and to examine how they are manifested in different relationships. This section identifies and describes what we consider to be the important dimensions of adult attachment. The characteristics we highlight are not necessarily orthogonal; in addition, none of these dimensions by themselves define healthy or problematic attachment. They do, however, reflect aspects of attachment relationships that have been viewed as important by researchers and clinicians who have observed or treated adults in attachment relationships.

Types of Adult Attachment Relationships

As noted above, there are many types of adult relationships, with differing degrees of importance to the individual (Kahn & Antonucci, 1980). Some of the adult relationships in our daily lives are close relationships, and a few of them can be characterized as "attachment relationships" in the sense that they provide the potential for security. These relationships typically include an adult's relationship with his or her parent(s), an adult's relationship with his or her child(ren), and one or a few love relationships that include security features. Most of the contributors to this book have addressed one of these types of relationships. Rothbard and Shaver (Chapter 2), Feeney, Noller, and Hanrahan (Chapter 4), and Hindy and Schwarz (Chapter 7) address attachment in love relations. Berman et al. (Chapter 8) address the related but distinct type of attachment in marriage. In comparison, Batgos and Leadbeater (Chapter 6), Adam (Chapter 11), and Parker (Chapter 12) address continued attachment to parents. There are occasional specialized relationships that may or may not be attachment relationships, including the psychotherapeutic relationship (see Sperling & Lyons, Chapter 14, and West & Keller, Chapter 13) and the mentoring relationship. Whether these latter two become attachment relationships depends on individual factors in the dyad, such as the intensity of the relationship, the duration of the relationship, and the significance of the relationship for the individuals involved.

Several other aspects of interpersonal functioning have been suggested to be attachment-based, including peer relationships (Greenberg, Siegal, & Leitch, 1984) and work functioning (Hazan & Shaver, 1990). These roles/relationships do not fit with the present definition of attachment relationships in this book. Attachment may have relevance to these domains of adult life, but the connection is less immediately evident, and inclusion of these domains within attachment theory would require extensive work to support it. Although some peer relationships may be considered attachment relationships, and one may feel quite comfortable and open with friends, the vast majority are based in an affiliative rather than an attachment domain. Many friendships, though important and valued, are not unique and irreplaceable (Ainsworth's [1989] criterion for affectional bonds) and do not create a substantial level of distress when disrupted (Ainsworth's [1985] and Berscheid's [1983] criterion for close relationships). Finally, when one is sick or threatened, one tends to be drawn to family members, to a spouse or partner, or perhaps to one long-term, very close friend.

Intensity of Attachment

The intensity or strength of an attachment relationship is difficult to quantify, although the intensity dimension is among the most important. Berscheid (1983) has proposed that the intensity of an intimate adult relationship can only be defined by one's reaction to the loss of the relationship. When a relationship is ongoing, the apparent emotion may not accurately convey the intertwining of the couple's lives. It is only when the intermingling is disrupted that the emotional intensity reveals the interdependence between the two. For example, a man may show little affect toward his wife throughout the marriage, but at her death he may exhibit very severe emotional and physical reactions to the loss, including depression, illness, or even death.

Although Berscheid was not suggesting the reaction to loss as a measure of attachment in itself, we believe that intensity of adult attachment is best understood by one's reactions to real, threatened, or imagined separations, as well as to long-term or more permanent losses. Intensity can be measured following a loss by the frequency of spontaneous, intrusive, or triggered thoughts about the attachment figure; efforts to seek or make contact with the attachment figure; and desire to or efforts to rejoin the attachment figure (Berman, 1988a; Berman et al., Chapter 8, this volume; Parkes, 1972; Weiss, 1975). It can also be evaluated by the strength of desires for merger and fusion (Sperling, 1988), or by the intensity of jealousy (Hazan & Shaver, 1987) or insecurity (Hindy, Schwarz, & Brodsky, 1989; Hindy & Schwarz, Chapter 7, this volume). Finally, intensity may be measured by one's self-report of the importance of the attachment figure to one's life (Feeney et al., Chapter 5, this volume; West et al., 1987; West & Keller, Chapter 13, this volume).

Intensity of attachment plays an important role in both Levitt et al.'s contribution (Chapter 9) and in Antonucci's discussion of attachment across the life span (Chapter 10). It is also implicitly involved in Sperling and Lyon's discussion of therapy within the context of attachment theory (Chapter 14).

Security/Reliability of Attachment

Security of attachment is probably the most commonly studied characteristic of attachment. The degree to which one experiences the attachment figure as reliable and responsive to one's needs has always defined the construct of security of attachment (Bowlby, 1969, 1982a; Ainsworth, 1982; Kobak & Hazan, 1991). In turn, security of attachment contributes to the degree to which negative affect states (anxiety, anger) are present in the context of the attachment relationship. Security of attachment in infancy has significant implications for adult social adjustment, and may be most closely related to later psychopathology through neurobiological mechanisms (Reite & Boccia, Chapter 4, this volume). The security-insecurity dimension has been the focus of studies of love relationships (Hindy et al., 1989; Hindy & Schwarz, Chapter 7, this volume; Shaver et al., 1988; Rothbard & Shaver, Chapter 2, this volume), marital relationships (Cohn et al., 1992; Berman et al., Chapter 8, this volume), and parent-child relationships in adolescence (Adam, Chapter 11, this volume, and Batgos & Leadbeater, Chapter 6, this volume). Parker (1979, 1983, and Chapter 12, this volume) has looked at the parental characteristics of availability and responsiveness in relation to depressive disorders, and West and Keller (Chapter 13, this volume) have examined it in relation to psychotherapy and personality disorders. The security-insecurity dimension appears to account for a great deal of differences in the nature of close relationships. People who appear to be insecure—that is, to experience to their attachment figure(s) as unreliable and unresponsive—have more interpersonal difficulties, experience greater depression and anxiety, and seek help from a variety of sources.

Sensitivity of Attachment

In addition to intensity and security, the ease with which an individual develops attachment relationships appears to be quite important, particularly in the clinical sphere. We are calling this characteristic "sensitivity," as a measure of how quickly an adult will experience a relationship as an attachment bond. Attachment relationships seem to develop more frequently in adults than in children. There are significant individual differences in the ease with which adults form attachment bonds with other adults. Although many adults conform to the classical attachment model of one or a few attachment relationships across the life span, some appear to form intense attachment relationships easily and to many individuals during their lives. These relationships are often dominated by issues of security and availability; they are typically very intense; and the loss of

these relationships is experienced as intensely disruptive for long periods of time. From a clinical perspective, patients diagnosed as having
borderline or dependent personality disorder would be extremely high
on this dimension, whereas those with schizoid or avoidant personality
disorder would be quite low (see West & Keller, Chapter 13, this volume).
In addition, the concept of "desperate love" characterizes the rapid, intense
development of attachment (Sperling, 1988; Sperling & Berman, 1989;
Sperling et al., 1992), and may in some cases reflect rapid formation of
an attachment relationship. How these attachment models are formed, and
what causes an individual to find multiple attachment relationships, are
some of the issues addressed by psychoanalytic theorists (see Diamond
& Blatt, Chapter 3, this volume).

Activation of Attachment

Within a given attachment relationship, the attachment behavioral system can be activated quickly across a wide range of situations, or may be
quite specific and delimited, emerging only at times of great stress or
threat. We have termed the degree to which the attachment behavioral
system can be engaged within an ongoing attachment relationship "activation." Enormous individual differences exist in the degree to which an individual or couple activates an attachment system. Activation on a moment-
to-moment basis is affected by the internal working models of each person,
by the environmental context of the relationship, and by aspects of the
interaction of the two (Berman et al., Chapter 8, this volume; Kelley et al.,
1983). Different determinants of availability are addressed by many of
these contributors. Activation is related to security, since insecure/ambiva-
lent and insecure/avoidant attachments are activated more easily than
secure attachments. However, other aspects of the internal model and the
relational context contribute to activation, as discussed by Diamond and
Blatt, by Berman et al., and by West and Keller in their chapters in this
book.
     Since activation is a new concept in adult attachment, an example
may be of benefit. A newly married husband and wife make contact frequently during the day, and spend a great deal of time together when both
arrive home in the evening. In addition, each reacts strongly to movements
away from the other, and requires time to "reconnect." When this same
couple is married for 20 years, the spouses may show minimal activation
of the attachment system in the context of their relationship; they experience tremendous security and safety, and the behaviors of each partner
are understood not to threaten that experience. A major disruption such
as illness, death, or job loss, however, may dramatically change the fre-

quency of attachment activation, returning the spouses to behaviors more like those at the beginning of their relationship. As a result, the attachment system becomes engaged repeatedly during the course of a week when minor instances of unavailability or responsiveness occur.

Frustration Tolerance (Role of Anger)

Perhaps one of the most complex and least clearly understood aspects of attachment in adults is the role of anger in close relationships. Bowlby (1973) explains how anger is an integral part of the attachment system. He provides numerous clinical vignettes describing the experience of anger in children as related to separation or threats of abandonment. Bowlby suggests that anger in close relationships can serve two functions: a facilitative function that activates the individual to overcome any barriers to reunion, and a coercive function that discourages further separations. Many have observed the common experience of the reunion of a lost child and his or her parent in a shopping mall; often the parent simultaneously berates the child and clings desperately to him or her—both actions that serve to regain and maintain proximity to the attachment figure.

Anger, however, serves a variety of both adaptive and maladaptive functions in adult close relationships. In many pathological relationships, anger becomes a central component of the relationship, often causing the demise of the bond. In many of these couples, the anger appears for reasons that are unclear or confusing, both to the individuals and to their therapists. Many clinicians believe, and some researchers have suggested, that anger in marriages fuels intimacy and serves to maintain a close and continuing bond between divorced ex-spouses.

In the case of divorce, Berman (1988a) found that anger was at times positively related to adaptation. That is, individuals who remained angry at their ex-spouses were at times less attached and better adjusted than those who experienced little anger, but continued attachment. It is possible that anger also serves an ego-protective function in some adults. The anger may serve to block feelings of attachment and hence anxiety, at least in adults with differentiated internal models of attachment. If one can feel anger toward attachment figures, then the experience of their unavailability is at least consistent with the emotional valence of the relationship. Other research has suggested that people with avoidant styles experience the most intense anger and loss, which may be expressed under periods of increased stress or decreased ego control (see Adam, Chapter 11, this volume). In some people, however, attachment and anger seem to coexist, being expressed simultaneously or alternating at a rapid rate (Sperling,

Sharp, & Fishler, 1991; Sperling et al., 1992; Melges & Swartz, 1989). Clearly, much more work is needed to clarify the role of anger in adult attachment.

CURRENT ISSUES AND PROBLEMS
IN ADULT ATTACHMENT

The chapters of this book address many issues that are central to the application of attachment to adults: issues of conceptualization, measurement, utility, and applicability to various stages and problems. Adult attachment is not yet a theory, in the sense of a limited set of propositions that can be used both to explain and to predict a wide range of events. For attachment to have conceptual value for adults, these issues must be addressed. The chapters in this text have been selected to do so. Part II deals with broad theoretical and conceptual questions that affect adult attachment. Parts III and IV address adult attachment, with relative emphases on normative and disturbed life-span development, respectively. In these latter two sections, theoretical issues are also addressed, but more specifically as they relate to a certain aspect of attachment.

The concept of attachment throughout the life cycle is, of course, central to our thesis. For those researchers and clinicians steeped in the theory, the relationship between childhood attachment experiences and adult behavior in close relationships seems intuitively obvious and needs no elucidation. The association is not nearly so clear-cut, however, and requires supporting documentation to be an acceptable heuristic model. Rothbard and Shaver confront this problem directly, and contribute a rich, thoughtful review of the literature in Chapter 2 on continuities of attachment. Their review provides those who are not "true believers" with a basis for accepting attachment as a useful model in understanding adult personality and relatedness, or at least for suspending judgment long enough to read further. It builds on Ainsworth's (1985) exploration of life-span attachment by examining the recent research on attachment in adults, as well as longitudinal studies of childhood attachment.

Just as the continuity of attachment from childhood to adulthood is crucial to a life-span attachment model, a clearer understanding of internal working models is also of central importance. With a few recent exceptions (Bretherton, 1991; Main et al., 1985), however, most theories of attachment have not elaborated either the nature or the development of these internal models. Psychoanalytic theory in general, and object relations theory in particular, have devoted considerable attention to internal models of the parent–child relationship. Attachment theory and psychoanalytic theory, however, have both parallels and divergences that make easy integration premature. Diamond and Blatt explore these common-alities and differences by a careful comparison of attachment theory and object relations theory in Chapter 3. It is an invaluable reference for ana-lytic thinkers interested in the contributions of attachment theory, and for researchers and clinicians interested in discovering existing contribu-tions from the psychoanalytic literature that elucidate early parent-child relationships. (Several of our other contributors also address aspects of mental representation of attachment: Berman et al. [Chapter 8], using an interpersonal perspective; Levitt et al. [Chapter 9], drawing from a social-cognitive perspective; and Sperling and Lyons [Chapter 14], integrating psychoanalytic and cognitive perspectives.)

The underlying basis of attachment has been assumed to be species survival, but this has not yet been well demonstrated. However, a physi-ological basis of attachment can have far-reaching theoretical implications in terms of continuity from childhood to adulthood, as well as implications for psychopathology. At this time, animal models of attachment provide the only feasible method of examining physiological bases of attachment. Martin Reite and his colleagues have devoted many years to researching the basic underpinnings of attachment theory by looking at changes in physiology and biochemistry in nonhuman primates as related to experi-mentally manipulated separation experiences. In Chapter 4, Reite and Boccia review the literature and discuss current and future directions in this area; they offer many possible associations between the earliest of social experiences and relatively permanent changes in physiological, bio-chemical, and immunological functioning.

How attachment is measured is crucial to a useful theoretical model. We have outlined some of the issues relevant to assessment in this chapter, including which attachment relationship is being studied, how attachment is conceptualized (state, trait, or interaction), and what components one wants to assess. These issues are further elucidated in Chapter 5 by Feeney et al. They highlight some of the major scales used to assess adult attach-ment, and identify their shortcomings. The chapter then presents a new scale for assessing adult attachment that has good psychometric proper-ties, is not limited to one attachment relationship, and is not dependent on having a current "attachment." This scale holds promise as an impor-tant methodological instrument. (Other assessment issues are addressed in several chapters, including those by Parker, Adam, and Berman et al.).

In Part III of this book, our contributors address the role of attach-ment at various stages of the life cycle. Normative interpersonal processes involve "the making and breaking of affectional bonds" throughout adult life. The stages of adolescence, young adulthood, middle adulthood, and late adulthood are all affected by these attachment bonds. Attention to attachment in each stage begins with the relationship of adolescent relations to parents and peers (Batgos & Leadbeater, Chapter 6), moves to the love relationships of late adolescence and early adulthood (Hindy & Schwarz, Chapter 7), and then goes on to attachment in marriage (Berman et al., Chapter 8). Attachment relationships may also be affected by important life transitions (Levitt et al., Chapter 9), as well as by continuities and discontinuities in the later stages of life (Antonucci, Chapter 10).

Adolescence has traditionally been viewed as a stage of increasing separation and differentiation. Recent research on adolescents has begun to consider that continued secure attachment to parents is central to healthy development. Batgos and Leadbeater (Chapter 6) connect the concepts of self-in-relation theory to attachment theory in adolescence, particularly in the sense that both theories support the continued interdependence with attachment figures throughout the life cycle. Batgos and Leadbeater suggest that the style of the attachment relationship to parents affects one's self-representation, and hence one's relationships with peers. When an adolescent has an insecure attachment, the style of attachment determines the type of dysphoria the adolescent experiences: An avoidant style leads to a self-critical orientation, whereas an ambivalent style leads to an interpersonal orientation, each with its own peer relational characteristics. The links among attachment, dysphoric style, and social competence in adolescents are important both to the development of attachments in later life and to the emotional and psychological vulnerabilities of adolescents.

Erikson (1963) noted that after the adolescent transition, the early adult stage presents the struggle for intimacy versus isolation. One of the most common areas of interest with regard to attachment style is its relationship to love and intimacy. In Chapter 7, Hindy and Schwarz offer their research on love relations as these are affected by attachment history. Their comprehensive studies have shown that an early history of parental rejection, parental aloofness, or hostility predisposes both males and females to anxious, preoccupied, or ambivalent love relationships. These findings have been supported in a number of other studies, including Hazan and Shaver (1987), Collins and Read (1990), and Feeney and Noller (1990).

Most people experience a number of love relationships in adult life. Only some of them become long-term relationships such as marriage. Berman and his colleagues argue in Chapter 8 that marital bonds are the most likely to be true attachment relationships. In the context of marital relationships, these authors explore the thorny problem of the relationship between internal working models of attachment and the nature of the interaction between the two members of a couple. They suggest a complex interactional relationship in which the nature of one person's mental model affects both his or her own behavior and the mental model and behavior of the partner. This interaction can account for many of the unusual patterns found in couples, including the tendency of some couples to "bring out the worst" in each person, while others "bring out the best."

One way of understanding the manifestations of internal working models of close relationships is through the expectations one person has regarding the other person and the self. Levitt et al. argue in Chapter 9 that the expectations of support, nurturance, and caretaking in connection with significant life events and life transitions causally influence the quality of close relationships. Using the life convoy model and social-cognitive theories of relational models, they emphasize the influence of "expectancy disconfirmation," or disappointment, on relationship quality and adjustment. They suggest that these expectancies mediate the relationship between mental models of close relationships and adaptation. Women's experience of childbirth is used as a test of their model, and they demonstrate that a woman's expectations regarding the close relationship affect the relationship quality, which in turn affects emotional and social adjustment.

The final chapter of this section explores in detail the role of attachment relationships throughout the latter part of the life cycle by using the convoy model of relationships (Antonucci, Chapter 10). Antonucci addresses the many developmental factors that affect close relationships, including intraindividual change and the integration of multiple attachment relationships across the life span. She also integrates concepts from other aspects of psychology to clarify the relevance of attachment to old age. The interaction of attachment with control and self-efficacy can help to understand the effects of attachment on both longevity and life satisfaction.

In the final section of the book, our contributors have sought to develop adult attachment theory as it relates to psychopathology and psychotherapy. Attachment researchers other than Bowlby have tended to emphasize healthy growth; psychopathology in general has been much less explored than Bowlby would have hoped (Bowlby, 1988b). As we have noted above, the original motivation for the theory was to explain adult psychopathology. Studies of suicide (Adam, Chapter 11), depression (Parker, Chapter 12; see also Batgos & Leadbeater, Chapter 6), and personality disorder (West & Keller, Chapter 13) help to develop this relationship. In the final chapters, West and Keller (Chapter 13) and Sperling and Lyons (Chapter 14) apply attachment theory to psychotherapy, with a particular emphasis on the interplay between the representational world and the experiential world.

In the first chapter of this third section, Adam (Chapter 11) presents data that strongly suggest a direct link among parenting behavior, parental trauma, and suicidal behavior. In this context, anger toward the parent plays a significant role in the attachment–suicide link. On the basis of this data, he presents a complex theory that identifies both distal (attachments) and proximal (family environment, family loss) causes of suicide, with both vulnerability and resiliency factors affecting the final expression (or nonexpression) of suicidal behavior.

In the second chapter, Parker (Chapter 12) reviews an extensive body of research indicating that problematic attachment bonds to one's parents are specific predisposing factors to depression in adult life. People with depressive disorders have been found to have significantly higher scores on the PBI, the instrument Parker and his colleagues developed to assess attachments to parents. The same effect has not been found in bipolar disorder. Moreover, Parker presents data supporting the belief that these are "real" descriptions of parents, rather than negatively perceived reconstructions.

West and Keller (Chapter 13) view the inability of individuals to recognize and mourn the failures of their caregivers to respond effectively and quickly as the central dynamic in patients with personality disorders. Both those who deny these chronic failures and those who seek to find in current relationships what was unavailable in past relationships enact in the therapeutic relationship the emotions and failures of the early attachment relationships. The principal goal of psychotherapy from an attachment perspective, according to West and Keller, is to identify this "feared loss dynamic" and to facilitate mourning, sadness, and anger in order to provide closure to the unresolved relationship longings with parental attachment figures.

Attachment provides for Sperling and Lyons (Chapter 14) a conceptual model for understanding the representational narratives invoked within psychotherapy. They use the notion of "mental representations" to integrate concepts from psychoanalytic, attachment, and cognitive theories relevant to therapeutic change. The majority of representationally formative relationships are attachment relationships. Over time, these attachment representations provide the narrative or schema by which one understands the interpersonal world. Psychotherapy can serve to modify these relational narratives in two ways: by providing a new relationship that forces accommodation of the existing schema, and by exploring and challenging existing schema through nonenactive transference manifestations. The relational and rational components work interactively to foster change in the patient without acting largely through the medium of the transference.

Taken *en masse*, these contributions reflect some of the most current thinking on the extrapolation of attachment to adult populations. Clearly, further research is needed, as well as additional theorizing. The more one moves away from the original population of study (infants and their mothers), the more difficult the project becomes. The connections between early attachment and the adult's internal models, interpersonal behaviors, and relationship capacities become more complex, affected by a variety of life events and personal capacities. The value of this book is not only in the contributions made, but in the questions that remain unanswered. Future directions will be limited only by the researchers and readers who ask these questions.

NOTE

1. It may be that even in parent-infant attachment, attachment and caregiving are part of the same nurturance system. The caregiving behaviors of the parent may also serve to foster the parent's attachment to his or her child (Weiss, 1988). For example, proximity to one's child gives a parent the experience of "felt security," even though safety of the *parent* is not relevant. Conversely, in the experience of parenting, one is often confronted with intense anxiety when one's child is inaccessible, whereas proximity is reassuring even in the face of real danger. Thus it is possible that in parent-infant attachment, the parents' caregiving is attachment behavior comparable to crying, calling, and clinging, rather than an analogous behavioral system. These behaviors are not seen in infants because of the limitations of their motor development. In somewhat older children, however, caregiving behaviors such as hugging or patting can also be observed toward attachment figures.

REFERENCES

Adam, K., Bouckoms, A., & Streiner, D. (1982). Parental loss and family stability in attempted suicide. *Archives of General Psychiatry, 39,* 1081-1085.

Ainsworth, M. D. S. (1967). *Infancy in Uganda: Infant care and the growth of attachment.* Baltimore: Johns Hopkins University Press.

Ainsworth, M. D. S. (1973). The development of infant-mother attachment. In B. M. Caldwell & H. N. Ricciuti (Eds.), *Review of child development research* (Vol. 3, pp. 1-94). Chicago: University of Chicago Press.

Ainsworth, M. D. S. (1982). Attachment: Retrospect and prospect. In C. M. Parkes & J. Stevenson-Hinde (Eds.), *The place of attachment in human behavior* (pp. 3-30). New York: Basic Books.

Ainsworth, M. D. S. (1985). Attachments across the life-span. *Bulletin of the New York Academy of Medicine, 61,* 792-812.

Ainsworth, M. D. S. (1989). Attachments beyond infancy. *American Psychologist, 44,* 709-716.

Ainsworth, M. D. S., Blehar, M. C., Waters, E., & Wall, S. (1978). *Patterns of attachment: A psychological study of the Strange Situation.* Hillsdale, NJ: Erlbaum.

Bartholomew, K., & Horowitz, L. M. (1991). Attachment styles among young adults: A test of the four-category model. *Journal of Personality and Social Psychology, 61,* 226-244.

Berman, W. H. (1988a). The role of attachment in the post-divorce experience. *Journal of Personality and Social Psychology, 54*(3), 496-503.

Berman, W. H. (1988b). The relationship of ex-spouse attachment and adjustment following divorce. *Journal of Family Psychology, 1*(3), 312-328.

Berman, W. H., & Sperling, M. B. (1991). Attachment and distress in the transition to college. *Journal of Youth and Adolescence, 20*, 427-440.

Berscheid, E. (1983). Emotion. In H. H. Kelley, E. Berscheid, A. Christensen, J. Harvey, T. Huston, G. Levinger, E. McClintock, A. Peplau, & D. Peterson, *Close relationships* (pp. 110-168). New York: W. H. Freeman.

Bloom-Feshbach, S. (1987). From family to classroom: Variations in adjustment to nursery school. In J. Bloom-Feschbach, & S. Bloom-Feschbach, (Eds.), *The psychology of separation and loss* (pp. 207-231). San Francisco: Jossey-Bass.

Bowlby, J. (1960). Symposium on "psycho-analysis and ethology": II. Ethology and the development of object relations. *International Journal of Psycho-Analysis, 41*, 313-317.

Bowlby, J. (1969). *Attachment and loss: Vol. 1. Attachment.* New York: Basic Books.

Bowlby, J. (1973). *Attachment and loss: Vol. 2. Separation: Anxiety and anger.* New York: Basic Books.

Bowlby, J. (1980). *Attachment and loss: Vol. 3. Loss: Sadness and depression.* New York: Basic Books.

Bowlby, J. (1982a). *Attachment and loss: Vol. 1. Attachment* (2nd ed.). New York: Basic Books.

Bowlby, J. (1982b). Attachment and loss: Retrospect and prospect. *American Journal of Orthopsychiatry, 52*, 664-678.

Bowlby, J. (1988a). Developmental psychiatry comes of age. *American Journal of Psychiatry, 145*, 1-10.

Bowlby, J. (1988b). *A secure base.* New York: Basic Books.

Bretherton, I. (1991). Pouring old wine into new bottles: The social self as internal working model. In M. R. Gunnar & L. A. Sroufe (Eds.), *Minnesota Symposia on Child Development: Vol. 23. Self processes and development* (pp. 1-41). Hillsdale, NJ: Erlbaum.

Cohn, D. A., Silver, D. H., Cowan, C. P., Cowan, P. A., & Pearson, J. (1992). Working models of childhood attachment and couple relationships. *Journal of Family Issues, 13*, 432-449.

Collins, N. L., & Read, S. J. (1990). Adult attachment, working models, and relationship quality in dating couples. *Journal of Personality and Social Psychology, 58*, 644-663.

Erikson, E. H. (1963). *Childhood and society.* New York: Norton.

Erickson, M. F., Sroufe, L. A., & Egeland, B. (1985). The relationship between quality of attachment and behavior problems in preschool in a high risk sample. In I. Bretherton & E. Waters (Eds.), Growing points of attachment theory and research. *Monographs of the Society for Research in Child Development, 50* (1-2, Serial No. 209), 147-186.

Feeney, J. A., & Noller, P. (1990). Attachment style as a predictor of adult romantic relationships. *Journal of Personality and Social Psychology, 58*(2), 281-291.

Glick, I. O., Weiss, R. S., & Parkes, C. M. (1974). *The first year of the bereavement.* New York: Wiley-Interscience.

Greenberg, M. T., Siegal, J., & Leitch, C. (1984). The nature and importance of attachment relationships to parents and peers during adolescence. *Journal of Youth and Adolescence, 12*(5), 373-386.

Hazan, C., & Shaver, P. (1987). Romantic love conceptualized as an attachment process. *Journal of Personality and Social Psychology, 52*, 511-524.

Hazan, C., & Shaver, P. (1990) Love and work: An attachment-theoretical perspective. *Journal of Personality and Social Psychology, 59*, 270-280.

Hinde, R. A. (1982). Attachment: Some conceptual and biological issues. In C. M. Parkes & J. Stevenson-Hinde (Eds.), *The place of attachment in human behavior* (pp. 31-53). New York: Basic Books.

Hindy, C. G., Schwarz, J. C., & Brodsky, A. (1989). *If this is love, why do I feel so insecure?* New York: Atlantic Monthly Press.

Kahn, R., & Antonucci, T. C. (1980). Convoys over the life course: Attachment, roles, and social supports. In P. Baltes & O. Brim (Eds.), *Life span development and behavior* (Vol. 3, pp. 253-286). New York: Academic Press.

Kelley, H. H., Berscheid, E., Christensen, A., Harvey, J., Huston, T., Levinger, G., McClintock, E., Peplau, A., & Peterson, D. (1983). *Close relationships*, New York: W. H. Freeman.

Kenny, M. (1987). The extent and function of parental attachment among first year college students. *Journal of Youth and Adolescence, 16*, 17-29.

Kernberg, O. (1976). *Object relations theory and clinical psychoanalysis*. New York: Jason Aronson.

Kobak, R., & Hazan, C. (1991). Attachment in marriage: Effects of security and accuracy of working models. *Journal of Personality and Social Psychology, 60*(6), 861-869.

Kobak, R., & Sceery, A. (1988). Attachment in late adolescence: Working models, affect regulation, and representation of self and others. *Child Development, 59*, 135-146.

Levitt, M. J., Weber, R. A., & Clark, M. C. (1986). Social network relationships as sources of maternal support and well-being. *Developmental Psychology, 22*(3), 310-316.

Main, M., Kaplan, N., & Cassidy, J. (1985). Security in infancy, childhood, and adulthood: A move to the level of representation. In I. Bretherton & E. Waters (Eds.), *Growing points of attachment theory and research. Monographs of the Society for Research in Child Development, 50* (1-2, Serial No. 209), 66-104.

Melges, F. T., & Swartz, M. S. (1989). Oscillations of attachment in borderline personality disorder. *American Journal of Psychiatry, 146*(9), 1115-1120.

Parker, G. (1979). Parental characteristics in relation to depressive disorders. *British Journal of Psychiatry, 134*, 138-147.

Parker, G. (1983). Parental "affectionless control" as an antecedent to adult depression. *Archives of General Psychiatry, 40*, 956-960.

Parker, G., Tupling, H., & Brown, L. B. (1979). A parental bonding instrument. *British Journal of Medical Psychology, 52*, 1-10.

Parkes, C. M. (1972). *Bereavement*. New York: International Universities Press.

Rutter, M. (1985). Resilience in the face of adversity: Protective factors and resistance to psychiatric disorder. *British Journal of Psychiatry, 147*, 598-611.

Shaver, P., Hazan, C., & Bradshaw, D. (1988). Love as attachment: The integration of three behavioral systems. In R. J. Sternberg & M. L. Barnes (Eds.), *The psychology of love* (pp. 68-99). New Haven, CT: Yale University Press.

Sperling, M. B. (1988). Phenomenology and developmental origins of desperate love. *Psychoanalysis and Contemporary Thought, 11,* 741-761.

Sperling, M. B., & Berman, W. H. (1989, April). *An attachment classification of desperate love: Preliminary findings.* Paper presented at the midwinter meeting of the Division of Psychoanalysis of the American Psychological Association, New York, NY.

Sperling, M. B., & Berman, W. H. (1991). An attachment classification of desperate love. *Journal of Personality Assessment, 56,* 45-55.

Sperling, M. B., Berman, W. H., & Fagen, G. (1992). Classification of adult attachment: An integrative taxonomy from attachment and psychoanalytic theories. *Journal of Personality Assessment, 59*(2), 239-247.

Sperling, M. B., Sharp, J. L., & Fishler, P. H. (1991). On the nature of attachment in a borderline population: A preliminary investigation. *Psychological Reports, 68,* 543-546.

Sroufe, L. A., Egeland, B., & Kreutzer, T. (1990). The fate of early experience following developmental change: Longitudinal approaches to individual adaptation in childhood. *Journal of Child Development, 61,* 1363-1373.

Stern, D. (1985). *The interpersonal world of the infant.* New York: Basic Books.

Von Bertalanffy, L. (1968). *General systems theory.* New York: George Braziller.

Weiss, R. S. (1975). *Marital separation.* New York: Basic Books.

West, M., & Sheldon, A. (1988). Classification of pathological attachment patterns in adults. *Journal of Personality Disorders, 2,* 153-159.

West, M., Sheldon, A., & Reiffer, L. (1987). An approach to the delineation of adult attachment. *Journal of Nervous and Mental Disease, 175,* 738-741.

West, M., Sheldon, A., & Reiffer, L. (1989). Attachment theory and brief psychotherapy: Applying current research to clinical interventions. *Canadian Journal of Psychiatry, 34,* 369-375.

PART II

Conceptual and Methodological Perspectives

CHAPTER 2

Continuity of Attachment across the Life Span

JULIE C. ROTHBARD

PHILLIP R. SHAVER

Bowlby's writings on attachment have inspired research in such diverse areas as social and cognitive development in childhood (e.g., Erickson, Sroufe, & Egeland, 1985), close relationships in adulthood (e.g., Bartholomew & Horowitz, 1991; Collins & Read, 1990; Hazan & Shaver, 1987), religiosity and sudden religious conversion (Kirkpatrick & Shaver, 1990, 1992), work and work satisfaction (Hazan & Shaver, 1990), and fear of death (Mikulincer, Florian, & Tolmacz, 1990). The widespread appeal of attachment theory stems from its ability to combine aspects of ethological, psychoanalytic, and social-cognitive perspectives into an integrative and rich, yet empirically testable, set of propositions concerning social behavior and personality. Attachment theory offers both distal and proximal explanations of the emergence and stability of personality; it suggests that an innate "attachment behavioral system," in combination with experience-based "internal working models," forms the basis for the various motivational, cognitive, emotional, and behavioral tendencies that constitute personality.

Bowlby's (1969/1982) theory portrays the mother–child (or caregiver–child) relationship as the root of both intra- and interpersonal functioning in later childhood and adulthood. Bowlby and others (e.g., Ainsworth, Blehar, Waters, & Wall, 1978; Bretherton, 1985; Main, Kaplan, & Cassidy, 1985) have suggested that as a result of early attachment experiences, a child accumulates knowledge and develops a set of expectations (known as "internal working models") about the self, significant others, and the larger social world. These working models regulate the attachment behavioral system and are, like all important affect-laden schemata, resistant though not impervious to change. Bowlby maintained that attachment behaviors "characterize human beings from the cradle to the grave" (1979, p. 129), and that "while attachment behavior is at its most obvious in early

31

childhood, it can be observed throughout the life cycle, especially in emergencies" (1989, p. 238). He also suggested that working models regulate attachment-related processes and personality dynamics throughout the life course (e.g., Bowlby, 1988).

The idea that individual differences in attachment patterns, or "attachment styles," might persist to some degree from infancy to adulthood continues to arouse controversy, although it is quite compatible with attachment theory's psychoanalytic roots. It seems to grate on our fellow social psychologists (e.g., Hendrick & Hendrick, 1994), and is perhaps the biggest stumbling block to applying Bowlby's and Ainsworth's ideas to the study of adult relationships. The purpose of the present chapter is to review the evidence for continuity and change in attachment styles during childhood and adulthood. The lack of a comprehensive review has allowed critics to form impressions of attachment research based on scanty or partial familiarity with the literature. We begin with a brief overview of attachment theory and its central constructs, including internal working models and individual differences in attachment styles. We then summarize the evidence for stability of attachment styles in both childhood and adulthood, and include a discussion of discontinuity and the factors affecting change. Throughout the review we address controversial issues in attachment research, such as methodological inadequacies and alternative interpretations of findings. In the end we evaluate the current status of attachment theory and research, especially as it applies to adults.

ATTACHMENT THEORY, WORKING MODELS, AND ATTACHMENT STYLES

Attachment Theory

The central tenet of attachment theory is that humans, like other primates, possess an evolutionarily adapted attachment behavioral system, the major goal of which is to keep vulnerable infants in close proximity to their caregivers, especially when danger threatens. The attachment system consists of a set of alternative behaviors (e.g., signaling, crying, clinging to the caregiver) that, through the process of natural selection, have become likely responses to threat or impending harm. (In what Bowlby called the "environment of evolutionary adaptedness," infants—and perhaps adults as well—who were better able to signal their needs and elicit protection from caregivers were more likely to survive to reproductive age.) According to Bowlby, the attachment system includes a variable "set goal" for proximity, which functions in homeostatic fashion to keep the infant within safe range of a caregiver. When danger seems unlikely, the attachment system recedes into the background and allows the child to learn through independent exploration of the environment. If, however, the caregiver's accessibility is questionable (thus exceeding the set goal for proximity), exploratory activity, which Bowlby considered necessary for healthy cognitive, social, and emotional development, is dramatically reduced.

A secure attachment relationship in infancy—the presumed norm according to which an infant displays "primary conditional strategies" (Main, 1990), such as proximity seeking under stressful conditions and exploration under conditions of safety—is by no means guaranteed. Such a relationship depends on the primary caregiver's sensitivity and responsiveness, and on the child's ability to trust in the caregiver's accessibility. When elements of sensitivity, reliability, or trust are missing in the relationship—for example, when the caregiver displays inconsistent accessibility, intrudes unpredictably or insensitively into the infant's activities, or rejects the infant's bids for physical contact—"secondary conditional strategies" (e.g., anxious clinging and vigilance or premature independence) become prominent. These secondary strategies are adaptive in the short run, given the child's nonoptimal caregiving environment, but may cause difficulty in subsequent relationships, as documented throughout this chapter.

Internal Working Models

Internal working models can be conceptualized as by-products of repeated attachment-related experiences. They are rooted in the same brain processes that generally construct schemata to organize and process information that otherwise would exceed cognitive capacity (Fiske & Taylor, 1991). Unlike simple cognitive schemata, however, working models are thought to include affective and defensive as well as descriptive cognitive components (Bretherton, 1985; Main et al., 1985). Working models consist of accumulated knowledge about the self, attachment figures, and attachment relationships. Functioning partially (perhaps largely) outside of awareness, they provide a person with heuristics for anticipating and interpreting the behavior and intentions of others, especially attachment figures.

Working models are considered the mechanisms through which continuity in the organization of attachment is achieved. During early childhood, the models are thought to be relatively flexible and impressionable—that is, responsive to a changing environment (hence the term "working"). Bowlby maintained, however, that repeated interactions of the same kind with one or more primary caregivers serve to structure and strengthen the emerging working models, rendering them increasingly resistant to change. It is useful to draw an analogy between this process and the Piagetian notions of "assimilation" and "accommodation." During early development, working models tend to accommodate (adjust themselves) to new information about attachment figures, the environment, and the self. Once more firmly established, however, they guide the processing of attachment-relevant information and tend to assimilate it to the existing structure, sometimes creating significant distortions. Only when the lack of fit between working models and reality becomes extremely apparent do working models change (Bretherton, Ridgeway, & Cassidy, 1990).

Attachment Styles

In a landmark study of Bowlby's ideas, Ainsworth et al. (1978) created a research paradigm known as the Strange Situation, which elicits an infant's attachment behaviors through repeated separations from an attachment figure and interactions with a stranger, and also elicits exploratory behavior by offering a multitude of attractive toys. On the basis of infants' reactions to separations and reunions in the Strange Situation, Ainsworth et al. identified three basic patterns of attachment, one secure and two insecure. Contemporary attachment researchers (e.g., Bartholomew & Horowitz, 1991; Main et al., 1985) generally believe that these attachment styles are organized around differing configurations of working models of self and others.

Infants classified as "secure" (denoted "B" by Ainsworth and others) fit Bowlby's conception of nature's prototype: They are distressed by separation, seek comfort upon reunion, and explore freely in their caregivers' presence. Ainsworth et al. (1978) concluded from a series of home visits that the primary caregivers of secure infants are generally sensitive and responsive to their infants' signals. In contrast, the typical mother of an "anxious/ambivalent" ("C") infant responds inconsistently to her infant's signals, being sometimes unavailable or unresponsive, and at other times intrusive or overly affectionate. (For additional findings concerning specific caregiver behaviors, see Crowell & Feldman, 1988, and Isabella & Belsky, 1991.) In the Strange Situation, these infants cry more than others, are distressed prior to separation, seem unable to be reassured or comforted, and are so preoccupied with their caregivers' availability as to reduce or preclude exploration.

Ainsworth et al. characterized the caregivers of "avoidant" ("A") infants as rejecting and tending to rebuff or deflect their infants' bids for proximity, especially for close bodily contact. In the Strange Situation, these infants exhibit little overt distress upon separation and do not seek contact upon reunion. Instead, they keep their attention directed toward toys or other objects, apparently to shift attention away from the wish to establish contact with their attachment figures. (Their hidden distress is suggested both by home observations and by laboratory measures of cardiac arousal; Ainsworth et al., 1978; Sroufe & Waters, 1977b.)

In recent years, researchers have become increasingly aware of a fourth attachment style, labeled "D" ("disorganized/disoriented") by Main and her colleagues (e.g., Main & Hesse, 1990; Main & Solomon, 1990; Main et al., 1985) and "A/C" (avoidant/ambivalent) by Crittenden (1985, 1988). Infants identified as D or A/C are not classifiable within the original Ainsworth et al. (1978) typology. During reunion episodes in the Strange Situation, these infants show signs of disorganized and contradictory behaviors, such as approaching the caregiver with head averted, crying for the caregiver during separation and then moving away from him or her during reunion, or approaching the caregiver and then falling to the floor or suddenly freezing in midapproach. Main and colleagues have discovered an association between an infant's D attachment status and a caregiver's unresolved feelings and incoherent thinking about attachment-related traumas and losses; Crittenden's research suggests that the A/C pattern arises when a primary caregiver is abused, depressed, disturbed, or extremely neglectful.

For the remainder of this chapter, except where otherwise noted, our discussion of differences among attachment styles refers mainly to the original three attachment patterns—secure, anxious/ambivalent, and avoidant—because there is still relatively little evidence concerning the fourth category. We suspect that most of the findings we discuss here would have been clearer and stronger if the four-category typology had been employed, because in many studies D children were inadvertently mixed with A, B, and C children. This suspicion remains to be tested in future research.

ATTACHMENT STYLES DURING CHILDHOOD

Following Ainsworth's pioneering work, numerous investigators eventually replicated her results, suggesting that the Strange Situation is a reliable procedure for assessing individual differences in the organization of attachment. In the 1970s, however, when the procedure was first gaining popularity among researchers interested in infant–parent relationships, the attachment construct came under fire from psychologists who subscribed to a behaviorist perspective (e.g., Masters & Wellman, 1974). Their criticisms centered around the lack of evidence for correlations among or stability of discrete, time-sampled attachment behaviors. Waters (1978;

Sroufe & Waters, 1977a) concurred that measures of discrete behaviors correlate poorly over a 6-month period, but noted that when attachment is operationalized in terms of the frequency with which smiling, crying, approaching, or other behaviors occur during a given time period, an erroneous assumption is made that "all instances of phenotypically similar behaviors are equivalent" (Waters, 1978, p. 492). Waters demonstrated that when attachment is viewed in terms of functional *categories* of behavior (secure, avoidant, anxious/ambivalent), substantial correspondence between attachment classifications at two points in time is obtainable. Of his 50 middle-class infant subjects, 48 (or 96%) received the same attachment classifications at 12 and 18 months of age. Using discriminant-function analyses, Main and Weston (1981) also found considerable stability between infant-father (81%) and infant-mother (73%) attachment classifications over a period of several months. Since the time of Waters's (1978) and Main and Weston's (1981) convincing demonstrations, use of the Strange Situation has become standard in studies of infant attachment styles and their sequelae in childhood. We turn now to an examination of this literature, which remains relatively unread by adult attachment researchers and their critics, even though most of the child findings can be (and now are being) reproduced with adult subjects.

Correlates of Attachment Classifications in Early Childhood and Preadolescence

Matas, Arend, and Sroufe (1978) examined the association between attachment classifications and later quality of play and problem solving in a randomly selected subset of a large middle-class sample. They hypothesized that children with secure attachment relationships, when compared to their insecure counterparts, would exhibit greater autonomy and self-confidence on problem-solving tasks and more affective sharing with their mothers. Quality of attachment was assessed at 18 months of age, with 23 infants classified as secure, 15 as avoidant, and 10 as anxious/ambivalent. (This distribution is similar to the ones obtained by other child development researchers and—as shown by Hazan & Shaver, 1987—to the distribution of adult versions of these styles.) At 24 months, the toddlers were observed during a free-play period, a clean-up period, and a problem-solving period during which they were presented with four increasingly difficult tasks. Secure toddlers engaged in more imaginative play than did toddlers in either of the two insecure groups. They were more enthusiastic, persistent, and compliant; made better use of their mothers' suggestions during problem solving; displayed more positive and less negative affect; and were less aggressive. According to Matas et al. (1978), these differences were not attributable to developmental quotient or temperament, on which the three groups did not differ. Differences in the quality of early attachment relationships seemed to explain these findings, which were subsequently replicated by Frankel and Bates (1990).

Arend, Gove, and Sroufe (1979) were also interested in the predictive validity of attachment classifications, but over a longer time period than studied by Matas et al. (1978). These researchers hypothesized that quality of attachment at 18 months would be significantly related to dimensions of ego resiliency and ego control between 4 and 5 years of age. "Ego resiliency" was defined as the ability to respond to problem situations with flexibility, persistence, and resourcefulness, rather than inflexibility and a tendency to become disorganized when stressed. "Ego control" was defined as the extent to which feelings, desires, impulses, and needs for gratification are kept under control. Moderate levels of ego control were considered to be most adaptive.

Using a subset of the sample studied earlier by Matas et al. (1978), Arend et al. (1979) found that securely attached infants were more ego-resilient than the two insecure groups, as rated on the California Child Q-Sort by nursery or kindergarten teachers. Although there were no significant group differences on a composite measure of ego control, a trend indicated that avoidant infants displayed the highest levels of ego control, anxious/ambivalent infants displayed the lowest levels, and secure infants fell in the moderate range. In addition, secure infants scored significantly higher than infants in the two insecure groups on an independent measure of curiosity.

In addition to studying cognitive correlates of early attachment relationships, researchers have been interested in the association between infant–mother attachment and later measures of sociability and social competence. Waters, Wippman, and Sroufe (1979) measured quality of attachment at age 15 months, and then related these differences to Q-sort measures of social competence and ego strength/effectance (similar to Arend et al.'s [1979] ego resiliency and ego control) at age 3½. The Q-sort data were based on extensive observations of the children in a preschool classroom, *without* mothers present. Results from the Peer Competence scale indicated that secure preschoolers were more likely to be leaders among their peers, to suggest activities, to be sympathetic to their peers' distress, and to be sought out as interaction partners. In contrast, insecure preschoolers were more likely to be socially withdrawn, hesitant with other children, spectators rather than participants in activities, and listeners rather than engagers. On the Ego Strength/Effectance scale, secure children were more likely to be self-directed, to enjoy learning new cognitive skills, and to "forcefully go after what [they] want," whereas insecure children tended to lack curiosity about the new and to be "unaware, turned off, or spaced out" (p. 827). These results are quite striking, particularly because mothers were absent when the assessments were made. They indicate that continuity can be demonstrated outside the realm of direct maternal influence; they also suggest that factors internal to the individual, as opposed to immediate environmental contingencies, are responsible for the observed behavior.

Pastor (1981) was also interested in sociability differences among the three attachment groups. Sixty-two infants were classified into attachment groups at 18 months of age. At approximately age 2, the toddlers were assigned to free-play dyads in such a way that members of each attachment group (designated "focal" children) were paired with securely attached playmates. Dyads were observed interacting in a laboratory playroom (with both mothers present) for 30 minutes, during which time each toddler was rated on a variety of dimensions. Results indicated that the secure focal children were significantly more sociable, more oriented toward both their mothers and their playmates, and more interested in engaging their playmates than were members of either of the insecure groups. They were also more likely than avoidant toddlers to redirect their play activities after struggling with their playmates over toys. Anxious/ambivalent toddlers were more likely than the other two groups to ignore offers made by the playmates, less likely to make social offers to the playmates, and less positive in their contacts with their mothers. According to Pastor, "the anxious group tended to be in close proximity to their mothers, whereas the avoidant group tended to be distant most often. Anxious children tended to look toward their mothers, avoidant toward objects, and securely attached toward their peers" (p. 331).

In a similar, subsequent study, Jacobson and Wille (1986) paired eight children (at both 2 and 3 years of age) from each attachment group (measured at 18 months) with same-sex, securely attached, unfamiliar playmates. Subjects and their partners were observed during a 25-minute free-play session, and interactive behavior was rated on six dimensions. Most interesting among the results of this study were several significant effects for secure playmates (also obtained by Pastor, 1981), suggesting that sociability differences related to the three attachment patterns can be attributed at least in part to subjects' attractiveness as interaction partners. At age 3, playmates paired with secure focal children responded more positively to their partners than did playmates paired with insecure focal children. Playmates paired with avoidant partners directed fewer positive initiations toward them. Playmates paired with anxious/ambivalent partners were more disruptive of their partners' play and initiated more conflictual encounters with them. Jacobson and Wille suggested that differences in early attachment relationships elicit differential responsiveness from interaction partners. It could be hypothesized that this differential responsiveness serves to confirm an individual's expectations about the social world and important others, thereby strengthening the character of existing working models and increasing the likelihood that early attachment styles will remain stable. Other researchers (e.g., Elicker, Englund, & Sroufe, 1992) draw similar conclusions from their work.

Renken, Egeland, Marvinney, Mangelsdorf, and Sroufe (1989) investigated early antecedents of elementary school aggression and passive withdrawal in a high-risk sample. Because the literature suggested that a history of abusive or punitive parental treatment is among the correlates of later aggressive behavior, Renken et al. hypothesized that children classified as avoidant at both 12 and 18 months of age would exhibit the most aggressive behavior, as rated by their school teachers. Among other predictors of aggression, such as stressful life circumstances and inadequate or hostile parental care, avoidant attachment was significantly related to aggressive behavior for boys but not for girls. Other researchers have found similar connections between avoidant attachment and preschool aggression (Egeland & Sroufe, 1981; Sroufe, 1983).

Related patterns emerged in the analysis of passive withdrawal. Renken et al. hypothesized that children classified as anxious/ambivalent at ages 12 and 18 months would exhibit the most passive withdrawal, because the quality of attachment for this group is characterized by parental behavior (such as intrusiveness or inconsistent responsiveness) that interferes with a child's sense of agency and resourcefulness. As expected, anxious/ambivalent attachment was significantly related to passive withdrawal, but only among boys. The authors suggested that the failure to find differences for girls could be attributed to the clustering of their scores at the low ends of the scales assessing aggression and passive withdrawal.

Erickson et al. (1985) also examined the relation between early attachment classifications and later social behavior in the school environment. Ninety-six infants were classified into attachment groups at 12 and 18 months of age. When the children were 4½ to 5 years old, they were observed in their respective preschool or day care settings, and three categories of behavior problems were identified (acting out, being withdrawn, and exhibiting attentional problems). Analyses indicated that insecurely attached children were significantly more likely than secure children to belong to any one of these groups. Additional results were quite striking. The behavior of children originally classified as avoidantly attached was judged to be the most discrepant from that of the secure children. Avoidant children were rated by observers as highly dependent, noncompliant, and incompetent in social interactions. Teachers rated these children as more hostile, impulsive, lacking in persistence, and withdrawn. (The high ratings on the hostility and noncompliance factors fit well with Renken et al.'s [1989] findings of increased aggressiveness among avoidant children.)

Anxious/ambivalent children also differed from secure children, although the differences were judged to be less striking than the ones for the avoidant group. Anxious/ambivalent children seemed to lack the agency, assertiveness, and confidence necessary for effective interaction with peers and the preschool environment. (Again, these findings fit well with Renken et al.'s [1989] study of passive withdrawal.)

Among the most impressive demonstrations of cross-age stability in the organization of attachment comes from the work of Main and Cassidy (1988) and its application by Grossmann and Grossmann (1991). Main and Cassidy devised an attachment classification system, similar to the Strange Situation, for 6-year-old children. Following a 1-hour separation from either mother or father, a child is rated as secure by this procedure if he or she "initiates conversation and pleasant interaction with the parent on reunion or is highly responsive to parent's own initiations. May subtly move into proximity or physical contact with parent, usually with rationale such as seeking a toy. Remains calm throughout episode" (Main & Cassidy, 1988, p. 420). Avoidant ratings are made if the child "minimizes and restricts opportunities for interaction with the parent on reunion, look[s] and speak[s] only briefly and minimally as required and remain[s] occupied with toys or activities. At extremes, moves away, but subtly, with rationale such as retrieving a toy" (p. 420). The child is classified as anxious/ambivalent if "in movements, posture, and tones of voice child appears to attempt to exaggerate intimacy with the parent as well as dependency on the parent. May seek proximity or contact, but shows some resistance or ambivalence . . . Moderately avoidant, signs of hostility [often subtle] are sometimes present" (p. 420). Grossmann and Grossmann (1991) used this classification system on a sample of 6-year-olds in Regensburg, Germany, obtaining 87% convergence between attachment ratings so derived and Strange Situation ratings of the same children during infancy.

Up to this point, we have reviewed several studies indicating short-term continuity in the developmental adaptation and attachment ratings of infants originally classified as secure, anxious/ambivalent, or avoidant. For obvious practical reasons, far fewer studies have been conducted on the relationship between infant attachment and later functioning in preadolescence or early adolescence. Among the exceptions are studies by Elicker et al. (1992) and Grossmann and Grossmann (1991), which suggest stability of attachment over a 10-year period.

Grossmann and Grossmann (1991) followed a sample of German children from infancy through 10 years of age and observed differences in adaptation at various ages similar to those found by previous researchers. At age 10, the children were interviewed about their peer relations and strategies for coping with stressful situations, among other topics. The children's response styles were noted. Most highly related to early attachment quality were the children's reports of relations with peers. Children originally classified as secure reported having at least one or a few good friends whom they considered reliable and trustworthy. Insecure children, especially those originally categorized as anxious/ambivalent, reported having either no good friends or many friends (the names of whom they were unable to provide). They also more often described themselves as exploited or ridiculed by peers and excluded from group activities.

In terms of coping with stress, only situations causing the children to feel afraid, angry, or sad significantly distinguished among the three attachment groups. Secure children reported coping with negative feelings by turning to others for help or comfort, whereas avoidant children more often attempted to work their problems out by themselves. (Very similar patterns have been observed in adults, as explained later in this chapter.) There were also some interesting differences in the children's social behavior during the course of the interview. According to Grossmann and Grossmann, insecure children either ignored the interviewer to the point of being rude or were inappropriately intimate or affectionate. The authors did not specify which inappropriate behaviors were more characteristic of which insecure group, but one might conjecture that the former behavior described avoidant children while the latter described anxious/ambivalent children.

Elicker et al. (1992) recruited 47 children from their original Minnesota high-risk sample to participate in a 4-week summer camp program, at which time extensive observations were made. The children had first been classified into attachment groups at 12 and 18 months of age. All participated in a preschool study at age 4. At the time of the summer camp study, the children were 10–11 years old. Approximately equal numbers of children from each attachment group were selected for participation. Data were collected at both a broad level (e.g., counselor ratings of social competence, emotional health, and self-confidence) and a more specific level (e.g., time-sampled observations of child–child and child–adult interactions), and the children were interviewed during the last week of camp to gain insight into their personal perspectives on the camp experience.

The results provided dramatic evidence that the quality of infant–mother attachment is an important predictor of competence and interpersonal relations in later years. Inter- and intrapersonal correlates of the attachment bond were evident 10 years after initial assessment, in the absence of direct maternal influence and away from familiar surroundings. Overall, children with secure attachment histories were rated as more emotionally healthy, self-assured, and competent, and those with insecure attachment histories were rated as more dependent on adults. Secure children spent significantly more time with peers and in groups of three or more, and significantly less time alone or with adults. They also received higher ratings than their insecure peers on popularity, sociability, and prosocial interaction skills. Furthermore, whereas secure children evidenced positive biases in evaluating the performance of their peers, insecure children displayed negative biases in their evaluations, with avoidant children showing the lowest levels of interpersonal understanding and sensitivity. In terms of cross-gender interactions, insecure children more often violated implicit rules of gender boundaries for 10-year-olds; that is, they engaged in cross-gender interactions more frequently than did children with secure attachment histories, and they more often sat next to members of the opposite sex when in group circles. Finally, secure children were more likely to have developed friendships (as determined by counselors' ratings as well as through nominations of friendship by the other children). They spent more time with their most frequent play partners and were more likely to befriend other secure children.

Attachment Styles and Internal Working Models in Childhood

Individual differences in the organization of attachment can be conceptualized not only as differences in infant reunion behavior (or the later correlates of such behavior), but as differences in mental representations of the self and others, particularly in the context of attachment relationships. Stated differently, behaviors associated with the three attachment styles can be conceptualized as the observable manifestations of internal working models. Several researchers have examined the relation between attachment classifications and children's working models, including Bretherton et al. (1990), Grossmann and Grossmann (1991), and Main et al. (1985).

The most impressive examination of working models in early childhood was conducted by Main et al. (1985), based on 40 families from the Berkeley Social Development Project who participated in the 6th-year phase of a longitudinal study. Subjects had been observed in the Strange Situation at both 12 and 18 months of age, and the quality of their attachment to their mothers and fathers, respectively, had been assessed. To facilitate correlational analyses, attachment classifications were transformed into continuous ratings running from very secure to insecure, such that the most secure infants (subcategory B3 in Ainsworth et al.'s [1978] detailed coding system) were assigned a value of 3, moderately secure infants (groups B2 and B1) were assigned a value of 2, and insecure infants (groups A, C, and D) were assigned a value of 1. At age 6, the children were observed participating in a variety of tasks designed to assess attachment styles and the nature of working models. Attachment classifications were obtained on the basis of the procedure designed by Main and Cassidy (1988) for use with 6-year-olds. Attachment to mother at age 6 proved to be highly related to attachment to mother in infancy ($r = .76$). Attachment to father at age 6 was also related to earlier attachment to father, but the continuity was not as strong as it was for mother ($r = .30$), perhaps because most of the children had spent much more time during the previous 5 years with their mothers than with their fathers.

Cognitive-representational measures of attachment were obtained as follows, with highly significant results:

1. Conversations between each parent and child following a 1-hour separation were analyzed, revealing very strong correlations between early attachment classifications to mother or father and fluency of discourse with the same parent at age 6. Secure children and their parents evidenced the greatest fluidity and balance in their conversational patterns, such that neither partner clearly led a conversation, a parent and child spoke directly to each other with little pause or difficulty in expressing information, and both addressed each other in a manner that promoted further conversation. Insecure children and their parents, especially those classified as disorganized/disoriented (category D) during infancy, displayed the greatest dysfluency of discourse. A typical conversation in the D group was characterized by frequent and awkward pauses, and was clearly led by the child, not the parent. At a lesser extreme, discourse between avoidant children and their parents also contained frequent pauses. Members of these pairs tended to talk, with limited elaboration, about impersonal topics (e.g., toys).

2. Responses to a series of pictures depicting a child's impending separation from parents were analyzed for evidence of subjects' emotional openness and ability to deal with separation. The results indicated a strong association between emotional openness and early security of attachment to mother. In addition, secure children, in contrast to insecure children, tended to respond to the hypothetical separation by dealing with it constructively and by expressing their feelings directly. (See Grossmann & Grossmann, 1991, for a German replication of these results.)

3. Early in the study session, a Polaroid photograph was taken of each child with his or her parents; each child was later presented with this family photograph. Secure children showed interest in the picture, smiled at it, and talked about it. Insecure children, especially those classified as avoidant, tended to look away from the photo when it was placed near them, or refused to accept the photo altogether. At the extreme, disorganized/disoriented children reportedly became suddenly depressed and disorganized when presented with the photo.

4. Overall functioning was rated in an unstandardized manner, with judges relying on their own notions of what constitutes social and emo-

tional adaptation. Interestingly, analyses revealed a strong, significant correlation between early attachment to mother and overall functioning, but not between overall functioning and early attachment to father.

Main et al. (1985) concluded that, in contrast to insecure children, "the secure 6-year-old seemed to have free ranging access to affect, memory, and plans, whether in forming speech in conversation with the parent or in discussing imagined situations relevant to attachment" (p. 95), suggesting that internal working models are quite different for children displaying secure and insecure attachment behavioral patterns. (Additional results indicated differences among the various insecure groups as well.)

Grossmann and Grossmann (1991) were likewise interested in internal working models in childhood. When subjects in their German sample reached the age of 6, each child was asked to draw a picture of his or her family. Results indicated that ratings of individualization significantly distinguished between children classified as secure and insecure in infancy, with secure children evidencing greater degrees of individualization in their pictures. These results are similar to those obtained by Kaplan and Main (1985, cited in Bretherton et al., 1990), who noted that secure 6-year-olds depicted family members as well individuated, close but not exaggeratedly close, and not always smiling. Pictures drawn by avoidant children tended to show increased distance between family members, and all family members were portrayed as smiling in similar, stereotyped ways. Avoidant children also tended to omit arms from their figures. Pictures drawn by disorganized/disoriented children tended to include unfinished or overly cheery elements that were not well integrated into the overall depiction. (See Fury, 1993, for a replication and extension of this work.)

Bretherton et al. (1990) studied internal working models of attachment in 3-year-olds. Subjects participated in a story completion task consisting of five story lines designed to elicit attachment-related thoughts and feelings. The stories dealt with spilled juice, a hurt knee, a monster in the bedroom, a parental departure, and reunion following a separation. Children were classified as secure if, in their story completions, (1) the juice was cleaned up with minimal parental anger; (2) parents responded to the hurt knee with hugs or by administering a Band-Aid; (3) the child approached the parents when frightened by the monster, or the parents attempted to deal in a constructive way with the child's fear; (4) the child suggested ways in which he or she might cope with the parent's departure; and (5) family members hugged each other and engaged in conversation or other activities upon reunion. Subjects were classified as insecure if they avoided the issue in the story line or otherwise responded in an odd or incoherent fashion. (According to Bretherton et al., and in accord with Main et al., 1985, evasive and incoherent responding is indicative of defensiveness.)

Subjects were also classified into attachment groups on the basis of a separation-reunion procedure similar to those used by other researchers (e.g., Main & Cassidy, 1988) in studies of older children. Correlations between concurrent attachment classifications were highly significant ($r = .49$). Correlations between 18-month attachment ratings and story completions at age 3 were weaker but still highly significant ($r = .33$).

Discontinuity and Factors Affecting Change

Although Waters (1978) and Main and Weston (1981), among others, were able to demonstrate substantial stability in attachment classifications over a 6-month period, not all researchers replicated those findings with equal strength. For example, Vaughn, Egeland, Sroufe, and Waters (1979) studied 100 mother-infant dyads from an economically disadvantaged sample. Although stability in attachment classifications at 12 and 18 months was significant, only 62% of their sample received the same classification at both assessments. Similarly, Thompson, Lamb, and Estes (1983) obtained only 58% stability between classifications at 12.5 and 19.5 months. In each of these studies, the occurrence of stressful life events or changes in family circumstances, respectively, seemed to influence stability in the caregiving environment, suggesting that such conditions influence stability versus change in children's attachment behavior.

In their comprehensive study, Erickson et al. (1985) examined the relationship between early attachment classifications and later behavior problems in a socioeconomically disadvantaged sample, where stressful life events or changes in family circumstances were expected to be common, resulting in less developmental stability among children. Although Erickson et al. were interested in the correlates of early attachment classifications (as described in a previous section), they also investigated factors that led securely attached infants to exhibit later behavior problems and insecurely attached infants to display later competent functioning.

Ninety-six children were observed in their preschool or day care settings, and three categories of behavior problems were identified. Although the majority of children with behavior problems were those originally classified as insecurely attached, a small number of insecure children were competent in preschool, and a handful of secure children manifested behavior problems. According to Erickson et al., secure children with behavior problems had mothers who seemed less supportive of the children's problem-solving efforts, less warm and encouraging, and less able to structure tasks or set limits when the children were 2 years old. At age 3½, the children's home environment seemed to lack age-appropriate toys, and when the children were 4 years old, their mothers reported feeling confused and disoriented, perhaps indicating an inability to deal with the demands of their growing children. Interestingly, these originally secure children were not statistically different at age 2 from secure children who did not manifest later behavior problems; however, by age 3½, they were less affectionate and more avoidant of their mothers. Similar patterns emerged among insecure children. At age 2, there were no differences between those who later exhibited either competence or behavioral problems. However, by age 3½, those without later problems had mothers who were respectful of their children's autonomy, warm and supportive, less intrusive, and able to structure tasks and set limits. These mothers also reported having better emotional and social support from friends and family members than did mothers of insecure children who exhibited behavior problems.

These important findings indicate that changes in the quality of caregiving produce changes in a child's behavioral profile (and, quite possibly, in the child's working models). Erickson et al. (1985) did not conclude, however, that shifts in parental sensitivity and competence obliterate the effects of earlier experience altogether. Instead, they suggested that despite improvements in the quality of caregiving, insecurity in infancy and early childhood may leave a child vulnerable for quite some time. Similarly, they suggested that securely attached infants who experience later deterioration in parental caregiving should be able to recover quickly if the attachment relationship once again becomes supportive. Recent studies (to be discussed shortly) provide empirical support for these ideas.

Other researchers have studied discontinuity in attachment styles and the factors influencing change. Egeland and Farber (1984) found that mothers of infants who were secure at 12 months but insecure at 18 months displayed caregiving skills similar to those shown by mothers of infants who remained secure, but that they differed in certain affective and personality characteristics. They seemed less delighted with their infants and scored higher on measures of hostility and suspiciousness administered prenatally and when the infants were 3 months old. Egeland and Farber suggested that whereas caregiving skills are critical in the early formation of a secure attachment, a mother's personality and affective characteristics play an increasingly important role in the *maintenance* of this security as a child grows older. Changes from insecure to secure tended to be associated with the development of caregiving skills among young, originally immature or incompetent mothers. There were no differences across groups in the number of stressful life events encountered between the two assessments, suggesting that changes in life circumstances need not affect the attachment behavioral system unless they are first associated with changes in the quality of caregiving. Similarly, Frodi, Grolnick, and Bridges (1985) found that although major life events (e.g., illness, moving to a new home) were not associated with changes in attachment classifications, infants either remained or became secure at 20 months when their mothers were sensitive, nonpunitive, and supportive of the infants' developing autonomy. Those who remained or became insecure at 20 months had mothers who were less sensitive and more punitive and controlling.

Easterbrooks and Goldberg (1990) examined correlates of and discontinuity in attachment when their young subjects reached kindergarten, following assessment of attachment quality to both mother and father during toddlerhood. Of greatest relevance here, these researchers found significant interactions between stability of home environment (as operationalized by the extent to which maternal work patterns—and hence the time a mother spent with her child—remained stable) and quality of attachment. Specifically, stability in family life was significantly associated with higher scores on ego resiliency, and instability was associated with lower such scores for children classified as secure at 20 months of age. The opposite pattern of effects emerged for children originally classified as insecurely attached; that is, increased stability was associated with lower ego resiliency.

Along similar lines, Lewis and Feiring (1991; Lewis, Feiring, McGuffog, & Jaskir, 1984) studied the interaction between early attachment classifications and later family cohesion and conflict as determinants of behavior and "psychopathology" at age 6. They proposed two attachment × environment interaction models of later emotional disturbances, labeled the "vulnerable child" and the "invulnerable child" model, respectively. When the infants in the study were 3 months old, their mothers were observed interacting with them, and various ratings of maternal responsivity and play behavior were made. Infants were classified into attachment groups at 12 months of age, on the basis of a modified version of the Strange Situation (only one separation–reunion episode was included). When the children were 6 years old, mothers completed the Family Environment Scale (FES) and the Child Behavior Profile, which measures school competence, peer behavior, and social activities, and allows for the differentiation of children with and without emotional problems.

The results, which were significant mainly for male subjects, suggested not only that security of attachment and environmental factors make independent contributions to later psychopathology, but that both the vulnerable child and invulnerable child attachment × environment models can account for significant portions of the observed variance. Specifically, only 5% of secure males showed signs of psychopathology at age 6, whereas 40% of insecure males showed signs of psychopathology. Also for males, 50% of the conflicted families (those scoring in the top 25% on the combined Cohesion and Conflict subscales of the FES) had children with signs of psychopathology, compared to 0% for nonconflictual families (those scoring in the bottom 25% on the combined subscales). Finally, later environmental stress had little effect on the development of psychopathology for secure ("invulnerable") males. For insecure ("vulnerable") males, however, psychopathology was dependent on exposure to poor environmental conditions.

The work of Lewis et al. (1984; Lewis & Feiring, 1991) indicates that measures of attachment style taken at a particular point in time might best be conceptualized as reflecting the interaction between early attachment (or working models) and current environment, not just the manifestations of one factor or the other, and that certain early experiences may leave a child either vulnerable or relatively invulnerable to later changes in attachment relationships. A recent article by Sroufe, Egeland, and Kreutzer (1990) provides additional compelling evidence that "adaptation is always a product of both developmental history and current circumstances" (p. 1363). Using hierarchical-regression analyses, these authors found that when two groups of children, originally classified as either secure or insecure in the Strange Situation, both evidenced poor adaptation in the preschool years, a significant rebound toward positive functioning in elementary school was experienced by those with more secure early attachment histories. In other words, the effects of early attachment relationships could be masked at a particular point in development, only to reassert themselves at a later point.

Summary and Implications

Individual differences in attachment classifications during infancy have been significantly associated with cognitive and socioemotional outcomes at subsequent ages and with theory-guided expectations concerning the character of internal working models. Moreover, changes in a child's caregiving environment can produce at least temporary discontinuity between early attachment style and expected childhood outcomes, suggesting that a stress-vulnerability model is applicable. At the heart of the attachment-theoretical perspective on personality development are internal working models, which can be conceptualized as playing a mediating role between environmental events and subsequent behavior. The research reviewed here indicates that children from the original three attachment groups maintain working models of self and attachment figures that differ across groups in theoretically consistent ways. Furthermore, indirect evidence for the existence of working models comes from behavioral differences noted in a wide range of settings *in the absence of a primary attachment figure*. This indicates that the child "carries" his or her cognitively represented caregiving environment into new situations. The process might be described as follows: Environmental factors (such as maternal caregiving behavior) influence the character of working models, which in turn direct and become manifest in observable behavior. Substantial changes in the caregiving environment lead to changes in working models, which then alter the behavioral profile. It cannot be assumed that the caregiving environment directly determines children's social behavior without the mediating effects of working models, because if this were true, cross-situational consistency in the absence of an attachment figure and cross-age resistance to change would be difficult to demonstrate.

Internal working models must be fairly complex structures. Research to date suggests that they include or influence social perception, symbolic representations of people and relationships, social behavior, affective predispositions, defenses, and forms of discourse. Among the biggest current challenges in the field of attachment research are clarifying the construct of working models and finding ways to assess it reliably.

Cross-situational and cross-age consistencies in attachment styles seem unlikely to be attributable primarily to innate temperament. The fact that many infants exhibit different attachment styles with their mothers and fathers, and that changes in attachment style track changes in parental or family environment, suggests that temperament is less important than parenting. A good way to explore this issue further would be to conduct large-scale studies of attachment with infant twins. When Ricciuti (1992) recently aggregated the existing small samples of twins who have been tested in the Strange Situation, she found no clear evidence for genetic differences in attachment patterns, but the issue deserves further study.

ATTACHMENT STYLES IN ADULTHOOD

Several investigators have been exploring the possibility that attachment styles like the ones identified by Ainsworth et al. (1978) in infancy continue to exist in adulthood and play a role in romantic and parenting relationships. Here we have space to mention only two such approaches—one developed by Main and her colleagues (e.g., Main et al., 1985), and one by Hazan and Shaver (e.g., 1987; Shaver & Hazan, 1993). (Other approaches are discussed elsewhere in the present volume.) Main et al.'s approach is based on an empirical search for adult interview correlates of a person's *infant child's* attachment classification in the Strange Situation. In the initial studies of this issue in Main's laboratory, adults with infant children were interviewed about their own childhood relationships with their parents, and the interviews were compared to see which features, if any, were related to the interviewees' infant children's attachment behavior. Hazan and Shaver's approach is based on a self-report questionnaire measure of adult *romantic* attachment styles. The purpose of their research was to see whether attachment theory in general, and the three patterns of attachment organization identified by Ainsworth et al. in particular, might help explain personality differences in the experience of romantic love.

There are at least two ways in which the findings summarized in the preceding sections are relevant to the study of adult attachment patterns (parenting patterns and romantic attachment patterns). First, attachment *dynamics* might be similar in childhood and adulthood, although the adult forms of attachment styles would presumably be more complex than the childhood forms. Second, the major *determinants* of attachment styles might be similar in childhood and adulthood; that is, the styles might originate in relationships with parents and then become elaborated and changed in the context of subsequent important close relationships. In general, the childhood origins of attachment styles should still be evident to some extent in psychological assessments of adults, because the influence of parents exerts itself in most people's lives for many years. These issues are explored in the following sections.

The Adult Attachment Interview

The Adult Attachment Interview (AAI) is coded in terms of two kinds of rating scales. One concerns the attachment-related *experiences* that adults recall having had with their parents during childhood—for example, the degree to which each of their parents was loving, rejecting, or role-reversing (demanding or needing care). The other kind of rating scale concerns the adults' *current state of mind*—for instance, the degree to which the adults seem to idealize their parents, fail to remember specific experiences with them, seem still to be angry with them, and have difficulty describing losses or abuse. For our purposes, the most important fact about the AAI is that it predicts quite well (with about 80% accuracy) how a parent's infant child will be classified in the Strange Situation (e.g., Ainsworth & Eichberg, 1991; Fonagy, Steele, & Steele, 1992; Grossmann & Grossmann, 1991; Main et al., 1985). This means that parents' organization of their thoughts and feelings about *their* parents is somehow directly related to the behaviors they exhibit when serving as attachment figures for their own children.

Adults whose infants are classified as secure in the Strange Situation generally describe their parents as loving, not rejecting, and so on, and exhibit what Main et al. (1985) call "coherence of discourse" and "coherence of mind" during the AAI. Security-providing adults seem to have no trouble recalling specific childhood incidents to support general statements about their parents, and they provide balanced and realistic descriptions. In short, their "state of mind with respect to attachment," which is thought to be a reflection of their internal working models, is similar to the state of mind exhibited by securely attached elementary school children, as documented by Bretherton et al. (1990), Grossmann and Grossmann (1991), and Main et al. (1985) (described earlier in this chapter). There are similar correspondences between childhood and adult versions of Main et al.'s other three attachment styles—the ones called A, C, and D in childhood and "dismissing of attachment," "preoccupied with attachment," and "evidencing unresolved attachment-related trauma," respectively, in adulthood.

The existence of similar dynamics makes it seem plausible that adult attachment patterns are developmental successors of childhood attachment patterns—an idea currently being tested with Sroufe's longitudinal sample in Minnesota. But continuity is not the entire story, as it was not the entire story in the longitudinal study of children's attachment patterns. Some adults recall insecure attachment relationships with at least one parent during childhood, which lowers their scores on AAI scales such as "loving mother" and increases their scores on scales such as "rejecting mother" or "role-reversing mother." Yet some of these adults with troubled histories are able to talk quite coherently about their childhood experiences; they have no difficulty retrieving specific examples from memory, do not idealize or denegrate their troublesome parent(s), and do not seem enmeshed, angry, or preoccupied. Such people make it seem likely that they would have appeared insecure if assessed during certain periods of childhood, although they seem relatively secure as adults; moreover, as expected given the empirical method of deriving the AAI categories, they are raising securely attached children now. An important topic for future research, then, is how such adults achieve "coherence of mind with respect to attachment" despite insecurity-producing experiences with one or both parents during childhood.

Further evidence concerning the personality correlates, communicative behavior, and psychophysiology of adults with different AAI scores has been reported by Kobak and his coworkers (e.g., Dozier & Kobak, 1992; Kobak & Sceery, 1988; Kobak, Cole, Ferenz-Gillies, Fleming, & Gamble, 1993). Kobak and Sceery, for example, found that college students' AAI classifications are related to measures of personality and ego resiliency in ways that closely parallel the findings reported earlier in this chapter for children. Moreover, Dozier and Kobak found that college students who score as more avoidant, or dismissing of attachment, on the AAI produce stronger skin conductance responses during the interview when providing the kinds of answers that Main and her colleagues view as defensive distortions or denials. This combination of autonomic arousal and denial of distress is reminiscent of Sroufe and Waters's (1977b) demonstration that avoidant infants in the Strange Situation are aroused (i.e., have a high heart rate) while acting behaviorally as if they are not bothered at all by their mothers' departure from the test room.

In general, AAI studies conducted to date are compatible with the notion that adult attachment patterns assessed in relation to a person's own parenting behavior are often fairly straightforward reflections of that person's prior attachment history. Such qualifications as "often" and "fairly" are needed, however, because some adults seem to have changed their attachment patterns between childhood and adulthood. We suspect that such changes are attributable to the impact of other close relationships, but so far this topic seems not to have been tackled by AAI researchers.

Adult Romantic Attachment and Memories of Childhood Relationships with Parents

In their theoretical writings, Hazan and Shaver (e.g., Shaver & Hazan, 1993; Shaver, Hazan, & Bradshaw, 1988) have identified parallels between the dynamics, feelings, and behavior associated with attachment between infant and caregiver on the one hand, and those associated with the experience of romantic love in adulthood on the other. These similarities include seeking and maintaining close physical proximity to one's partner; relying on the partner's continued availability; turning to the partner for comfort when threatened physically or emotionally; and being distressed by separations, threats to the relationship, and losses. Hazan and Shaver hypothesized that the three infant attachment styles identified by Ainsworth et al. (1978) correspond to three distinct styles of love in adulthood. They devised a simple single-item self-report measure to test their predictions, translating the infant patterns described by Ainsworth et al. into terms designed to capture the manifestations of these patterns in adulthood.

The three answer alternatives in the single-item measure (as revised slightly by Hazan & Shaver, 1990) read as follows:

> *Avoidant:* "I am somewhat uncomfortable being close to others; I find it difficult to trust them completely, difficult to allow myself to depend on them. I am nervous when anyone gets too close, and often, love partners want me to be more intimate than I feel comfortable being."
>
> *Anxious/ambivalent:* "I find that others are reluctant to get as close as I would like. I often worry that my partner doesn't really love me or won't want to stay with me. I want to get very close to my partner, and this sometimes scares people away."

> *Secure:* "I find it relatively easy to get close to others and am com-
> fortable depending on them. I don't often worry about being aban-
> doned or about someone getting too close to me."

Interestingly, without altering their original wording to create a particular
frequency distribution, Hazan and Shaver (1987) obtained percentages
for the three groups (56% secure, 25% avoidant, and 19% anxious/
ambivalent) that were roughly equal to those obtained in studies of infant–
parent attachment (e.g., Ainsworth et al., 1978; Campos, Barrett, Lamb,
Goldsmith, & Stenberg, 1983; Waters, 1978).

As explained earlier, differences in the organization of attachment in
infancy are thought to result from differences in the quality of the infant–
caregiver relationship. Ainsworth et al. (1978) observed that whereas the
primary caregivers of secure infants were generally sensitive and responsive to their infants' signals, primary caregivers of avoidant infants tended
to be emotionally distant and to reject or rebuff their infants' bids for
proximity. Primary caregivers of anxious/ambivalent infants typically
responded inconsistently to their infants' signals, being sometimes unavailable or unresponsive, and at other times intrusive or overly concerned.

Hazan and Shaver (1987) used a 37-item adjective checklist to retrospectively assess the attachment histories of college-age and older adult
subjects. Participants in the studies were also asked whether "they had
ever been separated from their parents for what seemed like a long time"
(p. 516). Although there were no differences in frequency of extended
separations from parents, recollections of childhood relationships with
parents differed systematically across the three attachment groups. Secure
subjects described respectful, responsive, caring, accepting, confident, and
undemanding mothers, whereas insecure (avoidant and anxious/ambiva-
lent) subjects described almost the opposite of this profile. As for differences between the avoidant and anxious/ambivalent groups, avoidant
subjects described their mothers as having been cold and rejecting, whereas
anxious/ambivalent subjects described their fathers as having been "unfair"
(which may mean inconsistent).

These results have been conceptually replicated by other researchers.
Using the single-item measure and an attachment history adjective checklist in a study of Australian adults, Feeney and Noller (1990) found that
secure subjects reported positive early family relationships, whereas anx-
ious/ambivalent subjects recalled a lack of supportiveness from their
fathers. A difference from Hazan and Shaver's (1987) findings, but a result
in line with theoretical expectations, was that avoidant subjects were significantly more likely than the other groups to recall separations from their
mothers during childhood. Similarly, using a sample of Israeli adults,
Mikulincer et al. (1990) found that avoidant subjects recalled childhood
relationships with their mothers in less positive terms than subjects in the

other two groups, whereas anxious/ambivalent subjects recalled fathers in less positive terms than did secure subjects. (To date, no one has explained the apparent importance of fathers in the lives of anxious/ambivalent subjects.)

Although these early results suggested that attachment histories have an influence on orientations to interpersonal relationships in adulthood, they were quite preliminary and based on rather primitive measures. For example, all of the studies discussed above used a checklist approach to assess the quality of the early attachment relationship. This method is problematic because it ignores distinctions of degree: All mothers may be responsive, critical, or intrusive at times (therefore allowing all three items to be endorsed by almost anyone), but the *extent* to which mothers possessed these characteristics during subjects' childhoods cannot be assessed. This problem may have resulted in a minimization of observed differences among the three attachment groups.

In a more recent study (Rothbard & Shaver, 1991), we devised a 180-item adjective *rating* list, based on subjects' open-ended descriptions of their mothers and fathers, to assess differences in attachment history across adult attachment groups. The adjective rating list contained two 90-item sets of attachment history adjectives (one set for mothers, one for fathers). When these sets were factor-analyzed, 15 highly reliable scales were produced, each of which pertained to a distinct aspect of attachment relationships during childhood. In addition to attachment histories, we were also interested in whether subjects would report differences in the nature and quality of *current* relationships with parents. Toward this end, we included modified versions of the Parental Attachment Questionnaire (Kenny, 1987) and the Inventory of Parent and Peer Attachment (Armsden & Greensberg, 1987). These measures factored into 16 highly reliable scales. In all, 31 scales were produced.

Statistical analyses of the scales yielded highly significant findings that were very much in line with theory-based predictions. In contrast to his or her insecure counterparts, the average secure subject described a mother who, during the subject's childhood, had been relaxed and fun-loving (humorous, confident, easy-going, patient) and dependable (reliable, not dishonest, not selfish). In the context of the present relationship, these qualities were reflected in the secure subject's description of the mother as available, emotionally supportive, warm, and respectful. Insecure (anxious/ambivalent and avoidant) subjects described mothers who had been troubled (nervous, depressed, frightened, worried, confused) during the subjects' childhoods, and reported feelings of discomfort and alienation in their mothers' presence now. For current relationships with their fathers, insecure subjects were more likely to describe the fathers as both physically and emotionally unavailable, and to report that, as with their mothers, they felt alienated in the fathers' presence. Insecure subjects were also more likely than secure subjects to report that, during their childhoods, their fathers had been difficult (not flexible, not patient, not reasonable, moody).

Avoidant subjects stood apart from the other two groups with respect to (1) lower levels of current parental communication and emotional support; (2) lower levels of confidence in fathers as trustworthy, good parents; and (3) lower ratings of fathers' dependability and attentiveness during the subjects' childhoods. Avoidant subjects also contrasted with the secure group by being relatively *less* likely to state that (1) they were *not* angry with their mothers now; (2) they relied on the mothers' decisions; (3) the mothers were trustworthy, good parents; (4) the mothers had been warm (expressive, sensitive, caring, comforting, close) during the subjects' childhoods; (5) they enjoyed their fathers' company; (6) the fathers had been fun-loving (humorous, enthusiastic, likable) during the subject's childhoods; and (7) the fathers had been sensitive (expressive, emotional, sympathetic). Avoidant subjects were *more* likely than secure subjects to report that (1) they were currently angry at their fathers; (2) the fathers had been abusive (hostile, hurtful, mean, hateful) during the subject's childhoods; (3) the fathers had been troubled (depressed, worried, nervous, frightened); and (4) the fathers had been manipulative (smothering, guilt-inducing, possessive, rejecting).

Anxious/ambivalent subjects were distinguished from secure subjects by their description of their mothers as intrusive at present ("Mother treats me like someone younger than I am," "Mother tries to control my life," "Mother imposes her ideas and values on me"), as well as having been intrusive in the past ("Mother was nosy, nagging, bothersome, guilt-inducing"). These findings are extremely consistent with Ainsworth et al.'s (1978) observation that mothers of anxious/ambivalent infants were often overly, intrusively affectionate or behaved in other ways that interfered with their infants' independent play. Also relative to the secure group, anxious/ambivalent subjects were more likely to report that their mothers had been angry (hateful, hostile) during their childhoods, and less likely to say that in the present their fathers promoted independence and self-efficacy.

The results of this study indicate strongly that members of the three adult attachment groups, as operationalized by Hazan and Shaver (1987, 1990), recall childhood relationships with parents (and describe current relationships with them) in ways that are predictable from the literature on infant–parent attachment. Despite these consistencies, however, Bartholomew (1990; Bartholomew & Horowitz, 1991) observed that Hazan and Shaver's (1987) avoidant category may obscure important differences between two distinct types of avoidant adults, which she calls "fearful" and "dismissing." This distinction suggests either that (1) divergent forms of avoidance emerge in later developmental periods from a single precursor in infancy; or (2) the fearful group represents the grown-up version of the D (disorganized/disoriented) or A/C (avoidant/ambivalent) classification in infancy (Brennan, Shaver, & Tobey, 1991). Bartholomew has provided compelling evidence that her four-category conceptualization is related to theory-relevant personality variables and is perhaps more compatible with adult interpersonal experiences than is Hazan and Shaver's three-category scheme. (See also Sperling, Berman, & Fagen, 1992.) Bartholomew's work suggests that the four attachment classifications—secure, preoccupied (equivalent to Hazan & Shaver's anxious/ambivalent category), fearful (similar to Hazan & Shaver's avoidant category), and dismissing (similar to Main et al.'s [1985] dismissing category)—can be distinguished from one another on the basis of differing configurations of working models of self and others. Differences in working models, in turn, may arise out of differences in attachment history.

Interview codes compared across Bartholomew's (1989) four attachment groups revealed that fearful adults, like Hazan and Shaver's (1987, 1990) avoidants, reported having experienced high levels of separation anxiety and parental rejection, and low levels of parental involvement, when they were children. In contrast, dismissing adults tended to voice idealized memories of their parents, while indirectly indicating that the parents were actually rejecting or emotionally cool. Preoccupied individuals, like Hazan and Shaver's anxious/ambivalent subjects, reported that their parents were overprotective and inept, but also responsive and accessible at least some of the time (i.e., unreliable and inconsistent, sometimes being loving and responsive and sometimes not). Finally, Bartholomew's secure adults recalled that though their parents occasionally made mistakes, they were generally supportive, warm, and accepting.

Summary of Self-Report Findings

Adult attachment studies based on a variety of retrospective self-report methodologies produce compatible findings. Regardless of which operationalization or approach is used, adults classified as secure describe their primary attachment figures in childhood as having been generally warm, responsive, available, and sensitive. Adults classified as insecure tend to portray their attachment figures as having provided less than optimal caregiving environments. Anxious/ambivalent (preoccupied) adults describe parents (at least the psychologically most important parent) as having been warm and loving part of the time, but also inaccessible, unresponsive, intrusive, and inconsistent. Issues related to the type of care they received as children continue to preoccupy them as adults; they seem both enmeshed in these issues and resentful or angry toward parents because of them. Compared to adults in the other groups, avoidant (fearful) adults describe parents as having been less warm or nurturant, relatively uninvolved, and at least somewhat rejecting when they were growing up. Dismissing adults, as classified using Main et al.'s or Bartholomew's procedures, remember parents as having been vaguely good, and yet cannot provide specific examples to support this generalization. (Actually, Bartholomew's results for dismissing adults are not quite so clear-cut. Dismissing subjects seem to provide a mix of positive and negative interview descriptions of both parents, generally stating that parents provided adequate, sometimes ideal care, but indirectly characterizing them as having been rejecting or otherwise less than optimal parents. The latter findings are compatible with studies using questionnaire measures, which sometimes produce mixed results for avoidant respondents. Because dismissingly avoidant individuals are especially well defended, they may be the most difficult to study with self-report measures.)

One criticism likely to be leveled at attachment history interviews and questionnaires is that retrospective self-reports cannot be trusted. First, it might be argued that subjects' memories of early relationship experiences are simply *reconstructions* of those events, not veridical characterizations; in other words, memories of childhood attachments may be filtered through cognitive–affective lenses that are affected by subsequent (including current) attachment experiences. On the other hand, as Collins and Read (1994) point out, we do not yet know that this is the case, and besides, "memories can provide valuable information about an individual's *current* organization and representation of attachment-related experience, which in itself is meaningful and informative." Second, it might be argued that in the studies described above, insecure adults were simply displaying generally negative self-report biases. Indeed, avoidant (fearful) and anxious/ambivalent (preoccupied) adults often did not differ in statistically significant ways. However, when each group was compared with the secure group, significant differences did emerge, suggesting that insecure groups *do* differ in terms of the caregiving they received as children. If the insecure groups were simply providing generalized negative descriptions, it seems unlikely that the factors differentiating each insecure group from the secure group would be both unique and theoretically predictable. Although longitudinal studies are clearly warranted (and are currently underway), available evidence suggests that the kinds of caregiving associated with the different attachment styles in infancy are also what the corresponding attachment groups recall or (in the case of dismissing individuals) inadvertently reveal as adults. This, in turn, suggests that systematic differences in the quality of early attachment relationships influence personality, attachment styles, and interpersonal relationships in adulthood.

Childhood Attachment and Adult Romantic Attachment: Similar Dynamics

Thus far, we have presented various kinds of evidence for the plausibility of the hypothesis that adult attachment patterns have their roots in childhood attachment relationships. In this section, we discuss a few of several available studies supporting the hypothesis that attachment dynamics are similar in childhood and adulthood.

The Strange Situation has been especially useful for assessing infant attachment patterns, because it raises infants' stress levels to the point where most infants are concerned about the availability and responsiveness of their primary caregiver. In a recent study of college students, Simpson, Rholes, and Nelligan (1992) tried to create a parallel situation for the female members of seriously dating couples. In particular, they examined the interaction between anxiety and avoidant attachment as determinants of both support seeking and support provision in an analogue of the Strange Situation.

Male and female dating partners came to a laboratory, where they were separated and asked to fill out questionnaires. On the way back to the waiting room, the female member of each couple was shown a darkened psychophysiology laboratory and told that the next phase of the experiment would involve an activity that creates considerable anxiety for most participants. Once in the waiting room, the two partners were unobtrusively videotaped for 5 minutes, and the tapes were later used to code couple members' verbal and nonverbal behavior. Analyses revealed that as observer-rated anxiety increased, secure women sought emotional and physical comfort from their partners, whereas avoidant women tended to distance themselves emotionally and physically from their partners. Specifically, avoidant women were significantly less likely than secure women to mention the anxiety-provoking situation to their partners. Furthermore, they scored significantly lower than secure women on the Comfort/Support Seeking factor, indexed by the extent to which they promoted physical contact and seemed comfortable with it. They were also more likely than secure women to resist their partners' attempts to touch and make physical contact with them. Similarly, secure male partners tended to provide more reassurance and emotional support as the females' anxiety level increased, whereas avoidant male partners were less inclined to provide such reassurances and support. These findings are consistent with patterns of proximity seeking and caregiving among infant–mother dyads in the Strange Situation (Ainsworth et al., 1978). Although it seems odd to untrained observers, avoidant parents actually become *less* emotionally and physically available to their infants when the infants become more visibly distressed, and avoidant infants are most likely to show extreme avoidance when they are anxious.

Several attachment studies of children, reviewed earlier in this chapter, indicate that secure children are emotionally open, empathic, and able to communicate coherently and sensitively in a variety of social situations. They also seem to prefer other secure children (i.e., children with the same communication preferences and skills) as close friends. In a related series of studies, Mikulincer and Nachshon (1991) found that three adult attachment groups (identified with a Hebrew translation of Hazan & Shaver's [1987] measure) could be distinguished from one another on the basis of feelings and behaviors related to self-disclosure. In one of the studies, subjects were read a personality description of an individual with whom they were (ostensibly) about to interact. In addition to receiving other relevant information, they were told that the person was someone who either liked to share personal thoughts and feeling with others (high-self-disclosing partner) or did not like to share thoughts and feelings (low-self-disclosing partner). Subjects were asked to rate both the extent to which they would like the partner and the extent to which they would disclose personal information to him or her. Analyses indicated that secure and anxious/ambivalent subjects reported greater likelihood of disclosing to a high-disclosing partner than to a low-disclosing partner, but avoidant subjects showed no differences in how much they would expect to disclose to either type of partner. Furthermore, in contrast to avoidant subjects, anxious/ambivalent and secure subjects were more attracted to the high-disclosing partner and were more likely to report that they would prefer the high-disclosing partner to the low-disclosing partner. Finally, avoidant subjects were more likely to report that they would feel more negative emotions when interacting with the high-disclosing partner than with the low-disclosing partner.

In another study in the same series, the three attachment groups' feelings and behaviors during real interactions with either high- or low-disclosing partners were observed and rated. Specifically, subjects' conversations were analyzed in terms of (1) the extent to which intimate information was disclosed, (2) the extent to which emotions or judgments were expressed, and (3) the extent to which subjects' statements referred back to something their partners had said. The results indicated that secure and anxious/ambivalent subjects revealed significantly more personal information to high- than to low-disclosing partners, and were significantly more disclosive to high-disclosing partners than were the avoidant subjects. Secure and anxious/ambivalent subjects were also more likely than avoidant subjects to express emotions and judgments during their inter-actions, although secure subjects were more likely than the other two groups to refer back to something their partners had said in conversation (suggesting that anxious/ambivalent and avoidant subjects are more self-involved or less other-oriented than secure subjects). In terms of affect, avoidant subjects were significantly more likely than secure or anxious/ambivalent subjects to report experiencing negative emotions while inter-acting with high-disclosing partners (perhaps because of norms of dis-closure reciprocity, which would be expected to make avoidant subjects uncomfortable), whereas secure and anxious/ambivalent subjects reported liking high-disclosing partners better than low-disclosing partners. In addition, they reported significantly greater liking for high-disclosing partners than did avoidant subjects.

Earlier, we mentioned that Grossmann and Grossmann (1991) fol-lowed a group of children from age 1, when they were assessed in the Strange Situation, to age 10, when they were given a broad-ranging inter-view about attachment-related feelings and experiences. Secure children were found to be more likely than insecure children to turn to others when feeling afraid, sad, or angry; avoidant children were more likely to attempt to work their problems out for themselves. Mikulincer, Florian, and Weller (1993) conducted a parallel study in connection with the Iraqi Scud mis-sile attacks on Israel during the Gulf War. These researchers interviewed secure, avoidant, and anxious/ambivalent Israelis shortly after the war and administered several stress, coping, and health questionnaires. Secure Israelis (again, measured with a Hebrew translation of Hazan & Shaver's [1987] measure) were more likely than their insecure counterparts to have sought social support and coped effectively, with no signs of prolonged distress. Avoidant subjects used denial and other avoidant coping strate-gies during the war, but after the war seemed angrier about the missile attacks and more troubled by psychosomatic symptoms. Anxious/ambiva-lent subjects became the most intensely upset during the attacks and were inclined to use what coping researchers call "emotion-focused" coping strategies. Interestingly, in line with Simpson et al.'s (1992) evidence that attachment style interacts with degree of threat, Mikulincer et al. found an interaction between attachment style and the distance a person lived from the areas where missiles actually hit.

Hazan and Shaver (1990) conducted a study of attachment style and feelings and behaviors at work, reasoning that work is the equivalent for many adults of what Bowlby called "exploration" in infancy. Their results indicate that secure adults get along well with coworkers, are generally satisfied with their jobs, and make a reasonable amount of money given their level of education. Avoidant adults get along less well with coworkers, prefer to work alone, and feel that work provides a good excuse to avoid social relations. They make as much money, on average, as secure adults. (A subsequent study [M. Hutt, personal communication, 1992] has indicated that avoidant business owners have a relatively high employee turnover rate, but this does not keep them from making a good profit, evidently because they do much of the work themselves.) Anxious/ambivalent workers feel overinvolved and underappreciated at work, and they make less money than secure and avoidant workers even when relevant variables such as education and gender are controlled. These results closely parallel the results of many studies of attachment and problem solving in early childhood.

Other studies have shown that secure adults, like secure children, are more emotionally positive than insecure adults (Simpson, 1990) and more trusting (Collins & Read, 1990). Like secure children, secure adults seem slightly more likely to pair up with secure relationship partners (e.g., Brennan & Shaver, 1994; Collins & Read, 1990; Kirkpatrick & Davis, 1994; Senchak & Leonard, 1992). Like anxious/ambivalent children, who seem to suffer from unusually conflictual peer relationships, anxious/ambivalent college students are especially likely to experience rapid relationship breakups (Shaver & Brennan, 1992; Kirkpatrick & Davis, 1994). The list of parallels between childhood and adult attachment dynamics continues to grow, increasing our confidence that attachment is fundamentally similar in childhood and adulthood.

Throughout this chapter, we have argued that internal working models mediate the connection between previous attachment experiences and subsequent personality and associated behaviors. As a final step in evaluating attachment theory's ability to predict and explain personality across the life span, it is important to show that members of different adult attachment categories possess different internal models of self, others, and attachment relationships—models that have emerged out of previous relationships with important attachment figures and may now account for the emotional and behavioral differences among adult attachment groups. In general, it would be expected that secure adults view others as trustworthy and dependable, the self as lovable and worthy, and relationships as a source of support and comfort. Avoidant (fearful, dismissing) adults would be expected to view others as generally untrustworthy and undependable, the self as either unlovable or (defensively) "too good" for others, and relationships as either threatening to one's sense of control, not worth the effort, or both. Anxious/ambivalent (preoccupied) adults would be expected to view others as desirable relationship partners but as largely unpredictable (sometimes available, sometimes not) and difficult to understand (Collins & Read, 1994). They should view the self as generally unlovable, and close relationships as the primary way in which people can achieve a sense of felt security. Hence, attaining intimate relationships with others should be a chronic, preoccupying goal for anxious/ambivalent adults.

Does research on working models in adulthood support these hypotheses? Hazan and Shaver (1987) found that secure subjects viewed themselves as likable, appreciated, and easy to get to know, and viewed other people as generally well-intentioned and good-hearted. Their love experiences were most often characterized as friendly, happy, and trusting. In addition, in an older, more romantically experienced sample (recruited via a newspaper questionnaire), secure subjects proved more likely than insecure subjects to believe that romantic love can last. Insecure subjects (avoidant and anxious/ambivalent) were less likely than secure subjects to view themselves as likable, self-confident, or appreciated, and less likely to view others as well-intentioned. They were also less likely to believe that Hollywood-style, happily-ever-after love can exist in real life or that it is easy for a person to find someone with whom to fall deeply in love. However, whereas avoidant subjects tended to associate relationships with fear of closeness, anxious/ambivalent subjects associated relationships with jealousy, extreme emotions, and strong desires for reciprocation.

Similar results have been obtained by other researchers. In a study by Feeney and Noller (1990), secure subjects stood apart from insecure subjects by virtue of higher scores on social, personal, and family-related self-esteem, and lower scores on self-conscious anxiety and unfulfilled hopes about love. Avoidant subjects were less likely than the other two groups to idealize their love relationships and were more likely to experience relationships in terms of intimacy avoidance. Anxious/ambivalent subjects had lower family-related self-esteem than the other two groups and were more likely to experience love in a neurotic fashion, characterized by idealization, mania, preoccupation, dependence, and heavy reliance on partners. Similarly, Collins and Read (1990) found that secure subjects had higher self-esteem than insecure subjects and felt more self-confident in social situations. Furthermore, secure subjects were more likely than avoidant subjects to describe themselves as expressive. Among insecure groups, avoidant subjects were more likely than anxious/ambivalent subjects to score high on a measure of agency and self-assertiveness (instrumentality). With respect to models of others, secure subjects were more likely than insecure subjects to believe in the trustworthiness of human motives. Avoidant subjects were less likely than the other groups to believe in the dependability of people or the integrity of social agents (parents, authorities, public figures). Finally, anxious/ambivalent subjects were less likely than secure subjects to see others as altruistic or possessing strength of will, and more likely than avoidant subjects to believe in the complexity of human nature (suggesting that they see others as difficult to understand).

In a separate study, Collins (1991; Collins & Read, 1994) hypothesized that adults with different attachment styles would explain events occurring within a hypothetical dating relationship in ways reflecting their working models of self and others. According to Collins and Read (1994),

> the explanations of secure subjects, compared to those of avoidant subjects, reflected stronger perceptions of love and security in their relationships, greater confidence in the partner's responsiveness, and stronger belief in the partner's warmth and desire for closeness. In contrast, anxious subjects were more likely to explain events in ways that revealed low self-worth and self-reliance, less confidence in their partner's love and in the security in their relationship, less trust, and a belief that their partner is not dependable and is purposely rejecting closeness. (p. 74)

Finally, Bartholomew and Horowitz (1991) interviewed members of the different attachment groups and obtained results consistent with those already reported. For models of self, secure and dismissing subjects (hypothesized to have positive models of self) scored significantly higher than fearful and preoccupied subjects (hypothesized to have negative models of self) on measures of self-esteem and self-confidence, and significantly lower on measures of personal distress (anxiety, sadness, and anger). In contrast, secure and preoccupied subjects (hypothesized to have positive models of others) scored significantly higher than fearful and dismissing subjects (hypothesized to have negative models of others) on measures of sociability and pleasure in interacting with other people. These self-reported orientations were corroborated by friends' reports.

Discontinuity of Attachment Styles in Adulthood

In contrast to the large body of literature on continuity and discontinuity of attachment styles during infancy and childhood, virtually nothing is known about stability of attachment styles across the life span, or about factors that may precipitate shifts during adulthood from one attachment style to another. Several studies have shown fairly high reliabilities for adult attachment measures compared over periods of several months and up to a few years (e.g., Brennan & Shaver, 1994; Kirkpatrick & Davis, 1994; Shaver & Brennan, 1992), but no one has conducted a long-term stability study. Hints about the likely outcome of such studies come from a retrospective interview study by Hazan and Hutt (1993), in which Sroufe et al.'s (1990) observation, quoted earlier, that "adaptation is always a product of both developmental history and current circumstances" (p. 1363) and Lewis and Feiring's (1991; Lewis et al., 1984) attachment × environment models of adjustment may find their parallels in adulthood. To examine the issue of stability from an adult viewpoint, Hazan and Hutt identified two groups of adults (averaging 38 years of age)—one group whose beliefs and expectations about relationships had been fairly stable, and one group who had experienced change (hereafter referred to as the "no-change" and "change" groups, respectively).

Consistent with Bowlby's claim that working models of relationships tend to be stable, change was less common than stability (22% vs. 78%). Also consistent with the theory-based assumption of an innate tendency to seek security, change was more likely to occur in the direction of security than of insecurity (98% vs. 2%). When a change occurred from one insecure type to another, it was much more likely to be from avoidant to preoccupied (100%) than from preoccupied to avoidant (0%)—a finding consistent with Bowlby's (1969/1982) observations of "detached" children who became suddenly anxious and clingy after concluding that their formerly absent mothers were now home to stay. Finally, when describing their close relationships (with friends, romantic partners, and other important adults), the change subjects were significantly more likely than the no-change subjects to have experienced relationships that *disconfirmed* their former models (e.g., 67% vs. 21% for romantic, 100% vs. 36% for important adult). The results suggest that one way in which working models of relationships change is through model-disconfirming social experiences.

These findings (and interpretations) are consistent with examinations of attachment style discontinuity in childhood (e.g., Lewis & Feiring, 1991; Sroufe et al., 1990); they suggest that changes in environment and/or repeated interactions with model-disconfirming relationship partners force the individual to accommodate working models to current experiences instead of assimilating these experiences to existing representational structures. These findings also suggest that therapy aimed both at altering attributional styles (or explanations for events) and at changing behaviors that result in self-fulfilling prophecies (e.g., driving relationship partners away through jealousy-induced behaviors) may be successful in bringing about changes in working models and expectations of others. This may be especially true if, in conjunction with using these techniques, a therapist actively and consistently behaves in a security-inducing manner that cannot be assimilated by existing working models (see Bowlby, 1988).

CONCLUDING REMARKS

The purpose of this chapter has been to evaluate the utility of an attachment-theoretical framework for understanding personality and personality development across the life course. After reviewing the literature on (1) the attachment behavioral system; (2) the role of early experiences with primary caregivers; (3) the development and maintenance of internal working models; (4) the stability and instability of attachment classifications; (5) the behavioral, cognitive, and emotional correlates of attachment styles in both childhood and adulthood; and (6) alternative explanations of attachment-related phenomena, what can we conclude about the attachment-theoretical perspective on personality? Throughout these pages, we have shown that attachment styles, as first assessed during infancy, maintain measurable cross-situational and cross-age continuity and are associated with theory-consistent psychological and interpersonal correlates in later childhood and adolescence. In addition, evidence based on working models, self-reported memories of parents, behavioral observations, and reports from peers suggests that attachment styles continue to exist in adulthood. Attachment styles are not fixed in stone, and seem not to be as stable as genetically based personality traits; nonetheless, they are consistent enough, and in some cases dysfunctional and troubling enough, to warrant both researchers' and clinicians' attention.

Despite the success of attachment theory and research, certain aspects of the attachment-theoretical approach to personality need further work. One problem, as indicated in other chapters of the present volume, is measurement. It seems unlikely that simple self-report measures of adult romantic attachment and complex interview measures of the attachment orientations of young parents will automatically converge. It will take a great deal of comparative work to discover what is tapped by each of these kinds of measures. A second target for future research should consist of factors that influence stability and instability of attachment styles, particularly in adulthood. Are members of the insecure attachment groups in adulthood largely doomed to lives of negative interpersonal expectations and unfulfilling relationships? Although research suggests that change toward attachment security is possible, the factors underlying this change need to be specified. To what extent and in what manner do current attachment relationships influence attachment styles? What proportion of the variance in adult attachment can be accounted for by experiences occurring subsequent to the relationship between young children and their primary caregivers (e.g., during adolescent and early adult friendships and romantic relationships)? Do these experiences also influence the manner in which individuals represent early attachment experiences? That is, can a person's memories of early relationships be revised? An examination of naturally occurring change may be useful not only for evaluating the attachment-theoretical perspective on personality and for understanding life-span attachment processes, but for developing therapeutic intervention strategies. There is obviously a need for life-span longitudinal studies of attachment-related phenomena. Fortunately, participants in some of the best-known infant attachment studies (e.g., the studies directed by Grossmann & Grossmann, Main, and Sroufe) will soon be entering adulthood. Let us hope that this milestone in their personal development will represent a concomitant milestone in the elaboration and validation of attachment theory.

ACKNOWLEDGMENT

Preparation of this chapter was facilitated by Grant No. BSN-8808736 from the National Science Foundation.

REFERENCES

Ainsworth, M. D. S., Blehar, M. C., Waters, E., & Wall, S. (1978). *Patterns of attachment: A psychological study of the Strange Situation.* Hillsdale, NJ: Erlbaum.

Ainsworth, M. D. S., & Eichberg, C. (1991). Effects on infant-mother attachment of mother's unresolved loss of an attachment figure, or other traumatic experience. In C. M. Parkes, J. Stevenson-Hinde, & P. Marris (Eds.), *Attachment across the life cycle* (pp. 160–183). London: Tavistock/Routledge.

Arend, R., Gove, F. L., & Sroufe, L. A. (1979). Continuity of individual adaptation from infancy to kindergarten: A predictive study of ego-resiliency and curiosity in preschoolers. *Child Development, 50,* 950–959.

Armsden, G., & Greenberg, M. T. (1987). The Inventory of Parent and Peer Attachment: Individual differences and their relationship to psychological well-being in adolescence. *Journal of Youth and Adolescence, 16,* 427–454.

Bartholomew, K. (1989). *Attachment styles in young adults: Implications for self-concept and interpersonal functioning.* Unpublished doctoral dissertation, Stanford University.

Bartholomew, K. (1990). Avoidance of intimacy: An attachment perspective. *Journal of Personal and Social Relationships, 7,* 147–178.

Bartholomew, K., & Horowitz, L. M. (1991). Attachment styles among young adults: A test of a four-category model. *Journal of Personality and Social Psychology, 61,* 226–244.

Bowlby, J. (1979). *The making and breaking of affectional bonds.* London: Tavistock.

Bowlby, J. (1982). *Attachment and loss: Vol. 1. Attachment* (2nd ed.). New York: Basic Books. (Original work published 1969)

Bowlby, J. (1988). *A secure base: Parent–child attachment and healthy human development.* New York: Basic Books.

Bowlby, J. (1989). The role of attachment in personality development and psychopathology. In S. Greenspan & G. Pollock (Eds.), *The course of life: Vol. 1. Infancy* (pp. 229-270). Madison CT: International Universities Press.

Brennan, K. A., & Shaver, P. R. (1994). Dimensions of adult attachment, affect regulation, and romantic relationship functioning. *Personality and Social Psychology Bulletin.*

Brennan, K. A., Shaver, P. R., & Tobey, A. E. (1991). Attachment styles, gender, and parental problem drinking. *Journal of Personal and Social Relationships, 8,* 451-466.

Bretherton, I. (1985). Attachment theory: Retrospect and prospect. In I. Bretherton & E. Waters (Eds.), Growing points of attachment theory and research. *Monographs of the Society for Research in Child Development, 50*(1-2, Serial No. 209), 3-35.

Bretherton, I., Ridgeway, D., & Cassidy, J. (1990). Assessing internal working models of the attachment relationship: An attachment story completion task for 3-year-olds. In M. T. Greenberg, D. Cicchetti, & E. M. Cummings (Eds.), *Attachment in the preschool years: Theory, research, and intervention* (pp. 273-308). Chicago: University of Chicago Press.

Campos, J. J., Barrett, K., Lamb, M. E., Goldsmith, H. H., & Stenberg, C. (1983). Socioemotional development. In M. M Haith & J. J. Campos (Eds.), *Handbook of child psychology* (4th ed.): *Vol. 2. Infancy and developmental psychobiology* (pp. 783-915). New York: Wiley.

Collins, N. L. (1991). *Adult attachment styles and explanations for relationship events: A knowledge structure approach to explanation in close relationships.* Unpublished doctoral dissertation, University of Southern California.

Collins, N. L., & Read, S. J. (1990). Adult attachment, working models, and relationship quality in dating couples. *Journal of Personality and Social Psychology, 58,* 644-663.

Collins, N. L., & Read, S. J. (1994). Cognitive representations of adult attachment: The structure and function of working models. In D. Perlman & K. Bartholomew (Eds.), *Advances in personal relationships* (Vol. 5, pp. 53-90). London: Jessica Kingsley.

Crittenden, P. M. (1985). Maltreated infants: Vulnerability and resilience. *Journal of Child Psychology and Psychiatry and Allied Disciplines, 26,* 85-96.

Crittenden, P. M. (1988). Relationships at risk. In J. Belsky & T. Nezworski (Eds.), *Clinical implications of attachment* (pp. 136-174). Hillsdale, NJ: Erlbaum.

Crowell, J., & Feldman, S. (1988). The effects of mothers' internal working models of relations and children's developmental and behavioral status on mother-child interactions. *Child Development, 59,* 1273-1285.

Dozier, M., & Kobak, R. R. (1992). Psychophysiology and adolescent attachment interviews: Converging evidence for repressing strategies. *Child Development, 63,* 1473-1480.

Easterbrooks, M. A., & Goldberg, W. A. (1990). Security of toddler-parent attachment: Relation to children's sociopersonality functioning during kindergarten. In M. T. Greenberg, D. Cicchetti, & E. M. Cummings (Eds.), *Attachment in the preschool years: Theory, research, and intervention* (pp. 221-244). Chicago: University of Chicago Press.

Egeland, B., & Farber, E. A. (1984). Infant–mother attachment: Factors related to its development and changes over time. *Child Development, 55,* 753–771.

Egeland, B., & Sroufe, L. A. (1981). Attachment and early maltreatment. *Child Development, 52,* 44–52.

Elicker, J., Englund, M., & Sroufe, L. A. (1992). Predicting peer competence and peer relationships in childhood from early parent-child relationships. In R. Parke & G. Ladd (Eds.), *Family–peer relations: Modes of linkage* (pp. 77–106). Hillsdale, NJ: Erlbaum.

Erickson, M., Sroufe, L., & Egeland, B. (1985). The relationship between quality of attachment and behavior problems in preschool in a high-risk sample. In I. Bretherton & E. Waters (Eds.), Growing points of attachment theory and research. *Monographs of the Society for Research in Child Development, 50*(1–2, Serial No. 209), 147–166.

Feeney, J., & Noller, P. (1990). Attachment style as a predictor of adult romantic relationships. *Journal of Personality and Social Psychology, 58,* 281–291.

Fiske, S. T., & Taylor, S. E. (1991). *Social cognition* (2nd ed.). New York: McGraw-Hill.

Fonagy, P., Steele, H., & Steele, M. (1991). Maternal representations of attachment during pregnancy predict the organization of infant–mother attachment at one year of age. *Child Development, 62,* 891–905.

Frankel, K. A., & Bates, J. E. (1990). Mother–toddler problem solving: Antecedents in attachment, home behavior, and temperament. *Child Development, 61,* 810– 819.

Frodi, A., Grolnick, W., & Bridges, L. (1985). Maternal correlates of stability and change in infant–mother attachment. *Infant Mental Health Journal, 6,* 60–67.

Fury, G. S. (1993). *The relation between infant attachment history and representation of relationships in school-aged family drawings.* Paper presented at the 60th anniversary meeting of the Society for Research in Child Development, New Orleans.

Grossmann, K. E., & Grossmann, K. (1991). Attachment quality as an organizer of emotional and behavioral responses in a longitudinal perspective. In C. M. Parkes, J. Stevenson-Hinde, & P. Marris (Eds.), *Attachment across the life cycle* (pp. 93–114). London: Tavistock/Routledge.

Hazan, C., & Hutt, M. J. (1993). *Continuity and change in inner working models of attachment.* Unpublished manuscript, Cornell University.

Hazan, C., & Shaver, P. R. (1987). Romantic love conceptualized as an attachment process. *Journal of Personality and Social Psychology, 52,* 511–524.

Hazan, C., & Shaver, P. R. (1990). Love and work: An attachment-theoretical perspective. *Journal of Personality and Social Psychology, 59,* 270–280.

Hendrick, C., & Hendrick, S. S. (1994). Attachment theory and close adult relationships: Reflections on Hazan and Shaver. *Psychological Inquiry, 5,* 38–41.

Isabella, R. A., & Belsky, J. (1991). Interactional synchrony and the origins of infant–mother attachment: A replication study. *Child Development, 62,* 373–384.

Jacobson, J. L., & Wille, D. E. (1986). The influence of attachment pattern on developmental changes in peer interaction from the toddler to preschool period. *Child Development, 57,* 338–347.

Kenny, M. (1987). The extent and function of parental attachment among first-year college students. *Journal of Youth and Adolescence, 16,* 17–29.

Kirkpatrick, L. A., & Davis, K. E. (1994). Attachment style, gender, and relationship stability: A longitudinal analysis. *Journal of Personality and Social Psychology, 66.*

Kirkpatrick, L. A., & Shaver, P. R. (1990). Attachment theory and religion: Childhood attachments, religious beliefs, and conversion. *Journal for the Scientific Study of Religion, 29*, 315-334.

Kirkpatrick, L. A., & Shaver, P. R. (1992). An attachment-theoretical approach to romantic love and religious belief. *Personality and Social Psychology Bulletin, 18*, 266-275.

Kobak, R. R., Cole, H. E., Ferenz-Gillies, R., Fleming, W., & Gamble, W. (1993). Attachment and emotion regulation during mother-teen problem solving: A control theory analysis. *Child Development, 64*, 231-245.

Kobak, R. R., & Sceery, A. (1988). Attachment in late adolescence: Working models, affect regulation, and perceptions of self and others. *Child Development, 88*, 135-146.

Lewis, M., & Feiring, C. (1991). Attachment as personal characteristic or a measure of environment. In J. L. Gewirtz & W. M. Kurtines (Eds.), *Intersections with attachment* (pp. 3-21). Hillsdale, NJ: Erlbaum.

Lewis, M., Feiring, C., McGuffog, C., & Jaskir, J. (1984). Predicting psychopathology in six-year-olds from early social relations. *Child Development, 55*, 123-136.

Main, M. (1990). Cross-cultural studies of attachment organization: Recent studies, changing methodologies, and the concept of conditional strategies. *Human Development, 33*, 48-61.

Main, M., & Cassidy, J. (1988). Categories of response to reunion with the parent at age 6: Predictable from infant attachment classifications and stable over a 1-month period. *Developmental Psychology, 24*, 415-426.

Main, M., & Hesse, E. (1990). Parents' unresolved traumatic experiences are related to infant disorganized status: Is frightened and/or frightening parental behavior the linking mechanism? In M. T. Greenberg, D. Cicchetti, & E. M. Cummings (Eds.), *Attachment in the preschool years* (pp. 161-184). Chicago: University of Chicago Press.

Main, M., Kaplan, N., & Cassidy, J. (1985). Security in infancy, childhood, and adulthood: A move to the level of representation. In I. Bretherton & E. Waters (Eds.), Growing points of attachment theory and research. *Monographs of the Society for Research in Child Development, 50*(1-2, Serial No. 209), 66-104.

Main, M., & Solomon, J. (1990). Procedures for identifying infants as disorganized/disoriented during the Ainsworth Strange Situation. In M. T. Greenberg, D. Cicchetti, & E. M. Cummings (Eds.), *Attachment in the preschool years* (pp. 121-160). Chicago: University of Chicago Press.

Main, M., & Weston, D. (1981). Quality of attachment to mother and to father: Related to confict behavior and the readiness for establishing new relationships. *Child Development, 52*, 932-940.

Masters, J. C., & Wellman, H. M. (1974). The study of human infant attachment: A procedural critique. *Psychological Bulletin, 81*, 218-237.

Matas, L., Arend, R. A., & Sroufe, L. A. (1978). Continuity of adaptation in the second year: The relationship between quality of attachment and later competence. *Child Development, 49*, 547-556.

Mikulincer, M., Florian, V., & Tolmacz, R. (1990). Attachment styles and fear of personal death: A case study of affect regulation. *Journal of Personality and Social Psychology, 58*, 273-280.

Mikulincer, M., Florian, V., & Weller, A. (1993). Attachment styles, coping strategies, and post-traumatic psychological distress: The impact of the Gulf War in Israel. *Journal of Personality and Social Psychology, 64,* 817-826.

Mikulincer, M., & Nachshon, O. (1991). Attachment styles and patterns of self-disclosure. *Journal of Personality and Social Psychology, 61,* 321-331.

Pastor, D. L. (1981). The quality of mother-infant attachment and its relationship to toddlers' sociability with peers. *Developmental Psychology, 17,* 326-335.

Renken, B., Egeland, B., Marvinney, D., Mangelsdorf, S., & Sroufe, L. A. (1989). Early childhood antecedents of aggression and passive-withdrawal in early elementary school. *Journal of Personality, 57,* 257-281.

Ricciuti, A. E. (1992). *Child-mother attachment: A twin study.* Unpublished doctoral dissertation, University of Virginia.

Rothbard, J. C., & Shaver, P. R. (1991). *Attachment styles and the quality and importance of attachment to parents.* Unpublished manuscript, State University of New York at Buffalo.

Senchak, M., & Leonard, K. E. (1992). Attachment styles and marital adjustment among newlywed couples. *Journal of Social and Personal Relationships, 9,* 51-64.

Shaver, P. R., & Brennan, K. A. (1992). Attachment styles and the "big five" personality traits: Their connections with each other and with romantic relationship outcomes. *Personality and Social Psychology Bulletin, 18,* 536-545.

Shaver, P. R., & Hazan, C. (1993). Adult romantic attachment: Theory and evidence. In D. Perlman & W. Jones (Eds.), *Advances in personal relationships* (Vol. 4, pp. 29-70). London: Jessica Kingsley.

Shaver, P., Hazan, C., & Bradshaw, D. (1988). Love as attachment: The integration of three behavioral systems. In R. J. Sternberg & M. L. Barnes (Eds.), *The psychology of love* (pp. 68-99). New Haven, CT: Yale University Press.

Simpson, J. A. (1990). The influence of attachment styles on romantic relationships. *Journal of Personality and Social Psychology, 59,* 971-980.

Simpson, J. A., Rholes, W. S., & Nelligan, J. S. (1992). Support-seeking and support-giving within couple members in an anxiety-provoking situation: The role of attachment styles. *Journal of Personality and Social Psychology, 62,* 434-446.

Sperling, M. B., Berman, W. H., & Fagen, G. (1992). Classification of adult attachment: An integrative taxonomy from attachment and psychoanalytic theories. *Journal of Personality Assessment, 59,* 239-247.

Sroufe, L. A. (1983). Infant-caregiver attachment and patterns of adaptation in preschool: The roots of maladaptation and competence. In M. Perlmutter (Ed.), *Minnesota Symposia in Child Psychology* (Vol. 16, pp. 41-83). Hillsdale, NJ: Erlbaum.

Sroufe, L. A., Egeland, B., & Kreutzer, T. (1990). The fate of early experience following developmental change: Longitudinal approaches to individual adaptation in childhood. *Child Development, 61,* 1363-1373.

Sroufe, L. A., & Waters, E. (1977a). Attachment as an organizational construct. *Child Development, 48,* 1184-1199.

Sroufe, L. A., & Waters, E. (1977b). Heart rate as a convergent measure in clinical and developmental research. *Merrill-Palmer Quarterly, 23,* 3-27.

Thompson, R. A., Lamb, M. E., & Estes, D. (1983). Harmonizing discordant notes: A reply to Waters. *Child Development, 54*, 521-524.

Vaughn, B. E., Egeland, B. R., Sroufe, L. A., & Waters, E. (1979). Individual differences in infant-mother attachment at 12 and 18 months: Stability and change in families under stress. *Child Development, 50*, 971-975.

Waters, E. (1978). The reliability and stability of individual differences in infant-mother attachment. *Child Development, 49*, 483-494.

Waters, E., Wippman, J., & Sroufe, L. A. (1979). Attachment, positive affect, and competence in the peer group: Two studies in construct validation. *Child Development, 50*, 821-829.

CHAPTER 3

Internal Working Models and the Representational World in Attachment and Psychoanalytic Theories

DIANA DIAMOND
SIDNEY J. BLATT

Recently there has been an interest in the convergence of psychoanalytic theories of mental representation with empirical research and theory on attachment. Attachment theorists have turned their attention from an investigation of interactive attachment patterns to the representational world—the ways in which early attachment relationships are subjectively experienced and internally constructed. Internal working models of attachment have been compared to Kernberg's (1976, 1980, in press) self-object-affect units that form the basis of self and object representations; to Fairbairn's (1954) internal objects and associated portions of the ego; and to Sandler and Rosenblatt's (1962) representational world as an internal drama in which the individual enacts multiple roles, each of which represents a discrete self- or object image (Blatt, in press; Bretherton, 1990; Levy & Blatt, 1993).

Although there are many similarities between internal working models of attachment and psychoanalytic self- and object representations, it is important not to make reductionist comparisons, but instead to distinguish what is unique in the psychoanalytic and attachment perspectives on the representational world in order to facilitate a fruitful dialogue between the two perspectives. Accordingly, we briefly review the conceptualizations of the representational world in psychoanalytic object relations theory and attachment theory, and then consider the concept of internal working models of attachment from the vantage point of two psychoanalytic concepts that have been relatively neglected by attachment theorists: the theory of internalization, and the concept of evocative object constancy—both of which can illuminate and amplify the recent findings on internal working models of attachment. A number of recent papers have systematically compared concepts of self- and object representation in psychoanalytic and attachment theory (see Bretherton, 1987; Silverman, 1991; Slade & Aber, 1992; Zelnick & Buchholz, 1990). Recent formulations from both these theoretical perspectives highlight the need for us to understand modes and mechanisms of internalization and the role of evocative object constancy in the development of the representational world. Psychoanalytic object relations and attachment theorists have recognized that the infant internalizes not a static image or representation of the other (as traditionally thought in psychoanalytic theory), or the actual attachment-related transactions (as originally thought in attachment theory), but the affectively charged relationship between self and other (Behrends & Blatt, 1985; Bretherton, 1987; Kernberg, in press; Loewald, 1962; Zeanah & Anders, 1987).

THE FORMULATIONS OF PSYCHOANALYTIC THEORY

Psychoanalytic object relations theorists have explored the processes through which the earliest dyadic relationships are internalized and transmuted into intrapsychic structures, largely as these structures are activated in the clinical situation. The cognitive, affective, and experiential components of representations (or "schemata") of self and other are gradually built up in the course of development, as early affect-laden interactions with significant others are transformed into psychic structures (e.g., ego and superego functions, self- and object representations) (Beres & Joseph, 1970; Behrends & Blatt, 1985; Blatt, 1974; Blatt & Lerner, 1983; Meissner, 1981; Sandler & Rosenblatt, 1962; Schafer, 1968). Thus, self- and object representations bear the imprint of actual interpersonal transactions in interaction with the individual's developmental level, expressed in psychosexual-stage-related libidinal and aggressive impulses and conflicts (Kernberg, 1976, 1980; Jacobson, 1964; Mahler, Pine, & Bergman, 1975) and in other aspects of intrapsychic life, including idiosyncratic wishes, affects, and fantasies (Fairbairn, 1954; Sandler & Sandler, 1978; 1987; Stern, 1989). This representational world is multilayered, with conscious aspects that are relatively accurate depictions of consensual reality, and unconscious aspects that reflect fundamental needs or fantasies and primitive, idiosyncratic constructions of self and others, the latter being predominant in severe psychopathology (Blatt, Brenneis, Schimek, & Glick, 1976). Schafer (1968), Kernberg (1980), and others have distinguished between "secondary-process" representations, which are relatively accurate, stable, and firmly structured, and "primary-process" representations, which are relatively inaccurate, unstable, timeless, and often distorted. Self- and object representations span and often synthesize these two poles.

In psychoanalytic object relations theory, self- and object representations are considered as multidimensional and complex, and the emergence of any particular representational configuration reflects a synthesis of the imperatives of the internal and external world (Sandler & Rosenblatt, 1962). These self- and object representations, established in early childhood, function as templates that organize subsequent interpersonal interactions. New transactions, as well as developmentally determined shifts in self- and object representations, provide a revised matrix for interpersonal capacities and experiences (Blatt & Lerner, 1983).

The representational world is thus composed of multiple sets of self- and object representations linked by an affect disposition (Kernberg, 1976, 1980; in press). The representational world is not a set of veridical representations of relationships, past and present, but aspects of real and fantasied relationships as they are experienced by the child (Pine, 1990). Since early experiences are determined by a convergence of idiosyncratic wishes and affects with actual interpersonal transactions, these are essentially knowable as reconstructions in the psychoanalytic process (Blatt, 1974; Pine, 1990; Sandler & Rosenblatt, 1962; Schafer, 1968).

THE CONTRIBUTIONS OF ATTACHMENT THEORY

Bowlby (1977, 1980) and other attachment theorists have critiqued psychoanalytic models of the representational world as placing too much emphasis on fantasy, drive, and defenses (e.g., projection and introjection). Instead, they have proposed a model of the representational world that is built on information processing and generalized event theory, and that emphasizes how the representational world bears the imprint of actual interactions and events. "Internal working models" of attachment derive primarily from interactions centering around attachment-related events, and specifically from the child's experiences as he or she exercises the stable propensity to seek proximity to the primary caretaker. Internal working models formed in early childhood tend to shape the construction of subsequent relationships; they are structured processes that facilitate or limit access to information (Main, Kaplan, & Cassidy, 1985). Internal working models enable the individual to perceive and interpret interpersonal events, and they shape current and future interpersonal transactions and behavior.

Investigations of the representational world by attachment theorists have relied on concepts from cognitive psychology, such as "event schemata" (Mandler, 1979), "active structural networks" (Nelson & Grundel, 1981), and "scripts" (Schank & Abelson, 1977). The consensus among attachment theorists is that internal working models are composed of multilayered, hierarchical networks of representations. The most rudimentary layers involve event schemata derived from actual interactions with attachment figures, which generalize into higher-order, overarching global representations of the self in interaction with attachment figures as development progresses (Bretherton, 1990; Stern, 1989). The extent to which specific representations of events coincide with the derived global abstractions determines the coherence (Main et al., 1985) or adequacy (Bretherton, 1987) of a working model of attachment. Thus, for example, an individual who maintains a global representation of the mother as affectionate and available, but who manifests specific event schemata of the mother as unavailable or rejecting, will have an inconsistent working model of attachment.

Generalized event representations include affective and cognitive components as the average feeling states are integrated with attachment events (Bretherton, 1987). When basic attachment event schemata are imbued with painful affects, as with parental rejection or inconsistency, the associated affects may become disconnected from the event schemata; thus, the higher-level representations become discrepant with the lower-level event schemata. The individual may recall negative or rejecting attachment-related events, but may be unable to experience the associated affects of pain and anger. Conversely, the original generalized negative attachment event schemata may be repressed, so that the individual has limited access to attachment-related information and affects. These formulations have important implications for considering conscious and unconscious aspects of internal working models.

Almost from birth, the infant begins to construct internal working models of attachment, in which knowledge of self and others is "embedded in event-based relationships" (Main et al., 1985, p. 73). These interpersonal transactions begin to be consolidated into internal working models from 9 to 18 months of age, which coincides with the consolidation of object permanence (Piaget, 1954). Internal working models are initially organized as action schemata of attachment-related events, and this has implications for what is internalized. Internal working models encompass the history of parent–child transactions related to attachment, including the infant's attempts to re-establish contact with the parent in his or her absence; as such, "the working model . . . reflects not an objective picture of 'the parent,' but rather the history of the caregiver's responses to the infant's actions or intended actions with/toward the attachment figure" (Main et al., 1985, p. 85).

According to Bowlby (1969) and others (e.g., Main et al., 1985; Ainsworth, Blehar, Waters, & Wall, 1978), the individual internalizes dyadic attachment experiences with significant primary caretakers. If the individual is continually rebuffed or ridiculed when seeking comfort from an attachment figure, the internal working model will be composed of a representation of a rejecting parent interacting with a self that is unworthy or ineffective. Conversely, if the parent consistently offers comfort and support in stressful situations, the internal working model will be comprised of a loving parent in interaction with a worthy and effective self. Internal working models of attachment encompass aspects of both the self and the other in the dyadic attachment relationship.

The close linkage between attachment and object relations theory is evident in Bowlby's (1973) statement that "the concept of working models . . . is no more than a way of describing, in terms compatible with systems theory, ideas traditionally described in such terms as 'introjection of an object' (good or bad) and 'self image'" (p. 204). Bowlby (1977, 1988), Slade (1987; Slade & Aber, 1992), and others, however, have hypothesized that internal working models differ from the psychoanalytic representational world in that internal working models are not only crystallizations of past interpersonal transactions, but evolving, dynamic structures that forecast and guide the formation of future attachment experiences and relationships. Bretherton (1987) has observed that these internal working models need not be detailed or complex. Indeed, internal working models in attachment theory lack the intricacy, complexity, and detail of psychoanalytic concepts of the representational world, and instead are limited to representational schemata of certain prototypic attachment transactions.

Perhaps because of its ethological underpinnings, attachment theory defines the nature of the relational content of the representational world more specifically than psychoanalytic object relations theory does. Internal working models of attachment are constructed from experienced and generalized outcomes of individual actions, plans, and intentions related to attachment figures, and their content reflects certain behavioral prototypes. Research with the Ainsworth et al. (1978) Strange Situation, a laboratory-based separation and reunion task, documents that a finite number of attachment patterns result when children exercise their environmentally stable propensity to seek and maintain proximity to their primary caretakers. Thus, when a child's attachment-seeking behaviors are responded to and reciprocated, a secure mother–infant attachment pattern tends to result; when they are rebuffed or avoided, an insecure, avoidant pattern may emerge; when they are inconsistently rebuffed and reciprocated, an insecure, anxious/ambivalent attachment pattern may develop (Ainsworth et al., 1978). Main and colleagues have added a fourth category: When the child's attachment-seeking behaviors are responded to in a punitive, abusive, or frightening way, a disorganized/disoriented pattern may result (e.g., Main & Hesse, 1990). These environmentally consistent attachment patterns, represented in an enactive modality in infancy, come to define the parameters of the development of internal working models.

The correspondences and divergences between the internal working models of attachment theory and the representational world of psychoanalysis have inspired recent empirical investigations of the relationship between these two ways of conceptualizing the representational world. A recent study (Levine, Tuber, Slade, & Ward, 1991), for example, found significant correlations between the security of internal working models of attachment (as assessed through the Adult Attachment Interview) and the quality of object relations (as assessed through the Krohn Object Representation Scale for Dreams) in a sample of 42 pregnant adolescents. In addition, the security of the internal working models of attachment and the quality of object relations of the mothers correlated significantly with their children's attachment classification as assessed through the Ainsworth Strange Situation when the infants were 15 months of age. Thus, security of attachment in actual mother–child transactions and at the representational level has been found to be associated with the quality and developmental level of object relations of the mother (Levine et al., 1991).

Levy and Blatt (1993) also found correspondences between young adults' attachment styles and the structure of these individuals' mental representations of their parents. In a sample of 196 undergraduates, attachment was assessed through both Shaver and Hazan's (1987) single-item checklist and Likert scale measures of attachment styles and Bartholomew's (1990) four-category measure of adult attachment style; object representations were assessed through written descriptions of parents (Blatt, Chevron, Quinlan, & Wein, 1982; Blatt, Chevron, Quinlan, Schaffer, & Wein, 1992). The parental descriptions were then scored for both structural and qualitative dimensions (Blatt et al., 1992), as well as for the degree of self-other differentiation on a 10-point scale ranging from "self–other confusion" to "a cohesive sense of self and other" (Diamond, Blatt, Stayner, & Kaslow, 1992; Diamond, Kaslow, Coonerty, & Blatt, 1990). The findings indicated that the parental representations of securely attached young adults were both more differentiated and organized at a higher conceptual level than were the parental representations of their insecurely attached counterparts. Furthermore, insecurely attached young adults described their parents as more malevolent and punitive than did the securely attached subjects. These findings provide further support for the hypothesis that working models of attachment and object representations are overlapping, if not identical, modes of conceptualizing the internalized cognitive-affective schemata that form the bedrock of the intrapsychic world, and that in turn shape interpersonal relationships. These findings also suggest that the consolidation of insecure attachment styles in young adulthood may disrupt the capacity to internalize stable, cohesive, integrated representations of significant others.

MECHANISMS AND MODES OF INTERNALIZATION IN ATTACHMENT THEORY

Bowlby (1988) stated that he developed the theory of internal working models of attachment to account for the ways in which attachment patterns become internalized and come to constitute an aspect of the self, as well as a relational propensity. But Bowlby, like most developmental theorists, did not focus on the processes or mechanisms of internalization. He hypothesized that the innate predisposition of humans to form and maintain affectional bonds to significant others involves inherent structuring effects, but he did not explore the extent to which attachment patterns come to constitute representational structures. As Silverman (1991) pointed out, "the internalization of attachment patterns is the key to their significance because internalizations are considered pivotal processes in developmental theory" (p. 172). Thus, the conceptualization of internalization is crucial to understanding how habitually enacted mother–infant attachment transactions are transformed into representational structures.

In recent years, a number of studies have demonstrated linkages between attachment patterns as they are enacted in infancy and internal working models of attachment expressed in later perceptual and cognitive development—that is, through language and imagery in later childhood, adolescence, and adulthood (Main et al., 1985; Grossmann, Fremmer-Brombik, Rudolph, & Grossmann, 1988; Fonagy, Steele, Moran, Steele, & Higgitt, 1991; Ricks, 1985). A number of studies indicate that a mother's internal working models of attachment, as narrated in the intensive Adult Attachment Interview (George, Kaplan, & Main, 1985), are expressed in early transactional attachment patterns with her infant in the Ainsworth Strange Situation (Main et al., 1985; Fonagy, Steele, & Steele, 1991; Grossmann et al., 1988). These transactional attachment patterns are then internalized by the child and transmuted into comparable internal working models of attachment expressed through words and imagery in later childhood (Slade & Aber, 1986; George & Solomon, 1989; Zeanah, Benoit, Hirshberg, Barton, & Regan, 1991).

In interpreting these research findings, which are discussed in greater detail below, attachment researchers have focused on the impressive continuity in patterns of attachment both throughout the life cycle and across generations (Main et al., 1985; Fonagy, Steele, & Steele, 1991; Slade &

Aber, 1992; Slade & Cohen, 1993). This striking continuity of attachment patterns, however, has caused attachment investigators to overlook an essential aspect of their findings: that internal working models undergo developmental transformations in their modes of representation (Bruner, 1964; Blatt, 1974; Horowitz, 1972, 1983, 1988) as the individual matures. Many theorists, including Freud (1915/1957), Piaget (1954), Werner (1948, Bruner (1964), Horowitz (1970, 1983, 1988), and Blatt (1974), have hypothesized that there is a developmental sequence of modes of representation–from concrete, enactive representations to affectively laden, sensory, imagistic representations to more abstract, symbolic, verbally mediated representations.

We briefly explicate this developmental sequence in greater detail as a prelude to further developing the implications of attachment research findings for our understanding of such shifts in modes of representation. Horowitz (1972, 1983, 1988), using Bruner's (1964) work as a basis, defined three modes of representation: the enactive, expressed through movement; the imagistic, expressed through sensory images; and the lexical, expressed through verbal and symbolic modes. These three modes of representation differentially organize the way in which information is processed and a representational model of the world is constructed. Enactive representations involve motor actions or responses that may be modified by interaction with the environment. In the enactive mode, the represented information is communicated through facial expressions, bodily gestures, and posture. An example of an enactive representation is as follows: A young child reaches for a forbidden object, but then makes a stern, reproving face and grasps his or her hand with the other hand (Horowitz, 1988). Imagistic representations are primarily sensory in nature (e.g., visual, auditory, tactile, etc.) and remain close to affect and perception. The imagistic representation system appears to have dual input of information–both from the external world and from internal schemata and memory networks. In the course of development, as words come to signify both real objects and intense images of objects, a lexical mode of representation emerges. Although Horowitz (1972, 1988) has conceptualized lexical representation as a more advanced stage of development than enactive or imagistic representations, the acquisition of the lexical or symbolic capacity also catalyzes further evolution of the enactive and imagistic modes of representation as well, and fosters linkages among all three modes of representation.

As attachment researchers have increasingly focused on the variations of patterns of attachment in later childhood, adolescence, and adulthood, they have indirectly illuminated the ways in which enactive representations of early dyadic attachment patterns are transformed into imagistic and lexical modes of representation involving imagery and language. Main et al. (1985), for example, found that continuity in infant's security of attachment from 12 months to 6 years involved significant shifts in representational modes. Children classified as securely attached at 12 months in the Ainsworth Strange Situation, for example, who approached their mothers readily and with a range of positive and negative affect (enactive mode), also at age 6 readily accepted and perused a family photograph (imagistic mode) and responded with a balance of verbal self-exposure and self-containment to photographs of children undergoing separations from parents, elaborating frequently on their own separation experiences (imagistic and lexical modes). In contrast, children characterized by avoidant attachment at 12 months, who tended to turn away from their parents in the Ainsworth Strange Situation (enactive mode), also at age 6 spurned a family photograph (imagistic mode) and responded to the questions about parent-child separations in a emotionally constricted (avoidant) manner (often insisting, for example, that a child would feel nothing); they thus showed a failure to develop a lexical mode of representation. Children classified as anxiously/ambivalently attached at 12 months, who alternated between clinging to and pushing away their parents, also at age 6 responded to photographs depicting separations in a distressed manner. Finally, children classified as disorganized at 12 months, who responded to reunion tasks with chaotic, disoriented behaviors, also at age 6 responded to the separation photos in an irrational, controlling, or punitive manner, involving destructive and self-destructive verbal and nonverbal outbursts such as hitting a stuffed animal (Main et al., 1985).

In summary, Main et al. found that the three groups of insecurely attached children appeared to express themselves primarily through the enactive mode of representation when issues about separation or reunion with primary objects were evoked. They expressed themselves less successfully through the imagistic mode, and failed to make the transition to the lexical mode. The securely attached children, however, showed the capacity to verbally explore or visually represent their internal experience of separation and reunion vis-à-vis primary objects. Thus, we may conclude that transformations to more mature modes of representation (i.e., imagistic and lexical) occur primarily in securely attached children.

Furthermore, Main et al. (1985) found significant differences in the structure as well as the content of attachment histories related on the Adult Attachment Interview by the parents of children who had been assessed 6 years earlier in the Ainsworth Strange Situation. Specifically, the most significant correlate of a mother's attachment-related behavior toward her infant was not the extent to which her relationship with her parents was recollected in positive or negative terms, but the extent to which the mother's internal working model of attachment was coherent—that is, the extent to which it integrated positive and negative qualities (as opposed to being polarized between idealization and denigration), and the extent to which generalized evaluations of attachment relationships coincided with specific attachment memories. The mothers of securely attached infants provided coherent narratives of their attachment histories; they were able to integrate negative and positive attachment experiences, and were able to contextualize negative experiences by presenting them in the light of their own parents' limitations, dilemmas, and conflicts, about which they showed compassion and understanding. The parents of insecurely attached infants, on the other hand, were also able to present negative attachment experiences, but they did so in an unintegrated and incoherent manner, so that their interview transcripts showed marked inconsistencies, contradictions, dysfluencies, and discontinuities. Parents of avoidant infants (who were classified as "dismissing of attachment" on the Adult Attachment Interview) presented narratives of their own early attachment experiences that contained contradictions between general attachment memories, which were often quite positive or even idealized (e.g., a mother was described in a global way as all-giving or supportive), and episodic or specific attachment memories (elicited through specific probes), which were quite often negative (e.g., a mother was described as rejecting pleas for attention when a child had a physical injury). Parents of anxiously/ambivalently attached infants (who were classified as "preoccupied with attachment" on the Adult Attachment Interview) appeared to be flooded and overwhelmed by episodic or specific attachment memories, and were unable to structure these memories coherently or to provide semantic or general attachment memories. Finally, parents of disorganized infants were found to have unresolved mourning of past traumas, such as loss of attachment figures or experiences of physical or sexual abuse, indicated by signs of continuing cognitive disorganization when the attachment figures were discussed. Ultimately, Main et al. (1985) found that it was not the content of the mother's previous attachment relationships, but the narrative structure and overall coherence of the material obtained in the interview, that was related to the attachment pattern the mother established with her own infant.

These findings led Main et al. (1985) to conclude that the internal working model of attachment, established by the end of the first year of life, functions as a "template of previously unrecognized strength" (p. 94), which is "related not only to individual patterns in nonverbal behavior, but also to patterns of language and structures of mind" (p. 67). These and other studies indicate that internal working models of attachment show remarkable consistency within the individual over time, as well as within family generations in multiple cultures (Fonagy, Steele, & Steele, 1991; Fonagy, Steele, Moran, et al., 1991; Main et al., 1985; Ricks, 1985;

Grossmann et al., 1988; George & Solomon, 1991; Slade & Cohen, 1993; Zeanah et al., 1991). Even more impressive is the fact that the quality of the attachment appears to be related to the child's capacity to move to higher or more mature levels of representation and to utilize the symbolic or lexical mode of representation effectively in narrative construction.

As previously noted, attachment theorists hypothesize that instead of internalizing objects, individuals internalize sets of rules and expectations that enable them to interpret and anticipate the behavioral and emotional responses of attachment figures. More recent formulations stipulate that internal working models of attachment represent the infant's subjective experience of multiple aspects of mother–infant exchanges and relationship, and that these dyadic transactions come to constitute a part of the self (Zeanah & Anders, 1987; Bretherton, 1987). A number of studies provide support for this conceptualization. These studies indicate that by age 5 or 6, when identifications are being consolidated, early parent–infant attachment patterns are replicated not only in current attachment-related transactions, but also in a child's self-representation (Main et al., 1985; Main & Cassidy, 1988). Main and Cassidy (1988), for example, found that children identified as having a disorganized/disoriented pattern of attachment at 12 months presented by age 6 either as directly punitive or as highly controlling, often resorting to a pattern of role reversal in which they acted as caretakers by attempting to organize their mothers' behaviors. Such a child has internalized both a sense of self as disorganized and a sense of self as the compulsive caregiver of a disorganized parent. Furthermore, there is evidence that these disorganized patterns of attachment have intergenerational roots in parents' unresolved attachment-related traumas and losses (Main & Cassidy, 1988; Main & Hesse, 1990). On the Adult Attachment Interview, parents of disorganized infants who have such unresolved traumas and losses were also found to show signs of cognitive disorganization, including lapses in metacognitive monitoring of reasoning processes and discourse processes (e.g., denial of the death or the implications of the death, inappropriate guilt, slippage into a special state of mind or defensive breakdown when discussing the loss or abuse). Thus, in such a disorganized, parentified relationship, the parent's own attachment needs, psychological frailty, and cognitive disorganization are internalized by the child, forming the basis for an organization of self as a caregiver, even while other aspects of the child's self-organization in relation to attachment figures remain chaotic and confusing. This split in the child's self-organization reflects not only the parent's inability to respond with any consistency or continuity to the child's attachment needs and the reenactment of past traumas, often in the form of frightening an/or frightened behavior (Main & Hesse, 1990), but also the parents' inability to represent their experience through the symbolic or lexcial mode (Main & Goldwyn, in press; Main & Hesse, 1990; Zeanah & Zeanah, 1989).

Similarly, in an assessment of the self in relation to attachment figures in 6-year-olds through a puppet interview and story completion task, Cassidy (1988) found that the earlier attachment relationships had been preserved and transformed in the way in which the children depicted themselves. Children classified as securely attached, based on observations of mother-child interaction in a separation and reunion task, depicted themselves in subsequent puppet play in positive ways, and were also able to acknowledge imperfect or problematic aspects of themselves in verbal and nonverbal aspects of the play sequence. On the other hand, 6-year-olds classified as insecure in the separation-reunion task either showed no clear pattern of response (anxious/ambivalent), tended to depict the self as perfect (avoidant), or tended to depict the self in extremely negative ways (controlling/disorganized). Similarly, children classified as secure in the separation-reunion task tended to portray the child doll as worthy and as engaged in positive, gratifying interactions with the mother in the story completion task. Children classified as insecure either tended to depict the child doll as isolated or rejected by the mother (avoidant); as having no clearly defined coherent sense of self or relation to the mother (anxious/ambivalent); or as engaged in hostile, violent, bizarre, or disorganized transactions with the mother (controlling/disorganized). Cassidy's (1988) study and the others cited above thus indicate that by age 5 or 6 the child's working model of attachment involves a consolidated and specific representation of the self, the other, and their transactions, and that these mental structures are increasingly represented in imagistic and lexical rather than enactive modes, especially in securely attached children.

These studies also suggest that the failure to attain the lexical mode of representation may predispose the individual to repetitively re-enact maladaptive, unverbalized attachment patterns, particularly when unconscious defensive aims predominate. The most inchoate, unverbalized, and unverbalizable material may be represented through the gestures, facial expressions, and body posture of the enactive mode. Indeed, the enactive mode is characterized by Horowitz (1988) as "thought by trial action" (p. 158), whereas the imagistic mode is characterized as "thought by trial perception" (p. 158). According to Horowitz (1972), the imagistic mode of representation is the most potent and economical organizer of object relations, because aspects of the self, the other, and their interaction can be readily coded in a single image. When such imagistically encoded self-other transactions are fueled by significant conflicts, traumas, or drive derivatives, they tend to be repeated; such repetition fosters their consolidation into cognitive schemata, which then organize new information.

Although such schematic images contain representations of self and other, the self does not have a fixed identification with either role in the dyad; instead, it may shift fluidly from one role to another if either aspect of the dyadic experience evokes inordinate anxiety, guilt, fear, or frustration. The controlling/disorganized child who shifts between punitive and caretaking behaviors with the parent thus shows the structural fluidity inherent in enactive and imagistic modes of representation.

The development of lexical structures thus may serve the function of differentiating and consolidating discrete self- and object representations apart from their interaction, and may permit the capacity to reflect on and thus transform especially maladaptive attachment patterns. Placing partially articulated experiences into words facilitates a greater sense of control over experience. Words convey a sense of structure and direction to previously unarticulated experiences, so that one can begin to think about and understand them. Placing experiences into words leads to a sharper delineation between self and other, helps clarify cause-and-effect sequences, and contributes to and enhances the sense of self as an active and effective agent. Main et al. (1985) make a similar point when they hypothesize that the development of formal operations (Piaget, 1954) in adolescence, which involves the capacity to recognize, to reflect on, and thus potentially to reorganize one's abstract thought processes and meaning systems, entails new possibilities for the transformation of internal working models of attachment.

The research evidence for the continuity, complexity, and predictive power of internal working models of attachment has led attachment researchers to refine further the nature of the structures involved in the internalization of early attachment relationships. Fonagy and colleagues (Fonagy, Steele, Moran, et al., 1991; Fonagy, Steele, Steele, Moran, & Higgitt, 1991) have attempted to elaborate the concept of the coherence of representations by rating parental self-reflective capacity—that is, the capacity to understand aspects of the psychological states of self and other, including intentionality, feelings, beliefs, motivations, and desires. Assessing internal working models of attachment during the third trimester of pregnancy, Fonagy, Steele, Moran, et al. (1991) found that infant security of attachment during the first postnatal year was most strongly predicted by a rating of parental self-reflective function. The capacity of the parents to anticipate and respond to the mental state of their infants seemed to determine the infants' capacity "to organize defense, control affect, and build up a constant representation of the object" (p. 128)—all of which were related to the infants' security of attachment. Fonagy, Steele, Moran, et al. (1991) compare their findings with those of Main (1991) that at 6 years of age securely attached children have a more advanced and comprehensive theory of mind and a better comprehension and appreciation of the psychological world than do insecurely attached children.

The interconnection between security of attachment and the articulation of a self-reflective function in both 6-year-olds and adults, noted in the foregoing studies, provides further evidence for the linkages between security of attachment and the attainment of a lexical mode of representation. Horowitz (1972) hypothesized that the acquisition of lexical capacities catalyzes the maturation of schemata and their availability to organize information in all modes of representation. Thus parents with self-reflective capacities are able to comprehend, anticipate, and act on the mental state of their infants, which in turn provide the mental environment for the rudiments of a reflective self in the infants.

Although the findings of attachment researchers and theorists have contributed much to our understanding of the transformations of representations that occur in the internalization process, psychoanalytic theory can provide an even more complete understanding of the mechanisms of internalization.

MECHANISMS AND MODES OF INTERNALIZATION IN PSYCHOANALYTIC THEORY

A comprehensive discussion of the psychoanalytic understanding of the modes and processes of internalization is beyond the scope of this chapter, but the definition of internalization offered by Behrends and Blatt (1985) summarizes the dynamic relational mechanisms involved in this process: "Internalization refers to those processes whereby individuals recover lost or disrupted, regulatory, gratifying interactions with others, which may have been either real or fantasied, by appropriating those interactions and transforming them into their own, enduring, self-generated functions and characteristics" (p. 22). The initial substrate for internalizations is the formation of gratifying interactions with significant others; thus, attachment research and theory have contributed much to our understanding of these fundamental attachment bonds.

Internalization, as articulated by Behrends and Blatt (1985), Kernberg (1975, 1980), Loewald (1973), Meissner (1981), Schafer (1968), and others, depends upon the establishment and maintenance of human connectedness throughout the life cycle. However, it also depends upon the inevitable moments of separation and disruptions of attachment bonds in the course of the infant's development. A number of theorists, including Schafer (1968) and Behrends and Blatt (1985), have questioned whether gratifying involvement alone can provide the incentive or grounds for internalization. Behrends and Blatt (1985) hypothesized that internalization takes place through an ongoing dialectic between gratifying involvements with significant others and the inevitable incompatibilities (e.g., separations) experienced in the course of development. Such gratifying involvements entail not only pleasurable libidinal exchanges (with exquisite mutual cueing and communicative matching between mother and infant on the vocal, visual, and kinesthetic level), but also the mismatches, rifts, discontinuities, and disruptions that are the inevitable concomitants of separateness between self and other. These experienced incompatibilities, thought of as subtle gradations of separation, include not only actual losses of the objects or aspects of the self and its functions, but also the disruptions and shifts in relationships and self-identity that accompany ongoing developmental processes, as well as conflicts between idiosyncratic wishes and environmental demands. Internalizations throughout the life cycle evolve through a hierarchical spiral in which gratifying involvements are disrupted by experienced incompatibilities between self and primary objects; this disruption catalyzes the internalization of functions and aspects of the relationship, which then forms the basis for more complex interactions.

This model of internalization, which emphasizes the catalytic effects of separation within a matrix of ongoing attachment relationships, is compatible with attachment theory in several respects. First, gratifying involvements are the basis for the continuity and coherence of self and other that make unavoidable relational disruptions and incompatibilities tolerable. Second, ongoing relationships may contribute to the establishment of representational structures in a lifelong process in which the individual seeks and maintains affectional ties to others. Third, "aspects of relationships are internalized, not . . . fantasied objects or part objects which are replicas of people in the external world" (Behrends & Blatt, 1985, p. 23). Finally, the basic mechanisms that trigger internalizations are the same, regardless of developmental stage (Behrends & Blatt, 1985).

These formulations of the processes of internalization owe much to Mahler's (1963; Mahler et al., 1975) hypothesis that the infant has an innate propensity, at first motoric and later psychological, to seek separation and autonomy. These formulations are also consistent with the growing recognition of the importance of both attachment and autonomy/ separation (Blatt & Blass, 1990) in the development of human relatedness, as evident in the renewed emphasis on Bowlby's and Ainsworth's original observations that securely attached individuals had parents who not only were supportive and affectionate when called upon, but also promoted and maintained autonomy (Bretherton, 1987). Indeed, the paradox at the heart of attachment theory and research is that the task most commonly used for studying attachment is essentially a separation and reunion process (the Ainsworth Strange Situation) that evaluates the ways in which mother and infant negotiate two 3-minute separations. Bretherton (1987) comments that optimal attachment is observed when separation is tolerated and autonomy and exploration are promoted in stage-appropriate ways, without disrupting overall relatedness. These formulations are supported by recent research linking a child's security of attachment to the extent to which the mother's internal working model incorporates behavior that fosters autonomy and nonpunitive encouragement of competence and self-regulation in infancy (Cassidy, in press) and early childhood (age 6) (George & Solomon, 1989).

Bretherton (1987) and Slade and Aber (1992) have pointed out, however, that separation within attachment theory is conceptualized as an aspect of gratifying involvement rather than as an alternative to relatedness involving both physical and intrapsychic autonomy, as in separation-individuation theory. In attachment theory, the emphasis is on the internal working models of self and attachment figures that function as a guide to attachment-related interactions between mother and child, whether the mother is present or absent. In separation-individuation theory, the internal representation of the mother embodies the soothing, stabilizing functions of the maternal object, which may undergo further transformations even in the mother's absence. Attachment theorists (Slade & Aber, 1992; Bretherton, 1987) have remarked that the psychoanalytic conceptualization of libidinal object constancy, with its focus on the fate of the internal object relationship, eclipses the ongoing vicissitudes of the actual relationship and its perpetual contributions to psychic structure. However, it should be noted that the attainment of lexical representation involves words as a means of thought in the *absence* of actual objects, and thus necessitates a focus on the consolidation of the internal representation of the mother, apart from the vicissitudes of the actual relationship (Horowitz, 1972).

Attachment researchers are beginning to recognize the interconnection between separation and internal structure as evident in the fact that the only major catalyst for internalization noted in the attachment literature (beyond the inherent structuring effects of attachment bonds) is the development of the capacity for symbolic representation at age 18 months, which involves the consolidation of a sustaining internal image of the mother (Zeanah & Anders, 1987). Thus, an understanding of the mechanisms and processes of internalization necessitates a reconsideration of the importance of separation as well as relatedness for the development and consolidation of the internal object.

THE IMPORTANCE OF EVOCATIVE
OBJECT CONSTANCY

Critical to both attachment and psychoanalytic theory is the concept of object constancy, which is central to the development of mental representations. Fraiberg (1969) linked the concept of libidinal object constancy as the capacity for recognition memory to the development of object or evocative constancy (e.g., the capacity to evoke and sustain the image of the mother, independently of either external or internal stimuli). The capacity for evocative memory involves the ability to sustain an internal representation or image of the mother, regardless of the mother's actual moment-to-moment presence or of experiences of frustration and gratification. Fraiberg (1969) explored the convergence of evocative constancy with Piaget's schema for the acquisition of object permanence, both of which emerge around 18 months of age.

Although attachment theorists have forged similar linkages between Piagetian object permanence and the consolidation of internal working models of attachment (Main et al., 1985; Zeanah & Anders, 1987), they have largely neglected the implications of such a linkage for aspects of the internalization of secure versus insecure patterns of attachment, as well as its implications for subsequent development and modification of mental representations. Indeed, attachment theorists hypothesize that the cognitive capacity for object permanence entails the inscription of patterns of attachment on the intrapsychic level. In investigating variations in patterns of attachment, attachment researchers focused on variations in the content rather than the structure of internal working models. For example, Main and Hesse (1990) comment that the consistent responses of both securely and insecurely attached children bespeak a relatively well-organized and coherent attachment system, although those of insecurely attached children remain more vulnerable to disorganization. The one area in which attachment researchers have begun to forge linkages between attachment pattern and the structure (as opposed to the content) of the internal working model is in their investigations of the disoriented/disorganized pattern of insecure attachment (Main & Hesse, 1990; Slade & Aber, 1992). The conflicted and contradictory behaviors—including freezing of movement, rocking on hands and knees after an abortive approach to the parents, and screaming for the parents upon separation combined with moving silently away from them on reunion—of children classified as disorganized/disoriented in the Strange Situation suggest an absence of a coherent internalized attachment system. However, the implications of such differences in the behavioral organization of attachment and the structure of internal working models of attachment have not as yet been thoroughly investigated by attachment researchers.

Some investigations (Blatt & Homann, 1992; Blatt & Maroudas, 1992) suggest, however, that impairments or failures in libidinal (recognition) and evocative object constancy are expressed in impairments in the cognitive and affective aspects of internal working models of insecure attachment. These impairments of mental representations predispose the individual to various types of psychopathology, particularly depression

(Blatt, 1990). Bowlby (1977, 1980) and others (e.g., Sroufe, 1988) have commented that anxious/ambivalent and avoidant attachment occurs in a developmental context that puts the individual at risk for depression. Bowlby (1977, 1980, 1988) noted a vulnerability to depression in both anxiously/ambivalently attached individuals, who are overly dependent on interpersonal contact as a result of their experience of early caretakers as inconsistently and unreliably available, and compulsively self-reliant or avoidant individuals, who shun interpersonal contact or who assume the parental role vis-à-vis their own caretakers. Indeed, recent research has validated this link between the development of insecure styles of attachment and various forms of psychopathology, including depression (Armsden, McCauley, Greenberg, Burke, & Mitchell, 1990; Cole, 1991; Kobak, Sudler, & Gamble, 1991).

Blatt (1974; Blatt & Homann, 1992) has formulated two subtypes of depression that intersect with the insecurely attached patterns delineated above. "Anaclitic" or "dependent" depression, characterized by inordinate needs for direct physical and emotional contact with need-gratifying others and chronic fears of abandonment, corresponds to the anxious/ambivalent pattern of insecure attachment; and "introjective" (self-critical) depression, characterized by unrelenting self-criticism, chronic fears of loss of approval of valued others, social isolation, and feelings of unworthiness and guilt, corresponds to the avoidant pattern of insecure attachment.

It is possible that there are differential impairments in the mode or level of mental representation in these two types of depression and in the two insecure patterns of attachment that may form their developmental substrates. Blatt, Wein, Chevron, and Quinlan (1979) found that a key mediating factor in anaclitic versus introjective depression was the developmental or conceptual level of mental representation of parents, as assessed through parental descriptions rated on a developmental continuum from sensorimotor, to concrete perceptual images, to external and internal iconic representations, to complex and integrated conceptual representations. Parental descriptions by anaclitically depressed individuals were characterized primarily by sensorimotor preoperational representations, with little indication that the object tie could be sustained without direct immediate need-gratifying contact. Parental descriptions of introjectively depressed individuals indicated a capacity to sustain autonomous functioning apart from the object, as evident in their focus on external iconic or concrete physical and functional behavioral attributes. But the image of the parent as a harsh, critical, and intrusive inner presence curtailed the sense of an autonomous, competent self (Blatt & Homann, 1992).

The research investigations of Sperling, Sharp, and Fishler (1991) provide convergent findings linking insecure patterns of attachment (e.g., the patterns they label "avoidant" or "resistant/ambivalent," as well as an additional "hostile" attachment category) with severity of borderline pathology. The preponderance of resistant/ambivalent and hostile attachment styles among borderline inpatients is seen by Sperling et al. (1991) as consistent with various aspects of borderline organization, including splitting, affective polarities, and primitive aggression. These findings are also consistent with object relations aspects of borderline pathology, particularly the impairments in evocative object constancy and its associated developmental failures (Adler & Buie, 1979; Blatt & Auerbach, 1988; Kernberg, 1975, 1980). The linkage between attachment styles and personality disorders has also been investigated by Rosenstein and Horowitz (1993), who have found that insecure patterns of adult attachment (e.g., preoccupied or dismissing) involve maladaptive modes of affect regulation and defensive patterns, which were in turn associated with specific forms of personality disorders in a sample of 60 adolescent psychiatric inpatients. Specifically, adolescents who were classified as dismissing of attachment (on the Adult Attachment Interview), and who utilized defensive strategies of denial and exclusion of negative affects or negative aspects of parental introjects, tended to be diagnosed as having narcissistic or antisocial personality disorders. By contrast, adolescents who were classified as preoccupied with attachment, and who exaggerated their affect and were overwhelmed by negative aspects of parental introjects, tended to receive a diagnosis of histrionic, borderline, dependent, or schizotypal personality disorder.

DISCUSSION AND CONCLUSION

In the foregoing sections, we have discussed how transformations from prerepresentational, enactive, behavioral patterns of attachment to the development of mental representations of attachment relationships necessitate the concept of evocative object constancy evolving out of a process of internalization that encompasses both gratifying attachment and relational discontinuities (e.g., separations). Psychoanalytic object relations and attachment theories have important contributions to make to the understanding of the processes through which attachment transactions are transformed into mental representations.

Attachment theory and research on internal working models have contributed significantly to our understanding of the representational world. Most notably, observations from attachment research on aspects of internal working models have enabled us to appreciate how representational structures follow an epigenetic developmental sequence from enactive to imagistic to lexical modalities as they are transformed from preoperational, habitual motor patterns into symbolic, cohesive representations of self, other, and their interaction. Early attachment experiences and information are encoded during the first year in the enactive mode of representation. That is, the organization of movements of an infant's body in relation to a parent—particularly whether the infant spontaneously approaches and interacts with the parent in a securely attached dyad, or demonstrates some disruption of this pattern in an insecurely attached dyad—reveals the pattern of attachment that has developed. Internal working models of secure attachment in childhood and adulthood are increasingly represented in imagistic and lexical modes in the securely attached child. The securely attached 6-year-old child's ready and cheerful acceptance and perusal of the family photograph of separation, and the various disturbances of this pattern in insecurely attached children (Main et al., 1985), illustrate how internal working models of attachment influence the development of representational process from nonverbal to imagistic and verbal (lexical) modes. Finally, differences in the narratives of adults rated as secure, preoccupied with attachment, or dismissing of attachment on the Adult Attachment Interview (Main et al., 1985) demonstrate both the potentially integrative and synthesizing power of lexical representation (in securely attached individuals, who moved flexibly between generalizations about their attachment relationships and specific attachment memories and images), and the ways in which access to lexical representations may be restricted (in adults classified as dismissing or preoccupied with attachment).

The transformation of internal working models through different representational modalities necessitates further attention to the development of capacities for symbolic representation. Further research needs to explore the consolidation of evocative constancy in securely attached children at 18 months and its impact on the future development of lexical and symbolic capacities at ages 4 to 6, when triangular Oedipal identifications are consolidated (Blatt, 1990). Of particular importance is the role of language in the child's capacity to experience and represent others in verbal as well as nonverbal realms, as well as the ways in which expanded linguistic capacities facilitate shifts from enactive to imagistic and lexical modes of representation.

The study of infant attachment patterns was originally based on observations of the enactive (behavioral) mode of representation, expressed in different attachment patterns. The development of methods to assess attachment patterns through narrative reports has expanded the focus of attachment researchers to an exploration of the mental structures of attachment. Structural aspects of representation have been relatively neglected, because of fascination with the discovery of the continuity of behavioral expression of attachment patterns in later childhood, adolescence, and adulthood. This focus on the continuity in attachment behavior should form the basis for the study of transformations in the structure of internal working models in normal and deviant behavior. The findings of research employing the Adult Attachment Interview (e.g., Main et al., 1985) demonstrate that it is not the quality of the parents' reported behavior (i.e., whether the individuals perceive their own parents as rejecting or loving) that relates to attachment patterns, and to the transgenerational transmission of those patterns, but the coherence, consistency, and openness of the individuals' narratives about attachment experiences. These findings should redirect the focus of attachment theorists to the structure of the representational world, thereby offering new possibilities for an expanded and more productive dialogue with psychoanalytic theory.

ACKNOWLEDGMENT

Portions of this chapter were presented at the 100th Annual Convention of the American Psychological Association, Washington, DC, August 1992.

REFERENCES

Adler, G., & Buie, D. H. (1979). Aloneness and borderline psychopathology: The possible relevance of child development issues. *International Journal of Psycho-Analysis, 60,* 83-96.

Ainsworth, M. D. S., Blehar, M. C., Waters, E., & Wall, S. (1978). *Patterns of attachment: A psychological study of the Strange Situation.* Hillsdale, NJ: Erlbaum.

Armsden, G. C., McCauley, E., Greenberg, M. T., Burke, P. M., & Mitchell, J. R. (1990). Parent and peer attachment in early adolescent depression. *Journal of Abnormal Child Psychology, 18,* 683-697.

Bartholemew, K. (1990). *Attachment styles in young adults: Implications of self-concept and interpersonal functioning.* Unpublished doctoral dissertation, Stanford University.

Behrends, R., & Blatt, S. J. (1985). Internalization and psychological development throughout the life cycle. *Psychoanalytic Study of the Child, 40,* 11-39.

Beres, D., & Joseph, E. D. (1970). The concept of mental representation in psychoanalysis. *International Journal of Psycho-Analysis, 51*(1), 1-9.

Blatt, S. J. (1974). Levels of object representation in anaclitic and introjective depression. *Psychoanalytic Study of the Child, 24,* 107-157.

Blatt, S. J. (1990). Interpersonal relatedness and self-definition: Two personality configurations and their implication for psychopathology and psychotherapy. In J. L. Singer (Ed.), *Repression and dissociation: Implications for personality theory, psychopathology, and health* (pp. 299-335). Chicago: University of Chicago Press.

Blatt, S. J. (in press). Representational structures in psychopathology. In D. Cicchetti & S. Toth (Eds.), *Representation, emotion and cognition in developmental psychopathology.* Rochester, NY: University of Rochester Press.

Blatt, S. J., & Auerbach, J. (1988). Differential cognitive disturbances in three types of "borderline" patients. *Journal of Personality Disorders, 2,* 19-25.

Blatt, S. J., & Blass, R. B. (1990). Attachment and Separateness. A dialectic model of the products and processes of psychological development. *Psychoanalytic Study of the Child, 45,* 107-127.

Blatt, S. J., Brenneis, C., Schimek, J., & Glick, M. (1976). Normal and psychopathological impairment of the concept of the object on the Rorschach. *Journal of Abnormal Psychology, 85,* 364-373.

Blatt, S. J., Chevron, E., Quinlan, D. M., Schaffer, C., & Wein, S. (1992). *The assessment of qualitative and structural dimensions of object representations* (rev. ed.). Unpublished research manual, Yale University.

Blatt, S. J., Chevron, E., Quinlan, D. M., & Wein, S. (1982). *The assessment of qualitative and structural dimensions of object representations.* Unpublished research manual, Yale University.

Blatt, S. J., & Homann, E. (1992). Parent-child interaction in the etiology of depression. *Clinical Psychology Review, 12,* 47-91.

Blatt, S. J., & Lerner, H. D. (1983). Investigations in the psychoanalytic theory of object relations and object representation. In J. Masling (Ed.), *Empirical studies of object relations theories* (Vol. 1, pp. 189-249). Hillsdale, NJ: Analytic Press.

Blatt, S. J., & Maroudas, C. (1992). Convergences among psychodynamic and cognitive-behavioral theories of depression. *Psychoanalytic Psychology, 9,* 157-190.

Blatt, S. J., Wein, S. J., Chevron, E. S., & Quinlan, D. M. (1979). Parental representation and depression in normal young adults. *Journal of Abnormal Psychology, 88,* 388-397.

Bowlby, J. (1969). *Attachment and loss: Vol. 1. Attachment.* New York: Basic Books.

Bowlby, J. (1973). *Attachment and loss: Vol. 2. Separation: Anxiety and anger.* New York: Basic Books.

Bowlby, J. (1977). The making and breaking of affectional bonds: I. Aetiology and psychopathology in the light of attachment theory. *British Journal of Psychiatry, 30,* 201-210.

Bowlby, J. (1979). *The making and breaking of affectional bonds.* New York: Methuen.

Bowlby, J. (1980). *Attachment and loss: Vol. 3. Loss: Sadness and depression.* New York: Basic Books.

Bowlby, J. (1988). *A secure base.* New York: Basic Books.

Bretherton, I. (1987). New perspectives on attachment relations: Security, communication and internal working models. In J. D. Osofsky (Ed.), *Handbook of infant development* (2nd ed., pp. 1061-1100). New York: Wiley.

Bretherton, I. (1990). Communication patterns, internal working models, and the intergenerational transmission of attachment relationships. *Infant Mental Health Journal, 11,* 237-252.

Bruner, J. S. (1964). The course of cognitive growth. *American Psychologist, 19,* 1-15.

Cassidy, J. (1988). Child–mother attachment and the self in 6 year olds. *Child Development, 59,* 121-134.

Cassidy, J. (in press). Emotion regulation: Influences of attachment relationships. In N. Fox (Ed.), Biological and behavioral foundations of emotion regulation. *Monographs of the Society for Research in Child Development.*

Cole, H. E. (1991, April). *Worrying about parents: The link between preoccupied attachment and depression.* Paper presented at the biennial meeting of the Society for Research in Child Development, Seattle.

Diamond, D., Blatt, S. J., Stayner, D., & Kaslow, N. (1992). *Differentiation, cohesion and relatedness of self and other representations: A developmental scale.* Unpublished manuscript, Yale University.

Diamond, D., Kaslow, N., Coonerty, S., & Blatt, S. J. (1990). Changes in separation–individuation and intersubjectivity in long-term treatment. *Psychoanalytic Psychology, 7,* 399-422.

Fairbairn, W. R. D. (1952). *Psychoanalytic studies of the personality.* London: Routledge & Kegan Paul.

Fonagy, P., Steele, M., Moran, G., Steele, H., & Higgitt, A. (1991). Measuring the ghost in the nursery: A summary of the main findings of the Anna Freud Center–University College, London Parent–Child Study. *Bulletin of the Anna Freud Center, 14,* 115-131.

Fonagy, P., Steele, H., & Steele, M. (1991). Maternal representations of attachment during pregnancy predict the organization of infant–mother attachment at one year of age. *Child Development, 62,* 891-905.

Fonagy, P., Steele, M., Steele, H., Moran, G. S., & Higgitt, A. C. (1991). The capacity for understanding mental states: The reflective self in parent and child and its significance for security of attachment. *Infant Mental Health Journal, 13,* 200-217.

Fraiberg, S. (1969). Libidinal object constancy and mental representation. *Psychoanalytic Study of the Child, 24,* 9-47.

Freud, S. (1957). The unconscious. In J. Strachey (Ed. and Trans.), *The standard edition of the complete psychological works of Sigmund Freud* (Vol. 14, pp. 159-215). London: Hogarth Press. (Original work published 1915)

George, C., Kaplan, N., & Main, M. (1985). *The Berkeley Adult Attachment Interview.* Unpublished manuscript, University of California at Berkeley.

George, C., & Solomon, J. (1989). Internal working models of parenting and security of attachment at age six. *Infant Mental Health Journal, 10,* 222-237.

George, C., & Solomon, J. (1991, April). *Intergenerational transmission of the family system: Children's representations of the family in doll play.* Paper presented at the biennial meeting of the Society for Research in Child Development, Seattle.

Grossmann, K., Fremmer-Bombik, E., Rudolph, J., & Grossmann, K. E. (1988). Maternal attachment representation as related to patterns of mother–infant attachment and maternal care during the first year. In R. A. Hinde & J. Stevenson-Hinde (Eds.), *Relationships within families: Mutual influences* (pp. 241-260). Oxford: Clarendon Press.

Horowitz, M. J. (1972). Modes of representation of thought. *Journal of the American Psychoanalytic Association, 20,* 793-819.

Horowitz, M. J. (1983). *Image formation and psychotherapy* (rev. ed.). New York: Jason Aronson.

Horowitz, M. J. (1988). *Introduction to psychodynamics: A new synthesis.* New York: Basic Books.

Jacobson, E. (1964). *The self and the object world.* New York: International Universities Press.

Kernberg, O. (1975). *Borderline conditions and pathological narcissism.* New York: Jason Aronson.

Kernberg, O. (1976). *Object relations theory and clinical psychoanalysis.* New York: Jason Aronson.

Kernberg, O. (1980). *Internal world and external reality.* New York: Jason Aronson.

Kernberg, O. (in press). Psychoanalytic object relations theories. In B. E. Moore & B. Fine (Eds.), *Psychoanalysis: The major concepts.*

Klagsbrun, M., & Bowlby, J. (1976). Responses to separation from parents: A clinical test for young children. *British Journal of Projective Psychology, 21,* 7-21.

Klein, M. (1932). *The psychoanalysis of children.* London: Hogarth Press.

Kobak, R. R., & Sceery, A. (1988). Attachment in late adolescence: Working models, affect regulation, and representations of self and others. *Child Development, 59,* 135-146.

Kobak, R. R., Sudler, N., & Gamble, W. (1991). Attachment and depressive symptoms during adolescence: A developmental pathways analysis. *Development and Psychopathology, 3,* 461-474.

Levine, L., Tuber, S., Slade, A., & Ward, M. J. (1991). Mother's mental representations and their relationship to mother-infant attachment. *Bulletin of the Menninger Clinic, 55,* 454-469.

Levy, K. N., & Blatt, S. J. (1993). *Attachment style and mental representation in young adults.* Unpublished manuscript.

Loewald, H. (1962). Internalization, separation, mourning, and the superego. *Psychoanalytic Quarterly, 31,* 483-504.

Loewald, H. (1973). On internalization. *International Journal of Psycho-Analysis, 54,* 9-17.

Mahler, M. (1963). Thoughts about development and individuation. *Psychoanalytic Study of the Child, 18,* 307-224.

Mahler, M., Pine, F., & Bergman, A. (1975). *The psychological birth of the human infant.* New York: Basic Books.

Main, M. (1991). Metacognitive knowledge, metacognitive monitoring, and singular (coherent) vs. Multiple (incoherent) models of attachment: Findings and directions for future research. In C. Parkes, J. Stevenson-Hinde, & P. Marris (Eds.), *Attachment across the life cycle.* London: Routledge & Kegan Paul.

Main, M., & Cassidy, J. (1988). Categories of response with the parent at age six: Predicted from infant attachment classifications and stable over a one month period. *Developmental Psychology, 24,* 415-426.

Main, M., & Goldwyn, R. (in press). Interview based adult attachment classifications: Related to infant-mother and infant-father attachment. *Developmental Psychology.*

Main, M., & Hesse, E. (1990). Parents' unresolved traumatic experiences are related to infant disorganized attachment status: Is frightened and/or frightening parental behavior the linking mechanism? In M. T. Greenberg, D. Cicchetti, & E. M. Cummings (Eds.), *Attachment in the preschool years* (pp. 161-185). Chicago: University of Chicago Press.

Main, M., Kaplan, N., & Cassidy, J. (1985). Security in infancy, childhood, and adulthood: A move to the level of representation. In I. Bretherton & E. Waters (Eds.), Growing points of attachment theory and research. *Monographs of the Society for Research in Child Development, 50* (1-2, Serial No. 209), 66-104.

Mandler, J. H. (1979). Categorical and schematic organization in memory. In C. R. Puff (Ed.), *Memory organization and structure* (pp. 303-319). New York: Academic Press.

Meissner, W. W. (1981). *Internalization in psychoanalysis.* New York: International Universities Press.

Nelson, K., & Grundel, J. C. (1981). Generalized event representations: Basic building blocks of cognitive development. In M. E. Lamb & A. Brown (Eds.), *Advances in developmental psychology* (Vol. 1, pp. 131-158). Hillsdale, NJ: Erlbaum.

Piaget, J. (1954). *The construction of reality in the child.* New York: Basic Books.

Pine, F. (1990). *Drive, ego, object and self: A synthesis for clinical work.* New York: Basic Books.

Ricks, M. H. (1985). The social transmission of parental behavior: Attachment across generations. In I. Bretherton & E. Waters (Eds.), Growing points of attachment theory and research. *Monographs of the Society for Research in Child Development, 50*(1-2, Serial No. 209), 211-227.

Rosenstein, D. S., & Horowitz, H. A. (1993, March). *Working models of attachment in psychiatrically hospitalized adolescents: Relation to psychopathology and personality.* Paper presented at the biennial meeting of the Society for Research in Child Development, New Orleans.

Sandler, J., & Rosenblatt, B. (1962). The concept of the representational world. *Psychoanalytic Study of the Child, 17,* 128-145.

Sandler, J., & Sandler, A. M. (1978). On the development of object relationships and affects. *International Journal of Psycho-Analysis, 59,* 285-296.

Sandler, J., & Sandler, A. M. (1987). The past unconscious, the present unconscious and the vicissitudes of guilt. *International Journal of Psycho-Analysis, 68,* 331-342.

Schafer, R. (1968). *Aspects of internalization.* Madison, CT: International Universities Press.

Schank, R. C., & Abelson, R. P. (1977). *Scripts, plans, goals and understanding.* Hillsdale, NJ: Erlbaum.

Silverman, D. (1991). Attachment patterns and Freudian theory: An integrative proposal. *Psychoanalytic Psychology, 8,* 169-193.

Shaver, P. R., & Hazan, C. (1987). Being lonely, falling in love: Perspectives from attachment theory. *Journal of Social Behavior and Personality, 2*(2, Pt. 2), 105-124.

Slade, A. (1987). The quality of attachment and early symbolic play. *Developmental Psychology, 23,* 78-85.

Slade, A., & Aber, J. L. (1986, April). *The internal experiences of parenting toddlers: Towards an analysis of individual and developmental differences.* Paper presented at the International Conference of Infant Studies, Los Angeles.

Slade, A., & Aber, L. J. (1992). Attachment, drives and development: Conflicts and convergences in theory. In J. Barron, M. Eagle, & D. Wolitsky (Eds.), *Interface of psychoanalysis and psychology* (pp. 154-185). Washington, DC: American Psychological Association.

Slade, A., & Cohen, L. (1993, March). *Parenting and the remembrance of things past.* Paper presented at the biennial meeting of the Society for Research in Child Development, New Orleans.

Slade, A., Director, L., Huganir, L., Grunebaum, L., & Reeves, M. (1991, April). *Representational and behavioral correlates of prebirth maternal attachment.* Paper presented at the biennial meeting of the Society for Research in Child Development, Seattle.

Sperling, M., Sharp, J. L., & Fishler, P. H. (1991). On the nature of attachment in a borderline population: A preliminary investigation. *Psychological Reports, 68,* 543-546.

Sroufe, L. A. (1988). The role of infant-caregiver attachment in development. In J. Belsky & T. Nezworski (Eds.), *Clinical implications of attachment* (pp. 18-38). Hillsdale, NJ: Erlbaum.

Stern, D. (1989). The representation of relational patterns: Some developmental considerations. In A. Sameroff & R. N. Emde (Eds.), *Relationship disorders in early childhood* (pp. 52-69). New York: Basic Books.

Werner, H. (1948). *Comparative psychology of mental development.* New York: International Universities Press.

Winnicott, D. W. (1965). *Maturational processes and the facilitating environment.* New York: International Universities Press.

Zeanah, C. H., & Anders, T. F. (1987). Subjectivity in parent-infant relationships: A discussion of internal working models. *Infant Mental Health Journal, 8,* 237-250.

Zeanah, C. H., Benoit, D., Hirshberg, L., Barton, M., & Regan, C. (1991, October). *Classifying mothers' representations of their infants: Results from structured interviews.* Paper presented at the annual meeting of the American Academy of Child and Adolescent Psychiatry, San Francisco.

Zeanah, C. H., & Zeanah, P. (1989). Intergenerational transmission of maltreatment: Insights from attachment theory and research. *Psychiatry, 52,* 177-196.

Zelnick, L., & Buchholz, E. S. (1990). The concept of mental representations in the light of recent infant research. *Psychoanalytic Psychology, 1,* 29-58.

CHAPTER 4

Physiological Aspects of Adult Attachment

MARTIN REITE
MARIA L. BOCCIA

Jesus wept. And the Jews said, "Behold, how He loved the man."
—THE GOSPEL OF ST. JOHN

The presence of an attachment is often inferred from an individual's response to separation or loss. Although this response is not the only indicator of the nature and quality of the attachment, it is one important indicator. Gubernick (1981), for example, outlined criteria for recognizing the existence of an attachment to a particular figure. Three of the six criteria relate to the response to separation. Thus, an individual's behavioral and physiological response to separation from the attachment figure can indicate something of the nature and strength of the attachment bond. This chapter, examining the physiological correlates of adult attachment, considers the response to separation as one (but only one) measure of attachment.

We draw heavily in this chapter on the conceptual framework so eloquently outlined by John Bowlby (e.g., see Bowlby, 1988). We believe, in fact, that our data are directly relevant to testing the hypothesis articulated by Bowlby: "that each person's resilience or vulnerability to stressful life events is determined to a very significant degree by the pattern of attachment he or she develops during the early years" (Bowlby, 1988, p. 8).

To date, we have very few substantive data concerning the physiology of attachment in adult humans. There is however, an emerging body of data on nonhuman primate models that can contribute very directly to the way we conceptualize the physiology of attachment (and the disruption of attachment) in humans. In this chapter, we summarize these data and their implications for adult human attachment, and suggest areas of future research that may contribute more directly to our understanding of human attachment. This approach has special implications as well for our understanding of loss and bereavement, and attachment as viewed from that vantage point.

Nonhuman primates offer unique advantages as animal model systems in terms of central nervous system (CNS) structure, social behavior, and evidence of true social attachment. In addition to commonalities in the CNS, we believe it likely, on the basis of a common evolutionary history, that the neurobiological basis of social attachment is homologous in human and nonhuman primates. Primate models therefore have great relevance to the human condition. Another advantage of primate models is their variability. Humans demonstrate substantial individual variability in their response to separation, loss, and bereavement, and nonhuman primates demonstrate similar individual variability. A systematic investigation into the sources of such variability in nonhuman primates, including intrinsic (e.g., temperament and other neurobiological influences) and extrinsic (e.g., nature of the relationship disrupted, and associated social networks and social support) variables, may further enhance the utility of primate models in these areas, and add to our understanding of the mechanisms underlying the variability in human responses.

Our laboratory has been utilizing nonhuman primate social separation paradigms as models of human grief, bereavement, and the effects of disruption of attachment bonds. Included in this research have been studies designed to (1) examine the nature of the behavioral and physiological responses to separation; (2) examine how different types of attachment objects modulate these responses; (3) examine the role of the social environment, and in particular the availability of alternative attachments, in modulating the response to loss; (4) identify physiological predictors of individual differences in the response to loss; and finally (5) evaluate the possible value of treatment intervention in the face of loss. These data, as well as related findings from other laboratories using nonhuman primate models, are reviewed in the following sections.

On the basis of the animal model data and available human data, we propose below a model of the neurobiological basis of social attachment in primates, and suggest research paradigms that might be used to evaluate it.

ATTACHMENT FROM THE VANTAGE POINT OF SEPARATION IN NONHUMAN PRIMATES

Nonhuman Primate Models: Behavioral and Physiological Responses

Social separation paradigms in nonhuman primates have served as valuable animal models of human separation, loss, and bereavement

(McKinney, 1986), and as tools for the study of attachment. Early work by Seay and Harlow (1965), using rhesus macaque monkeys (*Macaca mulatta*), and Kaufman and Rosenblum (1967), using pigtail macaques (*Macaca nemestrina*), described a two-stage behavioral response in infant monkeys to separation from their mothers. This response is characterized by an initial agitation reaction with agitated behavior and increased distress vocalization, followed in these species by a so-called "depression" reaction consisting of decreased activity and social play, a slouched posture, and a characteristic sad facial expression similar to that described by Darwin (1872/1955) as characteristic of grief in animals, and universally recognized as sadness in humans (Ekman, Sorenson, & Fausen, 1969; Izard, 1971).

We developed a multichannel, implantable biotelemetry system capability that permitted the collection and analysis of multivariable physiological data concurrently with behavior in social-group-living monkey infants (Pauley & Reite, 1981; Reite, 1985), as well as methods for assessing immune function as a consequence of separation experiences (Reite, Harbeck, & Hoffman, 1981; Laudenslager, Held, Boccia, Reite, & Cohen, 1990). These methods have been used to examine the physiological and immunological correlates of the separation response in both pigtail and bonnet monkey (*Macaca radiata*) infants, as well as the moderating effects of several variables, including social context (Boccia, Reite, & Laudenslager, 1991; Caine & Reite, 1981) and autonomic reactivity (Boccia, Reite, Kaemingk, Held, & Laudenslager, 1991).

In typical maternal separation experiments, infants are born and raised in a social group. Pigtail mothers tend to be restrictive of their infants, and do not permit the infants to establish close social relationships (alternative attachments) with other adult females in the group. At about 4 to 6 months of age, when their mothers are removed (leaving the infants in their natal social groups), pigtail infants typically undergo the two-phase behavioral response described above. Initially the infants are very agitated, increasing their rates of locomotion and vocalizations, in apparently frantic attempts to relocate and re-establish contact with their missing mothers. This agitated behavior is associated with dramatic increases in both heart rate (HR) and body temperature (BT). After about 24–48 hours, the infants enter the second phase, depression or despair. They dramatically decrease their activity, increase their eating behavior, cease playing entirely, and exhibit the characteristic slouched posture. The period of behavioral depression or despair is accompanied by decreases in HR and BT (Reite, Seiler, & Short, 1978); disruptions of sleep patterns, including increased sleep latency, increased arousals and awake time, prominent increases in rapid eye movement (REM) latency, and decreases in total amount of REM sleep and number of REM periods (Reite & Short,

1978); and increases in cardiac arrhythmias (Seiler, Cullen, Zimmerman, & Reite, 1979). Phase delays are noted in HR and BT circadian rhythms (Reite, Seiler, Crowley, Hydinger-Macdonald, & Short, 1982), and immunological changes include reduced lymphocyte activation by mitogens (Laudenslager, Reite, & Harbeck, 1982; Laudenslager et al., 1990; Boccia, Reite, Kaemingk, Held, & Laudenslager, 1989; Reite et al., 1981), lower total plasma immunoglobulin antibody (IgM and IgG) levels (Scanlan, Coe, Latts, & Suomi, 1987), and reduced antibody response to a foreign protein antigen (keyhole limpet hemocyanin, or KLH) (Laudenslager, Boccia, & Reite, 1993). These findings are compatible with a disturbance of regulation of autonomic homeostasis precipitated by the separation experience.

Of note, and to be discussed in detail in sections following, is the observation that the adoption of a recently separated pigtail infant by another adult female in the social group—with whom the infant is familiar, but with whom no significant previous relationship existed—does not prevent the adverse physiological consequences of separation, even though the adoptive mother provides the separated infant with elements such as warmth, ventral-ventral contact, and protection (Reite, Seiler, & Short, 1978).

Other laboratories have examined other aspects of mother–infant separation in nonhuman primates. Separated rhesus monkeys have been shown to have an increase in adrenal catecholamine-synthesizing enzymes (Breese et al., 1973). Increases in cerebrospinal fluid (CSF) norepinephrine (NE) are found in rhesus infants following separation from either their natural mothers, or maternal surrogates, which may persist if the mothers are not returned (Kraemer, Ebert, Schmidt, & McKinney, 1989). We have also found evidence of a 30% increase in the CSF NE metabolite 3-methoxy-4-hydroxyphenylglycol (MHPG) in pigtail infants following maternal separation (Reite Cox, Laudenslager, Garrick, & Boccia, 1991). Recent evidence (Laudenslager, Boccia, Berger, & McFerran, 1993) also suggests elevations in cortisol and growth hormones during separation in pigtail infants. Studies from Levine's laboratory (Bayart, Hayashi, Faull, Barchas, & Levine, 1990; Weiner, Bayart, Faull, & Levine, 1990) have shown that the CSF amine metabolites MHPG and homovanillic acid (HVA) covary with serum cortisol as a measure of arousal associated with response to separation. Thus, in macaque infants, both monoamine and pituitary-adrenal systems are activated by maternal separation, although specifics of behavioral and physiological components of the response to separation are related to different aspects of the particular separation environment, in keeping with aspects of coping theory (Levine, 1983). Alpha-methylparatyrosine (AMPT), a tyrosine hydroxylase inhibitor that depletes CNS NE and dopamine (DA), potentiates the depressive response (as defined by decreases in locomotion and increases in huddle behavior) following peer separation (Kraemer & McKinney, 1979). Thus, evidence from a number of laboratories has highlighted the significance of brain catecholamine systems in the separation response. Other systems are likely to be involved in separation as well, as indicated by the work of Kalin and colleagues, who find evidence for opiate and endogenous benzodiazepine system involvement (Kalin, Shelton, & Barksdale, 1987, 1988).

In sum, the response to separation, of which one component is the disruption of an attachment bond or relationship, is a multifaceted bio-behavioral response suggesting dysregulation of multiple physiological systems. We have postulated that this represents a generalized dysregu-lation of autonomic function, with a relative parasympathetic predomi-nance (Reite & Capitanio, 1985). Note that this is not necessarily a tran-sient or evanescent phenomenon. Laudenslager, Capitanio, and Reite (1985) found evidence of diminished lymphocyte response to mitogen stimulation in pigtail macaques aged 3 to 6 years, following a 10-day maternal separation in infancy. Capitanio, Rasmussen, Snyder, Lauden-slager, and Reite (1986) found that, as adults, pigtail monkeys who had experienced a short maternal separation in infancy tended to have fewer adult friends, possibly reflecting impairment or alteration of adult social-ization.

How Can the Separation Response in Young Monkeys Be Modulated?

Separation from Objects Other Than the Mother

Studies conducted with other types of attachment objects in standardized environments suggest some interesting relationships between character-istics of the attachment object and the nature of the infant monkey's response to separation from the object. From these, inferences may be made about the nature of the attachment relationship itself.

We have studied surrogate-reared, socially isolated pigtail macaques (Reite & Short, 1977; Reite, Short, & Seiler, 1978). These infants were separated from their mothers within 24–48 hours of birth, and were raised on inanimate cloth surrogates, with no social contact with other monkeys. Although these infants exhibited the predictable behavioral abnormalities (such as high levels of self-orality, self-clasping, and rocking behaviors), their baseline physiological profiles were quite similar to those of mother-reared infants living in social groups. These infants exhibited attachment to their surrogates, in that they maintained high levels of contact with them and would retreat to them for comfort when threatened. The surrogate-reared infants, however, exhibited a much less dramatic response to separation than did mother-reared infants. Although they exhibited some behavioral agitation on the first day of separation from their surrogates, this was less than that seen in mother-reared infants. Furthermore, there was no evidence of the second (depressive) phase. At reunion, they also did not exhibit the typical increase in attachment behaviors.

In addition, surrogate-reared infants separated from their surrogates did not show the same physiological disruption seen in mother-reared infants. Initially, sleep latency and awake time increased, and total sleep and REM sleep decreased. By the fourth day of separation, however, all measures had returned to within one standard deviation of baseline. These infants also did not show changes in HR or BT. Thus, overall, these surrogate-reared infants did not exhibit the same type of attachment seen in mother-reared infants, as measured by these physiological responses to separation.

These studies suggest that although some form of an attachment develops between an infant and its surrogate, it is not the same as that between a mother and infant. There may be several contributions to these differences. Inanimate surrogates cannot provide a model of species-typical behaviors. More fundamentally, they lack many of the capacities that may serve as the basis of formation of an attachment, such as ability to support physiological synchrony and to provide species-typical contingent responses.

Another attachment modeling system that may discriminate some of these features is the peer-rearing paradigm, in which monkey infants are separated from their mothers within 24–48 hours of birth and raised only with other infants, and their behavioral and physiological development and response to separation are then examined. As with other species, peer-reared pigtail monkeys do not exhibit the profound behavioral disturbances evident in socially isolated, surrogate-reared infants. Except for self-orality, they do not exhibit the extensive self-directed behaviors, and they exhibit expected social behaviors, such as grooming, play, and sex (Reite, Kaemingk, & Boccia, 1984). Their sleep patterns are somewhat different from those of mother-reared infants, however. They exhibit more time awake and in stage 2 sleep, and less time in stages 3 and 4 and in REM sleep, suggesting that they have more disrupted sleep patterns (Reite & Kaemingk, 1987). These variables tend to correlate across the peer pairs, suggesting that the social environment unique to each pair is related to the sleep disruption. There is some evidence of synchrony in the HR and BT circadian rhythms of members of peer pairs living together (Reite & Capitanio, 1985).

When members of peer pairs are separated from each other, they exhibit initial behavioral agitation, but no subsequent depressive response. Agitation is evident in the increased activity on the first day of separation.

Although there is a decrease in play and increase in self-orality initially, these behaviors return to baseline by the second week of the separation (Boccia et al., 1989). There is no behavioral rebound in attachment-related behaviors during reunion.

Physiologically, separated peers exhibit a transient increase in HR and BT on the first day, which rapidly returns to baseline (Boccia et al., 1989). There is evidence of a diminution in synchrony between HR and BT rhythms during the period of separation, however (Reite & Capitanio, 1985). Among the sleep variables, only REM shows significant change (decrease), and this is confined to the first night of reunion, when the two members of the peer pair significantly disrupt each other's sleep. Separated peers both may show a decline in lymphocyte response to mitogen stimulation, suggesting an effect on immune system regulation (Reite et al., 1981; Boccia et al., 1989). Overall, peer-reared infants exhibit fewer separation-induced changes in behavior and physiology, suggesting differences in the nature of the attachment from that of mother-reared infants.

The environment of separation also figures prominently in the response to separation in peer-reared infants (Boccia, Reite, Kaemingk, et al., 1991). We studied four infants that were reared as two pairs of peers. One month before the separation, the two peer pairs were housed together. During the separation, one member of each pair was housed in social isolation and the other was housed socially (with the other, now familiar peer pair). The socially housed peer did not exhibit any noticeable response to the separation. This suggests that the agitation seen in response to peer separation in the original study may have been at least in part a response to social isolation, rather than to disruption of the peer-attachment bond per se.

Overall, these studies suggest that the quality of the attachment bond formed between peers may be quite different from that formed by an infant with an adult female. The many significant differences between an adult female and another infant include the ability to model mature social behavior, to provide behavioral and physiological regulation, and to provide appropriate contingent responsivity. It is significant to note that under conditions of social housing, the agitation response may be eliminated, suggesting an important role for social support. That the peer-reared infant can utilize this support to regulate itself in the face of loss suggests that the peer's infant attachment object (the other member of the peer pair) is able to provide some "scaffolding" for the development of physiological regulation. It may also be that exposure to species-typical behavior, however immature, facilitates behavioral and/or physiological development. Other investigators (Mason & Kenney, 1974) have found that rhesus monkeys reared on heterospecific attachment objects (dogs) show developmental behavioral deficits intermediate between those of monkeys reared in total social isolation and peer-reared monkeys; this suggests that the experiences of behavioral contingency, even in the absence of species-typical behavior, facilitate behavioral development.

Maternal Separation in Bonnet Monkeys: The Role of Alternative Attachments

Mother-reared bonnet monkey infants exhibit a pronounced agitation phase in response to separation, again with increases in both HR and BT, when separated in their natal social group; however, the subsequent depressive response is muted, with much less evidence of either behavioral or physiological change (Laudenslager et al., 1990; Reite, Kaemingk, & Boccia, 1989). We believe this results from the fact that under conditions of normal social group rearing, the infants have opportunities to interact with and develop relationships with other adult females. When their mothers are removed from the social group (the separation), bonnet infants are adopted by particular adult females in the group, with whom they have developed previous relationships (Reite et al., 1989). We believe the difference between the differential protective effect of adoptions in pigtails (no protective effect) and bonnets (protective effect) is related to the fact that bonnet infants have previously established close relationships (attachment-like) with these other adult females in the group who adopt them. Pigtail infants, although familiar with the other females in the group, have not been allowed to developed close relationships with the other adults (because of their mothers' restrictiveness). One might infer from these observations that more than one attachment relationship can have a protective or buffering effect in times of loss or stress.

This lack of a depressive response in bonnet monkey infants may be more a reflection of the availability of alternative attachments than of a difference in maternal attachment, since experimental elimination of the availability of alternative attachment objects results in a depressive response following maternal separation in bonnet infants. For example, if bonnet infants are raised in a mixed-species social group, with both bonnet and pigtail members, the pigtail monkey females do not develop relationships with the bonnet infants; when the bonnet mothers and all other conspecifics are removed, the bonnet infants exhibit a behavioral and physiological agitation–depression reaction quite as profound as that seen in separated pigtail infants (Reite & Snyder, 1982). This indicates that bonnet infants are quite capable of exhibiting the same biobehavioral response to disruption of an attachment bond if there are no mitigating circumstances present, such as alternative attachments.

Environmental Modification of the Development of Attachment

The development of attachment is fluid and can adapt to varying environments and conditions. We have found that experimental manipulation of the social environment of a bonnet monkey group can substantially alter the development of attachment in the infants. When competition for access to (but not amount of) food is experimentally induced, bonnet monkeys become aggressive (Boccia et al., 1989). As a consequence, mothers become restrictive with their infants, and the infants fail to develop alternative attachments in the group (Boccia, Laudenslager, & Reite, 1988). When the mother of such an infant is removed, even though the infant remains in its conspecific social group, it may exhibit a profound behavioral depressive response (Boccia, Reite, & Laudenslager, 1991).

In a related experiment, Rosenblum (1987) has raised bonnet infants in a variable-foraging-demand environment, where food, while equally plentiful, is more difficult to obtain, and the mother must spend considerable time searching for food hidden in piles of wood chips. This environmental experience alters the mother-infant relationship and results in an apparent "insecure attachment." Such an infant may exhibit evidence of depressive behaviors even in the presence of the mother, while the mother is involved in foraging tasks. Such observations demonstrate that patterns of early mother-infant attachment may be significantly influenced by the early social environment, with substantial effects on later response to separation or disruption of the bond, and perhaps the individual's vulnerability to loss generally.

In both these paradigms, experimental manipulations of the environment alter the developing infant's attachment relationships. We (Boccia et al., 1988, 1989) have focused on the alterations produced in alternative attachments, which appear also to affect the primary attachment to the mother. Rosenblum (1987) has focused on the primary attachment to the mother. Both these observations probably have implications for the social development of human infants. That is, the impact of a loss may be a function of both the availability of alternative attachments, and the ability of the individual sustaining the loss to benefit from these alternative attachments. Stressful environments may limit or alter the formation of attachments, and so may influence the vulnerability of the individual to subsequent adverse experience. Attachment formation, however, appears to be canalized and requires profound environmental disruption (e.g., see the discussion of the Ik later in this chapter) to be eliminated.

More generally, although the capacity to develop attachment probably represents the function of an inborn neurobiological system (as we discuss in more detail below), whether or how such attachments may develop can be substantially affected by the social environment in which the organism finds itself. The protective effect of adoption in bonnet infants suggests that certain types of social support may serve as protective influences in separation or loss-related stress. We believe that this is the case, and, furthermore, that aspects of social support may be mediated by attachment systems.

The Role of Social Support

The role of social support in health maintenance is a topic of considerable recent interest (Cohen, 1989). House, Landis, and Umberson (1988) conclude:

> Prospective studies, which control for baseline health status, consistently show increased risk of death among persons with a low quantity, and sometimes low quality, of social relationships. Experimental and quasi-experimental studies of humans and animals also suggest that social isolation is a major risk factor for mortality from widely varying causes. (p. 540)

Thomas, Goodwin, and Goodwin (1985), in a study of 256 elderly human adults, found that strong social support systems were associated with higher indices of immune function (mitogen response to phytohemagglutinin stimulation). More recently, Kamarck, Manuck, and Jennings (1990) have demonstrated that, in a human laboratory situation, the presence of social support reduced cardiovascular reactivity to stressful situations. These and other studies indicate that social support may be a significant factor in the health status of individuals facing major life stressors. Our data suggest that the efficacy of this social support may be based, at least in part, on its being a form of attachment.

Old World monkeys such as the macaques are social animals with complex social structures, and can serve as valuable models of social support in humans. Data from such animal models suggest that social support plays a significant role in the response to separation, and that the mechanisms of action may involve the attachment system. Caine and Reite (1981) found that pigtail infants separated in social groups containing peers had a less pronounced decrease in HR following maternal separation than those separated in groups without peers. We recently found that bonnet infants separated in the presence of social support (presence of juveniles to whom they were attached) exhibited a less pronounced alteration in lymphocyte activation and natural cytotoxicity after maternal separation than those separated in environments lacking such support (Boccia, Scanlan, Broussard, Laudenslager, & Reite, 1994).

Social relationships may exert their effects by promoting important regulatory influences on social organisms. This has been demonstrated to be the case for the mother–infant relationship in rodents (Hofer, 1981) and humans (Brazelton, Koslowski, & Main, 1974), and has been implicated in later development as well (Field, 1985). Social relationships have also been implicated as important regulators of circadian rhythms (Moore-Ede, Sulzman, & Fuller, 1982). It has been suggested that the adverse medical and psychological consequences of separation and loss are attributable to the withdrawal or loss of regulatory influences intrinsic to the relationship (Hofer, 1984). The extent to which social support functions as a main effect or as a buffering effect remains unresolved (Cohen, 1989).

Our observations above as to the role of adoption in moderating the effects of maternal separation in monkey infants suggest that social support may be mediated at least in part via the attachment system. Pigtail infants, which have not developed an attachment to their adoptive mothers, do not appear to benefit from adoption. Bonnet infants, which appear to be attached to their adoptive mothers, do benefit. The observations are consistent with a study reported by Brown, Bifulco, Harris, and Bridge (1986), who examined the role of social support in altering the risk of depression related to stress (usually loss) in a cohort of 400 working-class women. If support was received from a so-called "core" relationship, there was a diminished risk of depression. Support received from a "noncore" relationship was not helpful, however, indicating that it was not so much the presence of support as the kind or nature of the support that was the critical variable. A "core" relationship in this study was similar to what we might consider an attachment relationship; a "noncore" relationship did not include elements of attachment.

One implication of such observations is that the protective or beneficial effects of social support may occur to the extent that there is a prior attachment relationship present with the individual providing the support. If, then, we propose to provide social support in an effort to benefit individuals undergoing stressful experiences, we should include a careful assessment of the nature of that support, in terms of whether it might be expected to include elements of pre-existing attachment.

Individual Differences in the Response to Separation

Kraemer, Ebert, Lake, and McKinney (1983) found that in young rhesus monkeys, low CSF NE levels (either spontaneous or drug-induced) were associated with a more severe depression (depressive slouched posture) in response to peer separation. McKinney (1986) found that CSF NE varied with rearing condition, and that HVA, a metabolite of DA, and 5-hydroxyindoleacetic acid (5-HIAA), a metabolite of serotonin, varied with separation experience. He suggests from this that CSF NE may be a trait-related marker predicting a more severe response to peer separation, whereas CSF HVA and 5-HIAA may be state-related markers that reflect behavioral response to peer separation.

Kraemer et al. (1989) also found that rhesus infants raised with their mothers during the first 6 months of life had significantly higher CSF NE levels than did infants raised without mothers. These differences were apparent as early as 1 month of age. Month-to-month correlations were more stable in mother-reared infants as well. Nursery-reared infants also have lower growth hormone levels and higher cortisol levels than mother-reared infants (Champoux, Coe, Schanberg, Kuhn, & Suomi, 1989); it is not yet clear whether this is related to CSF amine measures.

Thus, aspects of early experience, especially the maternal rearing environment, appear capable of producing long-term alterations in CNS amine (NE) systems. These alterations may in themselves preferentially alter an individual's subsequent response to stress, as manifested by response to social separation experiences. Such physiological markers may be related to the development and expression of attachment.

Human data have suggested that HR variability may index a measure of responsivity to novel social situations, a facet of "temperament" (Kagan, Reznick, Clarke, Snidman, & Garcia-Coll, 1984; Rosenberg & Kagan, 1989). Stable individual differences are found in such measures in children. Recent data suggest that nonhuman primates may also demonstrate individual differences in HR, which may predict aspects of the response to a stress such as separation (Boccia, Laudenslager, & Reite, 1994). In a group of 29 pigtail monkey infants, we computed mean day HR for each subject, and a median split of subjects based on HR was performed: Subjects above the median were classified as "High HR" and those below as "Low HR." Behavioral responses to separation, including vocalizations, slouch, exploration, locomotion, and eating behaviors were analyzed via analysis of variance, with HR classification as a between-subjects variable, and separation phase (baseline, separation day 1 [SD1], and the remainder of separation [separation week 1, or SW1]) as a within-subjects variable. Subjects classified as High HR exhibited significantly more distress vocalizations on SD1, and spent more time in the depressive slouch posture during SW1, than subjects classified as Low HR. These data are illustrated in Figure 4.1. Subjects also differed in the degree to which typical sleep disruption occurred at separation, particularly for REM sleep variables.

These are the same behaviors that we have found to covary with immunological measures during separation (Laudenslager et al., 1990; Laudenslager, Held, Boccia, Gennaro, Reite, & Cohen, 1993). This relationship suggests that individual differences in autonomic variability may relate to the response to separation. Kagan (1982) also found evidence of HR's correlating with separation distress in the Ainsworth Strange Situ-

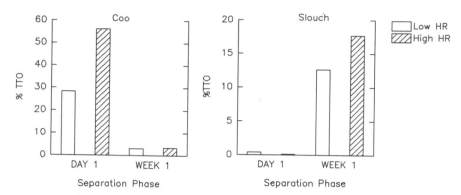

FIGURE 4.1. Coo behaviors on Day 1 of separation were significantly elevated in animals with high heart rates compared to animals with low heart rates (left panel, day 1). No differences was noted during the entire first week of separation (left panel, week 1). Slouch behaviors were virtually nonexistent on day 1 of separation (right panel, day 1). Slouch behavior was higher during the first week of separation in animals with higher heart rates (right panel, week 1). %TTO, percentage of total time observed (for behaviors).

ation in human infants between 5 and 29 months of age. The details of its interaction with attachment remain to be explored.

Nonhuman primate data also suggest that altered early rearing experience may induce changes in brain morphology. Siegel et al. (1993) found evidence that rhesus monkeys raised under conditions of social deprivation had increased amounts of nonphosphorylated neurofilament protein in cells of the dentate granule layer of the hippocampus, suggesting that aspects of the early social environment might contribute to altered development of the hippocampus. Such studies would suggest that developmental aspects of brain morphology may be sensitive to early rearing environment; such changes in turn may influence an individual's subsequent capability to adapt to stressful situations and experiences such as separation, or perhaps even to form attachments.

Summary

In summary, then, research on maternal attachment and separation in nonhuman primates suggests that the nature of the response to maternal separation, both behavioral and physiological, reflects in part the nature of the attachment relationship with the mother, and therefore the nature of the bond disrupted by the separation. In addition, intrinsic physiological factors (e.g., autonomic control of HR, CNS neurotransmitter systems) may be related to the variability seen in responses to separation. This research also demonstrates that the context of separation can have an impact on the expression of separation distress, and that the presence of alternative attachments or social support can ameliorate certain facets of the response. Significant alterations in early experience may themselves produce long-lasting changes in brain biochemistry and morphology, which may further influence subsequent behavior and response to stress.

SEPARATION AND ITS CONSEQUENCES IN HUMANS

In humans, separation and loss commonly lead to depression (Freud, 1917/1957; Paykel, 1983; Phifer & Murrell, 1986). There is a marked similarity between symptoms of uncomplicated bereavement and major depression. Clayton (1990) has presented data suggesting that over 40% of recently bereaved individuals exhibit symptoms that would support a diagnosis of a major depression within 1 year of the loss. Roy, Gallucci, Avgerinos, Linnoila, and Gold (1988) suggest that predisposed individuals may respond to bereavement with a depressive illness accompanied by dysregulation of the hypothalamic–pituitary–adrenal axis. Depression has been hypothesized to result from dysregulation of circadian and other biological systems (Wehr & Goodwin, 1983; Siever & Davis, 1985); Ehlers, Frank, and Kupfer (1988) specifically suggest that this dysregulation may be attributable to loss, or separation-induced removal, of social "zeitgebers" (external factors that affect or time circadian rhythms).

Other adverse health consequences may follow separation or loss. In a review of the literature on psychosomatic medicine, we found reference to several dozen medical illnesses or disorders thought to be caused or exacerbated by loss (Laudenslager & Reite, 1984; Lown, 1990). These may ensue at least in part from generalized dysregulation of autonomic physiology, as well as from alterations in immune function accompanying loss (Laudenslager, 1988).

Relatively few data are available on the specific physiological consequences of separation or loss in human beings, however. Grief is typically accompanied by a set of symptoms involving respiration, motility, sleep, cardiac activity, and appetite (Lindemann, 1944). A report by Jellinek, Goldenheim, and Jenike (1985) described abnormalities in ventilatory control in parents grieving over the death of an infant. Sleep patterns in bereaved elderly individuals exhibiting symptoms of major depression were similar to sleep changes in nonbereaved individuals with unipolar major depression, but sleep in nondepressed bereaved elderly persons was not significantly different from normal (Reynolds et al., 1992). The incidence of cardiac-related deaths is increased by bereavement (Lown, 1990). Bereavement may also be associated with alterations in immune system regulation (He, 1991; Reichborn-Kjennerud, 1990; Beutel, 1991; Irwin, Hauger, Brown, & Britton, 1988). The implication again is that in adult humans, the disruption of an attachment relationship leads to physiological (including immunological) dysregulation; this suggests that attachment per se plays some role in establishing/maintaining physiological regulation, as is also found in nonhuman primate studies.

TREATMENT OF SEPARATION EXPERIENCES

Loss experiences, such as bereavement, are accompanied by behavioral and physiological changes that may adversely affect individuals, and may have adverse public health implications as well. A question of considerable importance is whether the symptoms of loss should, or can, be treated.

Pharmacological treatment of grief in humans has in fact been suggested (Clayton, 1990; Jacobs, Nelson, & Zisook, 1987), in hopes of preventing or ameliorating certain of the adverse affective and medical consequences. One open (non-double-blind) study that involved treatment of a group of recently bereaved elderly individuals with the tricyclic antidepressant nortriptyline found evidence of significant improvement of symptoms of depression, sleep quality, and general level of functioning, although symptoms of grief were not significantly influenced; this suggested that psychological "grief work" might be separable from adverse physiological alterations (Pasternak et al., 1991).

Several nonhuman primate studies have shown that tricyclic antidepressant agents, which enhance activity of central catecholaminergic and/or serotonergic systems, appear to diminish the severity of the response to peer separation in rhesus monkeys (Suomi, Seaman, Lewis, DeLizio, & McKinney, 1978) and maternal separation in *Macaca fascicularis* monkeys (Hrdina, von Kulmiz, & Stretch, 1979) when administered orally. Physiological measures were not obtained in these studies, however.

In a recent study (Reite, Laudenslager, Garrick, Boccia, & Cox, 1991), we began treatment of a group of six pigtail infants with either the monoamine oxidase (MAO) inhibitor clorgyline (2 mg/kg) or a placebo during maternal separation, using an implantable osmotic minipump; their responses were compared to those of six unseparated controls. Clorgyline has been shown to be a clinically effective antidepressant in humans (Murphy et al., 1981), and has also been shown to produce significant inhibition of MAO in pigtail monkeys when administered by osmotic minipump at dose levels of 0.5-2 mg/kg (Cox, Garrick, Reite, & Gennaro, 1991). These infants were also immunized at the time of separation with KLH, a foreign antigen, to allow us to determine whether the expected separation-induced impairment of antibody formation to this foreign protein would be prevented or ameliorated by treatment with clorgyline.

Clorgyline-treated infants were found to have a less pronounced decrease in HR following separation than placebo-treated infants. HR in placebo animals decreased 32 ± 6 beats per minute (bpm) from baseline to SW2, whereas HR in clorgyline animals decreased only 17 ± 35 bpm, $F(1, 5) = 17.06$, $p = .009$. This suggests that the type of autonomic imbalance normally seen during separation may be altered or prevented by clorgyline treatment.

With respect to specific KLH antibodies, plasma IgM levels were not different among the three groups (placebo, clorgyline, unseparated control). Plasma IgG, however, was lower in the separated placebo group than in the separated clorgyline group or the control group, suggesting that the drug administration attenuated the impact of the separation experience on specific antibody levels. One implication of these findings is that the switch from IgM to IgG may be altered by the separation experience, but that clorgyline treatment may attenuate these changes. This preliminary study suggests that clorgyline treatment may prevent or ameliorate certain physiological and immunological consequences of separation.

The data above suggest that loss (e.g., bereavement) can be thought of as an event that may, in some cases, benefit from pharmacological treatment in order to prevent or ameliorate certain adverse physiological sequelae. Before such interventions can be formally recommended, however, more data are needed on specific physiological abnormalities that accompany grief in humans; a method is also needed to assess which individuals might benefit from treatment, and which particular agent, at what dose, is the most effective.

IMPLICATIONS OF SEPARATION STUDIES FOR MODELS OF ATTACHMENT

Overall, the evidence suggests that a separation experience is a potent disrupter of many physiological and behavioral systems in young monkeys and adult humans. Why should a loss or separation experience be associated with such physiological dysregulation? We believe that separation has these physiological consequences because one function of attachment is to promote concordant regulation of physiological and behavioral systems. The disruption of this attachment, then, permits dysregulation of the systems that it supports.

The earliest relationship, that of infant to mother, is clearly seen as containing a system of physiological and behavioral regulation. Several years ago we proposed a definition of attachment as "a neurobiologically based and mediated biobehavioral system, one of whose major functions is to promote the development and regulation (or modulation) of psychobiological synchrony between organisms" (Reite & Capitanio, 1985, p. 224). Such a definition presupposes several issues that are not always considered in thinking about attachment. First, it suggests that attachment is biologically based, with a phylogenetic history independent of a particular time and place in human culture. A biological system implies physiological events that can be monitored, and whose synchrony or concordant regulation can be measured in attached individuals. It implies a neurobiological basis in the structure and function of the nervous system, and an ontogenetic history in terms of maturational and experiential effects.

In rats, the role of the mother as a regulator of infant pup development is complex and multifaceted, as shown in the elegant series of studies by Hofer and colleagues (Hofer, 1981). We might not wish to conceptualize this as a manifestation of attachment, because "attachment," which involves recognition of a specific individual, may not characterize the rat pup–mother relationship—or, for that matter, social relationships in rodents generally. These data, however, clearly support the role of the mother–infant relationship in regulating the physiological development and functioning of the infant.

In primates, where attachment bonds *are* found, the mother also plays an intricate and enduring role in the development and maturation of the offspring. In humans, there is evidence of synchrony between certain activity, behavioral, and speech rhythms in mothers and infants (Sander, Stechler, Burns, & Julia, 1970; Condon & Sander, 1974; Bernieri, Resnick, & Rosenthal, 1988; Tronick, Ricks, & Cohn, 1982). Brazelton et al. (1974) found evidence for emergence of complex patterns of social interactions between mother and infant, concluding that "this interdependency of rhythms seemed to be at the root of their 'attachment' as well as communication" (Brazelton et al., 1974, p. 74). McKenna, Mosko, Dungy, and McAninch (1990) suggest that human mother–infant cosleeping during the first year or so of life may foster development of the important capability for appropriate spontaneous arousals, and in so doing may diminish the probability of sudden infant death syndrome.

Thus, one function of maternal behavior in primate species may be to foster the development of synchrony or concordant regulation with the developing offspring. This apparent concordant regulation between mother and offspring is an early form of physiological self-regulation, but in the context of a relationship. The promotion of physiological regulation, prominent in the early mother–infant bond, may well underlie concordant regulation associated with later-developing attachment bonds, including peer bonds and adult attachment relationships. The implicit assumption in such a construct is that when early relationships are deficient in such regulation-enhancing functions, older or adult individuals may be similarly deficient in exhibiting—and perhaps with their own subsequent offspring, entraining—such physiological (as well as behavioral) regulation.

Perhaps those systems and structures that underlie this aspect of maternal behavior in nonprimate mammalian species should be considered as candidate systems underlying similar behavior in primates, including humans. This would suggest that research on such regulatory systems in nonprimate mammals might serve as a knowledge base that can be used either to develop testable hypotheses about, or even possibly to explain, homologous regulatory systems in primates (both nonhuman and human).

A MODEL OF ATTACHMENT

The model we propose suggests that human attachment evolved from the relatively simpler (but by no means "simple") maternal regulation of and interaction with the development of the infant (perhaps any infant in rodents, or a specific infant in ungulates) observed in various nonprimate mammals and extending through the higher primates, wherein parental involvement with the developing offspring is long-lasting (lifelong in some cases), and where individual recognition and discrimination are the hallmarks of attachment. Within an individual organism, the maturation of attachment from infancy to adulthood is associated with predictive alterations in its nature and object, from infancy through childhood, adolescence, and adulthood. Again within an individual, and in accordance with the principle of Occam's Razor, we see no compelling need to postulate essentially different mechanisms underlying such normal maturational development; rather, we prefer to suggest that the system responsible matures with the developing organism, and incorporates species- and developmental-stage-appropriate experiences. Both neurobiological development and alterations in experience might be expected to shape the final form of attachment.

The model of attachment we propose is in fact quite similar to that of language in humans: It has a firm neurobiological basis, requires species-appropriate experience for proper development, and is strongly shaped by early experience, while having a profound impact on adult functions.

A primate attachment system elaborated upon the underlying maternal behavior in mammals generally would appear to be a reasonable starting point. Maternal behavior incorporates physiological and behavioral regulation—and, in primates, individual recognition by multisensory pathways and mechanisms. The mother-infant bond is the first manifestation of attachment; subsequent social bonds might be expected to develop by means of similar systems and mechanisms. Disturbances in biology and experience that interfere with such functions would be expected to interfere with attachment. Attachment is clearly manifested in bonds other than the mother-infant, such as father-infant, sibling, peer, and adult bonds; thus, the mother is not a *sine qua non* in the equation. Rather, the important issue is the development of those CNS systems subserving such behaviors, in which the primary attachment figure is highly significant, but not limited to one sex or age.

Neuroanatomy and Neurochemistry

There are relatively limited data on the specific neuroanatomical structures and systems that underlie maternal behavior, especially in primates. The existing data have recently been reviewed by Numan (1988). Even within rodents, where neuroanatomical and neurochemical mechanisms relating to maternal behavior have been examined in a number of species, quite substantial species differences are found.

Maternal behavior has been most extensively studied in rodent species, where subcortical hypothalamic and thalamic systems are important. Specifically, in rodents, medial preoptic area neurons and their projections to the ventral tegmental area are directly involved in neural mediation of maternal behavior (Numan, 1988). No substantive evidence relates function of cortical regions to maternal behavior.

With respect to neurochemistry of the onset of maternal behavior, Numan (1988) concludes that in the rat, "Estrogen and prolactin superimposed on progesterone withdrawal interact with an endogenous oxytocin system to facilitate maternal behavior" (p. 1622). Interestingly, oxytocin has recently also been found to be involved in the regulation or modulation of sexual behavior (Witt & Insel, 1991) and social affiliative behavior in the prairie vole (Carter, Williams, Witt, & Insel, 1992) and rat (Witt, Winslow, & Insel, 1992). Furthermore, there is some evidence that in rats, opiate systems may play an inhibitory role in maternal behavior (Rubin & Bridges, 1984).

In primates, it is not unreasonable to suppose that such systems remain important; in addition, however, the phylogenetically later-developing cortical regions that subserve individual recognition may also come into play. Several studies in nonhuman primates have suggested that temporal and frontal cortical regions as well as cingulate cortex may subserve important aspects of maternal behavior (Pechtel, McAvoy, Levitt, Kling, & Masserman, 1958; Franzen & Myers, 1973; Kluver, 1950; Bucher,

Myers, & Southwick, 1970; Myers, Swett, & Miller, 1973). Clearly, many of these effects might relate to an impairment of the mother's ability to recognize the infant for what it is. An important aspect of attachment resides in recognition of the individual. There is evidence that in adult monkeys, single neurons in the temporal cortex respond preferentially to specific individuals on the basis of facial structure (Perrett et al., 1988). This may not be limited to primates, for ungulates (sheep) appear to demonstrate similar neuronal preferences (Kendrick & Baldwin, 1987).

We would suggest, then, that the neurobiological root of attachment behavior might be found in those hypothalamic and midbrain systems supporting maternal behavior in lower mammals such as rodents, combined with the later-developing neocortical systems essential for individual recognition. Again, a clear caveat is that attachments form independently of the mother–offspring bond as well, (e.g., father–offspring, peer–peer, and adult–adult bonds). The extent to which similar mechanisms underlie all such attachments is yet unknown and awaits further study. There is also emerging evidence that specific neuroanatomical systems and mechanisms (which may or may not be similar to systems involved in maternal behaviors) may underlie social affiliative behavior in adult nonhuman primates. In a recent review, Steklis and Kling (1985) summarize evidence obtained from their own studies and those of others implicating three specific brain areas—the orbitofrontal cortex, anterior temporal cortex, and amygdaloid nuclei—as underlying social affiliative behavior in primates.

Malleability

This "attachment system" is exquisitely sensitive to experience, both early and late. The absence of appropriate social experiences permitting the development of social or attachment bonds in early infancy can significantly skew the developmental trajectory of the individual and compromise later social bonding as an adult. Primates (both human and nonhuman) that have been subjected to atypical early attachment experience, including separation and/or abuse, may become abusive parents themselves (Caine & Reite, 1983).

Typical mother–infant or parent–offspring attachment seen in contemporary Western cultures, where attachment research is concentrated, is not necessarily the norm for the species, but rather for this particular time and place. More typical, in fact, might be the child-rearing practices in Europe from the time of imperial Rome to the Renaissance, where it has been estimated that as many as one-fourth to one-third of all children were abandoned by their parents (Boswell, 1988).

To this day, severe stress—such as the chronic and unremitting starvation experienced by the Ik, a hunter-gatherer culture in Uganda relocated to an agricultural area to which they were neither disposed nor capable of accommodating (Turnbull, 1972)—can interfere with the development of those types of parent-offspring bonds seen in most cultures during times of well-being. The Ik had been forced to give up a nomadic existence for a sedentary farming life, just at the time when a severe drought lasting several years devastated crops and produced a famine. The response of the Ik was a total breakdown of their culture. The heart of their cultural breakdown was a total abandonment of social structure, institutions, and attachments in favor of a completely egocentric survivalist orientation. Marriage, community commitment, and attachment to their children all became irrelevant. Mothers resented infants as a drain on their energy and abandoned them as quickly as possible. If an infant survived to 3 years of age, he or she was thrown out of the family compound and left to survive on his or her own, or not. Turnbull (1972) reported the case of a child who refused to be rejected, and persisted in returning to the family compound. The parents locked her inside and did not return until she died, and then discarded her body.

The treatment of the children demonstrated how the Ik's new culture (or lack thereof) systematically destroyed the natural instinct of the infants to form attachments. Upon being thrown out of their parents' homes, the children joined juvenile bands. In these bands, they experienced a series of emotional rejections—forming attachments to older children, only to be rejected and attacked by those children subsequently. By the time these children reached adolescence, they had learned the lesson well: "Do not care for anyone but yourself." The consequences of this for the very survival of the Ik was profound: At the time of writing (1972), Turnbull reported their numbers to be reduced to only 2,000, and the population was still declining because of both high mortality and low birthrate.

One may look at this tragic situation and attribute it to the incredible strain on their culture that years of famine had produced. Two things mitigate against so simple an explanation. First, Turnbull returned a couple of years later and found the drought broken and the fields full of an abundant harvest. The Ik, however, had not changed; they remained the egocentric people they had become. Presumably only their social behavior had changed, and not their genotype. The genetic capacity for development of attachment surely persisted, but it was not expressed. Second, although similar breakdowns in social bonds have been described in other severely stressful situations (such as those involving starvation in concentration camps—Bettelheim, 1943, 1960), not all peoples in all stressful situations react in this way, for reasons not yet clear. The massive starvation associated with the Irish potato famine in the middle of the 19th century found families remaining and dying together (Scheper-Hughes, 1992).

The highly selective lack of parent-infant attachment recently described by Scheper-Hughes (1992) in certain contemporary cultures in northeast Brazil that are chronically severely impoverished indicates that attachment is fluid, and may not develop in social situations wherein the survival of a particular offspring may not be in the best interest of the parent or social group. In this culture, apparently in response to the stress of severe impoverishment, certain offspring may benefit from formation of parent–offspring bonds, whereas others are left (within the family home) to die.

Attachment is of clear benefit to the organism and the social group under some conditions (generally those of adequate resources to support all individuals), but perhaps not under other conditions (severe restriction of resources, threatening the integrity of individuals). In the latter situations, it may not develop or may dissipate. Overall, however, attachment processes are critical for social integrity at multiple levels. If attachment is not developed in an individual, the consequences for that individual and his or her offspring can be devastating. If attachment does not develop within a culture, the consequences for the culture can be catastrophic.

FUTURE DIRECTIONS

In summary, we hypothesize that specific neuroanatomical structures and neurochemical systems underlie the attachment formation process in primates, both human and nonhuman. These neuroanatomical structures are not yet clearly known, but probably include the medial preoptic nucleus of the hypothalamus, the anterior temporal cortex, and frontotemporal limbic areas. These structures and systems develop in interaction with species-expected early experiences (including cognitive, emotional, and physiological stimulation in the context of maternal attachment), which facilitate their development and ultimate degree of complexity. Later in life (through childhood, adolescence, and adulthood), these neurobiological structures serve in turn to support the development of new attachments. In the absence of species-expected experience (such as appropriate socialization), or in the presence of species-atypical experiences (such as extreme stress), the development of these centers and systems is deficient, with concomitant deficiencies in the ability to form and maintain attachment in later life. Once again, the system is not "written in stone"; indeed, it is malleable and open to change, whether through positive life experiences or (in humans) appropriate therapy (Bowlby, 1988).

These hypotheses suggest that we might benefit from designing experiments to elucidate in more detail which specific neuroanatomical and neurochemical mechanisms relate to the development, expression, and maintenance of attachment behavior. How such systems develop normally, how their development is altered by species-atypical early experience, and whether such changes are permanent or reversible—these are all relevant and testable questions. The issues of neurochemical systems underlying the development of attachment, their mutability in the face of stress, and their long-term influence if altered are similarly important, and now open to research. As corollaries, we might also look to dysfunction of such regions and/or systems as possibly being related to clinical instances of aberrant attachment or social affiliative behaviors, including atypical child-rearing practices (such as abuse or neglect) and difficulties in forming or sustaining social bonds (such as may be observed in various adult psychopathologies, including sociopathic, borderline, and schizophrenic disorders).

It seems clear that not only should the underlying neurobiology be intact, but that early social experience should also be within the limits of species-expected norms as well, for these complex behaviors to develop and function normally. Their malleability—as, for example in adult monkeys and humans experiencing various degrees of privation or restriction of resources—suggests that underlying mechanisms are fluid at some level, and that environment can still substantially alter the behavioral expression of the attachment system, even in adults. It is fair to say that few areas are of greater potential importance to the successful survival of our species than a better understanding of how and why attachments do or do not form.

ACKNOWLEDGMENTS

We would like to thank the Developmental Psychobiology Research Group in the Department of Psychiatry, University of Colorado School of Medicine, for helpful discussions in this topical area, as well as for providing financial support early in the course of our research. The research described in this chapter was supported by U.S. Public Health Service Grants Nos. MH19514 and MH44131, and by National Institute of Mental Health Research Scientist Award No. MH46335 to Martin Reite.

REFERENCES

Bayart, F., Hayashi, K. T., Faull, K. F., Barchas, J. D., & Levine, S. (1990). Influence of maternal proximity on behavioral and physiological responses to separation in infant rhesus monkeys. *Behavioral Neuroscience, 104*(1), 98-107.

Bernieri, F. J., Reznick, J. S., & Rosenthal, R. (1988). Synchrony, pseudosynchrony, and dissynchrony: Measuring the entraining process in mother-infant interactions. *Journal of Personality and Social Psychology, 54,* 243-253.

Bettelheim, B. (1943). Individual and mass behavior in extreme situations. *Journal of Abnormal and Social Psychology, 38*(4), 417-452.

Bettelheim, B. (1960). *The informed heart: Autonomy in a mass age.* Glencoe, IL: Free Press.

Beutel, M. (1991). Zur psychobiologie von trauer und verlustverarbeitung und befunde. *Psychotherapie, Psychosomatik, Medizinische Psychologie, 41*(7), 267-277.

Boccia, M. L., Laudenslager, M. L., & Reite, M. L. (1988). Food distribution, dominance, and aggressive behaviors in bonnet macaques. *American Journal of Primatology, 16,* 123-130.

Boccia, M. L., Laudenslager, M. L., & Reite, M. L. (1994). Intrinsic and extrinsic factors affect infant responses to separation. *Psychiatry: Interpersonal and Biological Processes, 57,* 43-50.

Boccia, M. L., Reite, M. L., Kaemingk, K., Held, P., & Laudenslager, M. L. (1989). Behavioral and autonomic responses to peer separation in pigtail infant macaque monkey infants. *Developmental Psychobiology, 22*(5), 447-461.

Boccia, M. L., Reite, M. L., Kaemingk, K., Held, P., & Laudenslager, M. L. (1991). Social context and reaction to separation in peer-reared pigtail macaques: Some preliminary observations. *Primates, 32*(2), 255-263.

Boccia, M. L., Reite, M. L., & Laudenslager, M. L. (1991). Early social environment may alter the development of attachment and social support: Two case reports. *Infant Behavior and Development, 14,* 252-260.

Boccia, M. L., Scanlan, J. A., Broussard, C. L., Laudenslager, M. L., & Reite, M. L. (1994). *Presence of juvenile "friends" mitigates behavioral and immunological response to maternal separation in bonnet macaque infants.* Manuscript submitted for publication.

Boswell, J. (1988). *The kindness of strangers.* New York: Vintage Books.

Bowlby, J. (1988). Developmental psychiatry comes of age. *American Journal of Psychiatry, 145*(1), 1-10.

Brazelton, T. B., Koslowski, B., & Main, M. (1974). Origins of reciprocity: The early mother-infant interaction. In M. Lewis & L. Rosenblum (Eds.), *The effect of the infant on its caregiver* (pp. 49-76). New York: Wiley.

Breese, G. R., Smith, R. D., Mueller, R., Howard, J. L., Prange, A. J., Lipton, M. A., Young, L. D., McKinney, W. T., & Lewis, J. K. (1973). Induction of adrenal catecholamine synthesising enzymes following mother-infant separation. *Nature New Biology, 246*(151), 94-96.

Brown, G. W., Bifulco, A., Harris, T., & Bridge, L. (1986). Life stress, chronic subclinical symptoms and vulnerability to clinical depression. *Journal of Affective Disorders, 11,* 1-19.

Bucher, K., Myers, R. E., & Southwick, C. (1970). Anterior temporal cortex and maternal behavior in monkeys. *Neurology, 20,* 415.

Caine, N., & Reite, M. (1981). The effect of peer contact upon physiological response to maternal separation. *American Journal of Primatology, 1,* 271-276.

Caine, N., & Reite, M. (1983). Infant abuse in captive pigtailed macaques: Relevance to human child abuse. In M. Reite & N. Caine (Eds.), *Child abuse: The non-human primate data* (pp. 19-27). New York: Alan R. Liss.

Capitanio, J., Rasmussen, K. L. R., Snyder, D., Laudenslager, M., & Reite, M. (1986). Long term follow-up of previously separated pigtail macaques: Group and individual differences in response to novel situations. *Journal of Child Psychiatry and Psychology, 27*, 531-538.

Carter, C. S., Williams, J. R., Witt, D. M., & Insel, T. R. (1992). Oxytocin and social bonding. *Annals of the New York Academy of Sciences, 652*, 204-211.

Champoux, M., Coe, C. L., Schanberg, S. M., Kuhn, C. M., & Suomi, S. J. (1989). Hormonal effects of early rearing conditions in the infant rhesus monkey. *American Journal of Primatology, 19*, 111-117.

Clayton, P. (1990). Bereavement and depression. *Journal of Clinical Psychiatry, 51* (Suppl.), 34-38.

Cohen, S. (1989). Psychosocial models of the role of social support in the etiology of physical disease. *Health Psychology, 7*, 269-297.

Condon, W. S., & Sander, L. W. (1974). Synchrony demonstrated between movements of the neonate and adult speech. *Child Development, 45*, 456-462.

Cox, M., Garrick, N., Reite, M., & Gennaro, M. (1991). Minipump clorgyline administration and CSF amine metabolites in unrestrained monkeys. *Pharmacology, Biochemistry and Behavior, 38*, 677-679.

Darwin, C. (1955). *The Expression of emotion in man and animals*. New York: Philosophical Library. (Original work published 1872)

Ehlers, C. L., Frank, E., & Kupfer, D. J. (1988). Social zeitgebers and biological rhythms. *Archives of General Psychiatry, 45*, 948-952.

Ekman, P., Sorenson, F. R., & Fausen, W. V. (1969). Pan-cultural elements in facial displays of emotions. *Science, 164*, 86-88.

Field, T. (1985). Attachment as psychobiological attunement: Being on the same wavelength. In M. Reite & T. Field (Eds.), *The psychobiology of attachment and separation* (pp. 415-454). Orlando, FL: Academic Press.

Franzen, E. A., & Myers, R. E. (1973). Neural control of social behavior: Prefrontal and anterior temporal cortex. *Neuropsychologia, 11*, 141-157.

Freud, S. (1957). Mourning and melancholia. In J. Strachey (Ed. and Trans.), *The standard edition of the complete psychological works of Sigmund Freud* (Vol. 14, pp. 237-260). London: Hogarth Press. (Original work published 1917)

Gubernick, D. J. (1981). Parent and infant attachment in mammals. In D. J. Gubernick & P. H. Klopfer, (Eds.), *Parental care in mammals* (pp. 243-305). New York: Plenum Press.

He, M. (1991). A prospective controlled study of psychosomatic and immunologic change in recently bereaved people. *Chinese Journal of Neurology and Psychiatry, 24*(2), 90-93.

Hofer, M. A. (1981). Toward a developmental basis for disease predisposition: The effects of early maternal separation on brain, behavior, and cardiovascular system. In J. Weiner, M. A. Hofer, & A. J. Stunkard (Eds.), *Brain, behavior, and bodily disease* (pp. 209-228). New York: Raven Press.

Hofer, M. A. (1984). Relationships as regulators: A psychobiologic perspective on bereavement. *Psychosomatic Medicine, 46*, 183-197.

House, J. S., Landis, K. R., & Umberson, D. (1988). Social relationships and health. *Science, 241,* 540-545.

Hrdina, P., von Kulmiz, P., & Stretch, R. (1979). Pharmacological modification of experimental depression in infant macaques. *Psychopharmacology, 64,* 89-93.

Irwin, M., Hauger, R., Brown, M., & Britton, K. (1988). CRF activates autonomic nervous system and reduces natural killer cytotoxixity. *American Journal of Physiology, 255,* R744-R747.

Izard, C. E. (1971). *The face of emotion.* New York: Appleton-Century-Crofts.

Jacobs, S. C., Nelson, J. C., & Zisook, S. (1987). Treating depression and bereavement with antidepressants. *Psychiatric Clinics of North America, 10*(3), 501-510.

Jellinek, M. S., Goldenheim, P. D., & Jenike, M. A. (1985). The impact of grief on ventilatory control. *American Journal of Psychiatry, 142,* 121-122.

Kagan, J. (1982). Heart rate and heart rate variability as signs of a temperamental dimension in infants. In C. E. Izard (Ed.), *Measuring emotions in infants and children* (pp. 38-66). New York: Cambridge University Press.

Kagan, J., Reznick, J. S., Clarke, C., Snidman, N., & Garcia-Coll, C. (1984). Behavioral inhibition to the unfamiliar. *Child Development, 55,* 2212-2225.

Kalin, N. H., Shelton, S. E., & Barksdale, C. M. (1987). Separation distress in infant rhesus monkeys: Effects of diazepam and Ro 15-1788. *Brain Research, 408,* 192-198.

Kalin, N. H., Shelton, S. E., & Barksdale, C. M. (1988). Opiate modulation of separation-induced distress in non-human primates. *Brain Research, 440,* 285-291.

Kamarck, T. W., Manuck, S. B., & Jennings, J. R. (1990). Social support reduces cardiovascular reactivity to psychological challenge: A laboratory model. *Psychosomatic Medicine, 52,* 42-58.

Kaufman, I. C., & Rosenblum, L. A. (1967). Depression in infant monkeys separated from their mothers. *Science, 155,* 1030-1031.

Kendrick, K. M., & Baldwin, B. A. (1987). Cells in temporal cortex of conscious sheep can respond preferentially to the sight of faces. *Science, 236,* 448-450.

Kluver, H. (1950). Discussion of cybernetics: Circular causal and feedback mechanisms in biological and social systems. In *Transactions of the Seventh Conference of the Josiah Macy, Jr. Foundation* (pp. 226-228). New York: Josiah Macy, Jr., Foundation.

Kraemer, G. W., Ebert, M. H., Lake, R., & McKinney, W. T. (1983). Neurobiological measures in rhesus monkeys: Correlates of the behavioral response to social separation and alcohol. In *Stress and alcohol use* (pp. 171-184). Amsterdam: Elsevier.

Kraemer, G. W., Ebert, M. H., Schmidt, D. E., & McKinney, W. T. (1989). A longitudinal study of the effect of different social rearing conditions on CSF norepinephrine and biogenic amine metabolites in rhesus monkeys. *Neuropsychopharmacology, 2*(3), 175-189.

Kraemer, G. W., & McKinney, W. T. (1979). Interactions of pharmacological agents that alter biogenic amine metabolism and depression: An analysis of contributing factors within a primate model of depression. *Journal of Affective Disorders, 1,* 33-54.

Laudenslager, M. L. (1988). The psychobiology of loss: Lessons from humans and nonhuman primates. *Journal of Social Issues, 44,* 19-36.

124 Conceptual and Methodological Perspectives

Laudenslager, M. L., Boccia, M. L., Berger, C. L., & McFerran, B. (1993). Intercorrelations of behavioral, endocrine, and immune parameters associated with brief maternal separations in young macaques. *American Journal of Primatology, 30,* 326.

Laudenslager, M. L., Boccia, M. L., & Reite, M. L. (1993). Biobehavioral consequences of loss in nonhuman primates: Individual differences. In M. S. Stroebe, W. Stroebe, & R. O. Hansson (Eds.), *Bereavement* (pp. 129-142). New York: Cambridge University Press.

Laudenslager, M., Capitanio, J. P., & Reite, M. (1985). Some possible consequences of early separation experiences on subsequent immune function. *American Journal of Psychiatry, 142,* 862-864.

Laudenslager, M., Held, P. E., Boccia, M. L., Gennaro, M. M., Reite, M. L., & Cohen, J. J. (1993). *Relationship of behavior to specific antibody levels in nonhuman primates.* Unpublished manuscript.

Laudenslager, M. L., Held, P. E., Boccia, M. L., Reite, M. L., & Cohen, J. J. (1990). Behavioral and immunological consequences of brief mother-infant separation: A species comparison. *Developmental Psychobiology, 23*(3), 247-264.

Laudenslager, M. L., & Reite, M. L. (1984). Losses and separations: Immunological consequences and health implications. *Review of Personality and Social Psychology, 5,* 285-312.

Laudenslager, M., Reite, M., & Harbeck, R. (1982). Suppressed immune response in infant monkeys associated with maternal separation. *Behavioral and Neurological Biology, 36,* 40-48.

Levine, S. (1983). A psychobiological approach to the ontongeny of coping. In N. Garmezy & M. Rutter (Eds.), *Stress, coping, and development in children* (pp. 107-131). New York: McGraw-Hill.

Lindemann, E. (1944). Symptomatology and management of acute grief. *American Journal of Psychiatry, 101,* 141-148.

Lown, B. (1990). The Mikamo Lecture: Role of higher nervous activity in sudden cardiac death. *Japanese Circulation Journal, 54*(6), 581-602.

Mason, W. A., & Kenney, M. D. (1974). Redirection of filial attachments in rhesus monkeys: Dogs as mother surrogates. *Science, 183,* 1209-1211.

McKenna, J. J., Mosko, S., Dungy, C., & McAninch, J. (1990). Sleep and arousal patterns of co-sleeping human mother/infant pairs: A preliminary physiological study with implications for the study of sudden infant death syndrome (SIDS). *American Journal of Physical Anthropology, 83,* 331-347.

McKinney, W. T. (1986). Primate separation studies: Relevance to bereavement. *Psychiatric Annals, 16,* 281-287.

Moore-Ede, M. C., Sulzman, F. M., & Fuller, C. A. (1982). *The clocks that time us.* Cambridge, MA: Harvard University Press.

Murphy, D. L., Lipper, S., Pickar, D., Jimerson, D., Cohen, R. M., Garrick, N. A., Alterman, S., & Campbell, I. C. (1981). Selective inhibition of monoamine oxidase type A: Clinical antidepressant effects and metabolic changes in man. In M. B. H. Youdim & E. S. Paykel (Eds.), *Monoamine oxidase inhibitors: The state of the art* (pp. 189-205). New York: Wiley.

Myers, R. E., Swett, C., & Miller, M. (1973). Loss of social group affinity following prefrontal lesions in free-ranging macaques. *Brain Research, 64,* 257-269.

Numan, M. (1988). Maternal behavior. In E. Knobil & J. Neill (Eds.), *The physiology of reproduction* (pp. 1569-1645). New York: Raven Press.

Pasternak, R. E., Reynolds, C. F., Schlernitzauer, M., Hoch, C. C., Buysse, D. J., Houck, P. R., & Perel, J. M. (1991). Acute open-trial nortriptyline therapy of bereavement-related depression in late life. *Journal of Clinical Psychiatry, 52,* 307-310.

Pauley, J. D., & Reite, M. L. (1981). A microminiature hybrid multichannel implantable biotelemetry system. *Biotelemetry and Patient Monitoring, 8,* 163-172.

Paykel, E. S. (1983). Recent life events and depression. In J. Angst (Ed.), *The origin of depression: Current concepts and approaches* (pp. 91-106). Berlin: Springer-Verlag.

Pechtel, C., McAvoy, T., Levitt, M., Kling, A., & Masserman, J. H. (1958). The cingulate and behavior. *Journal of Nervous and Mental Disease, 126,* 148-152.

Perrett, D. I., Mistlin, A. J., Chitty, A. J., Smith, P. A. J., Potter, D. D., Broennimann, R., & Harries, M. (1988). Specialized face processing and hemispheric asymmetry in man and monkey: Evidence from single unit and reaction time studies. *Behavioral Brain Research, 29,* 245-258.

Phifer, J. F., & Murrell, S. A. (1986). Etiological factors in the onset of depressive symptoms in older adults. *Journal of Abnormal Psychology, 95*(3), 282-291.

Reichborn-Kjennerud, T. (1990). Tap, depresjon og immunitat. *Tidsskr Nor Laegeforen, 110*(15), 1965-1967.

Reite, M. (1985). Implantable biotelemetry and social separation in monkeys. In G. Moberg (Ed.), *Animal stress* (pp. 141-160). Bethesda, MD: American Physiological Society.

Reite, M., & Capitanio, J. (1985). On the nature of social separation and social attachment. In M. Reite & T. Field (Eds.), *The psychobiology of attachment and separation* (pp. 223-255). Orlando, FL: Academic Press.

Reite, M. L., Cox, M., Laudenslager, M. L., Garrick, N., & Boccia, M. L. (1991). Effects of monoamine oxidase-A inhibitor on maternal separation in pigtail monkey infants (*Macaca nemestrina*). *American Journal of Primatology, 24,* 130.

Reite, M., Harbeck, R., & Hoffman, S. (1981). Altered cellular immune response following maternal separation. *Life Sciences, 28,* 1133-1136.

Reite, M., & Kaemingk, K. (1987). Social environment and nocturnal sleep: Studies in peer reared monkeys. *Sleep, 10,* 542-550.

Reite, M. L., Kaemingk, K., & Boccia, M. L. (1984). *Behavior of peer-reared pigtail macaque infants.* Unpublished data.

Reite, M., Kaemingk, K., & Boccia, M. (1989). Maternal separation in bonnet monkey infants: Altered attachment and social support. *Child Development, 60,* 473-480.

Reite, M., Laudenslager, M., Garrick, N., Boccia, M., & Cox, M. (1991). Clorgyline effects on maternal separation in pigtail (*M. nemestrina*) monkey infants. *Psychosomatic Medicine, 53,* 233-234.

Reite, M., Seiler, C., Crowley, T. J., Hydinger-MacDonald, M., & Short, R. (1982). Circadian rhythm changes following maternal separation in monkeys. *Chronobiologica, 9,* 1-11.

Reite, M., Seiler, C., & Short, R. (1978). Loss of your mother is more than loss of a mother. *American Journal of Psychiatry, 135,* 370-371.

Reite, M. L., & Short, R. (1977). Nocturnal sleep in isolation-reared monkeys: Evidence for environmental independence. *Developmental Psychobiology, 10*(6), 555-561.

Reite, M., & Short, R. (1978). Nocturnal sleep in separated monkey infants. *Archives of General Psychiatry, 35,* 1247-1253.

Reite, M. L., Short, R., & Seiler, C. (1978). Physiological correlates of maternal separation in surrogate-reared infants: A study in altered attachment bonds. *Developmental Psychobiology, 11*(5), 427-435.

Reite, M. L., & Snyder, D. S. (1982). Physiology of maternal separation in a bonnet macaque infant. *American Journal of Primatology, 2,* 115-120.

Reynolds, C. F., Hoch, C. C., Buysse, D. J., Houck, P. R., Schlernitzauer, M., Frank, E., Mazumdar, S., & Kupfer, D. (1992). Electroencephalographic sleep in spousal bereavement and bereavement-related depression in late life. *Biological Psychiatry, 31*(1), 69-82.

Rosenberg, A. A., & Kagan, J. (1989). Physical and physiological correlates of behavioral inhibition. *Developmental Psychobiology, 22*(8), 753-770.

Rosenblum, L. A. (1987). Influences of environmental demand on maternal behavior and infant development. In N. A. Krasnegor (Ed.), *Perinatal development: A psychobiological perspective* (pp. 377-393). New York: Academic Press.

Roy, A., Gallucci, W., Avgerinos, P., Linnoila, M., & Gold, P. (1988). The CRH stimulation test in bereaved subjects with and without accompanying depression. *Psychiatry Research, 25*(2), 145-156.

Rubin, B. S., & Bridges, R. S. (1984). Disruption of ongoing maternal reponsiveness in rats by central administration of morphine sulfate. *Brain Research, 307,* 91-97.

Sander, L., Stechler, G., Burns, P., & Julia, H. (1970). Early mother-infant interaction and 24-hour patterns of activity and sleep. *Journal of the American Academy of Child Psychiatry, 9,* 103-123.

Scanlan, J. M., Coe, C. L., Latts, A., & Suomi, S. J. (1987). Effects of age, rearing, and separation stress on immunoglobulin levels in rhesus monkeys. *American Journal of Primatology, 13,* 11-22.

Scheper-Hughes, N. (1992). *Death without weeping: The violence of everyday life in Brazil.* Berkeley: University of California Press.

Seay, B., & Harlow, H. F. (1965). Maternal separation in the rhesus monkey. *Journal of Nervous and Mental Disease, 140*(6), 434-441.

Seiler, C., Cullen, J. S., Zimmerman, J., & Reite, M. L. (1979). Cardiac arrhythmias in infant pigtail monkeys following maternal separation. *Psychophysiology, 16*(2), 130-135.

Siegel, S. J., Ginsberg, S. D., Hof, P. R., Foote, S. L., Young, W. G., Kraemer, G. W., McKinney, W. T., & Morrison, J. H. (1993). Effects of social deprivation in prepubescent rhesus monkeys: Immunohistochemical analysis of the neurofilament protein triplet in the hippocampal formation. *Brain Research, 619,* 299-305.

Siever, L. J., & Davis, K. L. (1985). Overview: Toward a dysregulation hypothesis of depression. *American Journal of Psychiatry, 142,* 1017-1031.

Steklis, H., & Kling, A. (1985). Neurobiology of affiliative behavior in nonhuman primates. In M. Reite & T. Field (Eds.), *The psychobiology of attachment and separation* (pp. 93-161). Orlando, FL: Academic Press.

Suomi, S., Seaman, S. F., Lewis, J. K., DeLizio, R. D., & McKinney, W. T. (1978). Effects of imipramine treatment of separation-induced social disorders in rhesus monkeys. *Archives of General Psychiatry, 35,* 321-325.

Thomas, P. D., Goodwin, J. M., & Goodwin, J. S. (1985). Effect of social support on stress-related changes in cholesterol level, uric acid level, and immune function in an elderly sample. *American Journal of Psychiatry, 142*(6), 735-737.

Tronick, E. Z., Ricks, M., & Cohn, J. F. (1982). Maternal and infant affective exchange: Patterns of adaptation. In T. Field & A. Fogel (Eds.), *Emotion and early interaction* (pp. 83-100). Hillsdale, NJ: Erlbaum.

Turnbull, C. M. (1972). *The mountain people.* New York: Simon & Schuster.

Wehr, T. A., & Goodwin, F. K. (1983). Biological rhythms in manic-depressive illness. In T. A. Wehr & F. K. Goodwin (Eds.), *Circadian rhythms in psychiatry* (pp. 129-184). Pacific Grove, CA: Boxwood Press.

Weiner, S. G., Bayart, F., Faull, K. F., & Levine, S. (1990). Behavioral and physiological responses to maternal separation in squirrel monkeys (Saimiri sciureus). *Behavioral Neuroscience, 104*(1), 108-115.

Witt, D. M., & Insel, T. R. (1991). A selective oxytocin antagonist attenuates progesterone facilitation of female sexual behavior. *Endocrinology, 128*(6), 3269-3276.

Witt, D. M., Winslow, J. T., & Insel, T. R. (1992). Enhanced social interactions in rats following chronic centrally infused oxytocin. *Pharmacology, Biochemistry and Behavior, 43*(3), 855-861.

CHAPTER 5

Assessing Adult Attachment

JUDITH A. FEENEY

PATRICIA NOLLER

MARY HANRAHAN

During the last decade, the concept of attachment has been applied by several groups of researchers to the study of adults' intimate relationships. Approaches to the measurement of adult attachment reveal a diversity of content and assumptions, however. The Interview Schedule for Social Interaction (Henderson, Byrne, & Duncan-Jones, 1981), for example, assesses the availability and perceived adequacy both of attachment (support from intimates) and of "social integration" (support from the wider social network), using a highly structured format that focuses on current patterns of social interaction. The Adult Attachment Interview (George, Kaplan, & Main, 1984), on the other hand, was designed to tap memories of childhood relationships with parents, together with assessment of the influence of these early relationships on adult personality. Administration and scoring of this instrument require in-depth training—a factor that clearly limits its accessibility.

Recognizing the desirability of deriving simpler and more economical forms of assessment of adult attachment, researchers have developed a number of self-report questionnaires in recent years. Like the interviews designed to assess attachment variables, however, these measures are diverse in terms of theoretical focus and item content. West and Sheldon have devised a questionnaire measuring key features of adult attachment, based on concepts of attachment theory (e.g., proximity seeking, separation protest; West, Sheldon, & Reiffer, 1987), as well as scales that focus exclusively on pathological patterns of adult attachment (West & Sheldon, 1988). Parker and his colleagues have developed two instruments designed to assess the quality of close relationships. The Parental Bonding Instrument (Parker, Tupling, & Brown, 1979) assesses subjects' retrospective memories of their parents in terms of two major dimensions of parenting: care and control. The Intimate Bonds Measure (Wilhelm & Parker, 1988) assesses the extent to which the dimensions of care and control characterize the behavior and perceived attitudes of an intimate (adult) relationship partner.

Yet another approach to the conceptualization of adult attachment is evident in the forced-choice measure developed by Hazan and Shaver (1987), which is based on the assumption that parallels of the major infant-caregiver attachment styles identified by Ainsworth and her colleagues ("secure," "avoidant," and "anxious/ambivalent"; see Ainsworth, Blehar, Waters, & Wall, 1978) can be found among adult lovers. The measure consists of a single item that presents simple descriptions of the three adult attachment styles, based on extrapolation from the features of the corresponding infant styles. Each description contains a number of themes, and subjects are required to select the description most applicable to their feelings about close relationships generally (see Table 5.1).

As this brief review suggests, the variety of attachment measures employed by researchers and clinicians has mitigated against the development of a cohesive body of empirical findings. The available instruments differ in their fundamental approach to attachment issues. The Adult Attachment Interview, for example, focuses on attachment bonds within the family of origin; the Intimate Bonds Measure focuses on subjects' perceptions of the behavior and attitudes of their relationship partners, rather than the subjects' own needs; the forced-choice measure of Hazan and Shaver adopts a "style"- or "type"-based approach, attempting to identify romantic relationship styles that parallel the major attachment styles discussed in the infant literature. Because of the intense interest generated

TABLE 5.1. Hazan and Shaver's (1987) Descriptions of the Three Attachment Styles

Style	Description
Secure	I find it relatively easy to get close to others and am comfortable depending on them and having them depend on me. I don't often worry about being abandoned or about someone getting too close to me.
Avoidant	I am somewhat uncomfortable being close to others; I find it difficult to trust them completely, difficult to allow myself to depend on them. I am nervous when anyone gets too close, and often, love partners want me to be more intimate than I feel comfortable being.
Anxious/ambivalent	I find that others are reluctant to get as close as I would like. I often worry that my partner doesn't really love me or won't want to stay with me. I want to merge completely with another person, and this desire sometimes scares people away.

by the work of Hazan and Shaver (1987), and because the present work is one of a number of attempts to overcome the limitations of their forced-choice measure, we briefly outline the directions that researchers have subsequently taken in conceptualizing and measuring adult attachment styles.

DEVELOPMENTS BASED ON THE WORK
OF HAZAN AND SHAVER

Despite the success of the initial studies in relating the forced-choice measure of attachment style to remembered relationships with parents, beliefs about romantic love, patterns of feelings in love relationships, and vulnerability to loneliness (Hazan & Shaver, 1987), researchers (including Hazan & Shaver themselves) have been quick to point out the limitations of the forced-choice measure. In particular, the measure is likely to possess limited reliability, especially in view of the forced-choice format and the number of themes addressed in each description. It should be noted that Hazan and Shaver have made several minor revisions to the content of the forced-choice measure, in order to improve its psychometric properties.

Subsequent developments in the measurement of adult attachment style have taken one of three major forms. First, some researchers have retained (intact) the three component descriptions of the forced-choice item, while requiring subjects to rate the applicability of each description using a Likert-type format. This approach overcomes the problem of assuming that the three attachment styles are mutually exclusive, and that subjects can readily classify themselves into one of the three styles. Empirical data based on this approach (e.g., Feeney, 1991; Levy & Davis, 1988) suggest that such an assumption is, in fact, unfounded: Ratings of secure attachment show a strong negative correlation with avoidant attachment and a weak negative correlation with anxious/ambivalent attachment, whereas ratings of avoidant and anxious/ambivalent attachment are virtually uncorrelated (hence, subjects can be high on both avoidant and anxious/ambivalent attachment).

Second, researchers have presented measures composed of more fine-grained items, usually based on the individual statements of the original forced-choice measure. Such an approach not only moves beyond forced-choice classification, but also allows an assessment of the dimensions underlying attachment items, and hence the development of empirically derived scales. The structure underlying the items remains a subject of controversy, however; although we and other researchers have reported a two-dimensional structure, defined by "comfort with closeness" and "anxiety" (Feeney, Noller, & Callan, 1994; Simpson, 1990; Strahan, 1991), others have advocated a three-dimensional structure (e.g., see Collins &

Read, 1990). Difficulty in obtaining agreement on the appropriate number of dimensions stems in part from minor variations in the item pool across studies, with some researchers adding items designed to represent themes not addressed explicitly in the original measure.

Third, and in parallel with the two developments outlined above, important conceptual issues have emerged concerning the number of attachment styles required to explain adult attachment behavior. Bartholomew (1990; Bartholomew & Horowitz, 1991) has argued on theoretical grounds that attachment styles are defined by two underlying dimensions: models of the self (positive-negative) and models of others (positive-negative). These dimensions define four possible attachment styles: "secure" (positive models of self and others); "preoccupied" (cf. anxious/ambivalent; negative models of self and positive models of others); and two "avoidant" styles—"dismissing" (positive models of self and negative models of others) and "fearful" (negative models of both self and others) (see Table 5.2). Bartholomew has developed self-report prototypes of the four attachment styles, similar in format to the attachment descriptions of Hazan and Shaver's forced-choice measure; these prototypes are pre-

TABLE 5.2. **Bartholomew's Four-Group Model of Attachment**

Model of other (avoidance)	Model of self (dependence)	
	Positive (low)	Negative (high)
Positive (low)	*Secure* It is relatively easy for me to become emotionally close to others. I am comfortable depending on others and having others depend on me. I don't worry about being alone or having others not accept me.	*Preoccupied* I want to be completely emotionally intimate with others, but I often find that others are reluctant to get as close as I would like. I am uncomfortable being without close relationships, but I sometimes worry that others don't value me as much as I value them.
Negative (high)	*Dismissing* I am comfortable without close emotional relationships. It is very important to me to feel independent and self-sufficient, and I prefer not to depend on others or have others depend on me.	*Fearful* I am somewhat uncomfortable getting close to others. I want emotionally close relationships but I find it difficult to trust others completely, or to depend on them. I sometimes worry that I will be hurt if I allow myself to become too close to others.

sented in Table 5.2. (Bartholomew has also developed interview schedules that yield ratings on each of the four prototypes.) A comprehensive data set based on these measures has been presented (Bartholomew & Horowitz, 1991), but it must be recognized that the obtained results hinge closely on the wording of the four prototype statements. Strong negative correlations are reported, for example, between attachment ratings in "opposing" positions of the model (i.e., between secure and fearful attachment, and between dismissing and preoccupied attachment)—a pattern that is interpreted as supporting the model. The wording of the prototypes almost ensures such a result, however, since prototypes in opposing positions contain (by definition) contrary themes.

The controversy surrounding the number of attachment styles and the use of categorical versus continuous measures has continued to hamper attempts to integrate findings on adult attachment. Moreover, one feature of all of the "style"-based measures (including the original forced-choice measure) limits their applicability: Specifically, these instruments depend on subjects' being in an intimate relationship, or at least having had significant experience of such a relationship (as indeed do all available questionnaire measures of adult attachment). This focus effectively precludes the study of individuals who do not regard themselves as having experienced adult attachment relationships; however, such individuals may be of considerable theoretical interest to attachment researchers, and the personal and relationship concerns of these individuals (independent of actual relationship involvement) should be amenable to investigation. For example, there may be many older avoidant individuals whose mental models of others are so negative that they have had little involvement in close relationships.

Moreover, although the three-style model of Hazan and Shaver has stimulated considerable research, and although clear differences have been found among the three groups defined by their measure, there has been little attempt to ensure that these styles are the ones most logically derived from empirical data. Although we (Feeney & Noller, 1991) found that the forced-choice attachment measure was related in theoretically expected ways to individuals' open-ended descriptions of their relationships, this work was designed to assess the existing model, rather than to address questions about such basic issues as the number of attachment styles.

DEVELOPMENT OF THE
ATTACHMENT STYLE QUESTIONNAIRE

We had three interrelated goals in setting up a new measure of attachment style: (1) to develop a broad-based measure that could be used to clarify issues concerning the dimensions central to adult attachment and the number of styles needed to define essential individual differences; (2) to design a measure suitable for young adolescents; and (3) to design a measure suitable for those with little or no experience of romantic relationships. Sixty-five items were developed, based on the constructs presented in Table 5.3. These constructs cover the major features described in both three- and four-group models of adult attachment, together with the basic themes of infant attachment theory. Although some items came from the forced-choice measure of attachment or from earlier measures of self-esteem, most were written especially for this measure. Items were rated on a 6-point scale from 1 = "totally disagree" to 6 = "totally agree."

The 65 items were administered to 470 young adults, who were all university students. Of these, 175 were second-year students who completed the measure as part of a class exercise; the other 295 were introductory students who participated in the study for course credit. In order to reduce the item set, a principal-components analysis was performed, and items with low communalities were removed. Principal-components analysis was then performed on the reduced item set, with orthogonal rotation. Initially, on the basis of an examination of eigenvalues and the scree plot, three-, four-, and five-factor solutions were examined. On the criterion of interpretability, only the three- and five-factor solutions are presented here.

TABLE 5.3. **Constructs Used in the Development of the Attachment Style Questionnaire**

	Positive view of self	Negative view of self
Positive view of other	Self-esteem Comfort with closeness Trust Healthy dependence	Overdependence Interpersonal anxiety Aloneness Desire for approval Lack of confidence Preoccupation with relationships
Negative view of other	Avoidance of intimacy Lack of trust Value on independence Compulsive self-reliance Emphasis on achievement	Low self-esteem Lack of trust Interpersonal anxiety Desire for contact and intimacy Need for approval Aloneness Anger/hostility

Three-Factor Solution

The three-factor solution accounted for 35.7% of the total variance, and yielded factors that could be labeled Security, Avoidance, and Anxiety. See Table 5.4 for sample items. These results indicate that the three constructs central to Hazan and Shaver's (1987) conceptualization of adult attachment are clearly present in this measure.

Five-Factor Solution

The five-factor solution accounted for 43.3% of the total variance, and yielded the factors of Confidence (in self and others), Discomfort with Closeness, Need for Approval, Preoccupation with Relationships, and Relationships as Secondary (to achievement). See Table 5.5 for sample items.

Although Confidence is clearly a factor representing secure attachment, each of the other four scales represents a particular aspect of insecure attachment. Discomfort with Closeness is central to Hazan and Shaver's (1987) conceptualization of avoidant attachment. According to Bartholomew's model (Bartholomew & Horowitz, 1991), Need for Approval characterizes both the fearful and preoccupied groups, and reflects individuals' need for others' acceptance and confirmation. Preoccupation with Relationships, which involves an anxious reaching out to others in order to fulfill dependency needs, is central to the original conceptualization of anxious/ambivalent attachment (Hazan & Shaver, 1987) and to Bartholomew's description of the preoccupied group. The Rela-

TABLE 5.4. Sample Items from Three-Factor Solution

Factor	Item
Security	I find it relatively easy to get close to other people. I find it easy to trust others. I feel confident about relating to others.
Avoidance	Achieving things is more important than building relationships. I am too busy with other activities to put much time into relationships. I worry about people getting too close.
Anxiety	I worry that I won't measure up to other people. I worry a lot about my relationships. Sometimes I think I am no good at all.

TABLE 5.5. Sample Items from Five-Factor Solution

Factor	Item
Confidence	I am confident that other people will like and respect me. I find it relatively easy to get close to other people. I feel confident that other people will be there for me when I need them.
Discomfort with Closeness	I find it difficult to depend on others. I find it hard to trust other people. While I want to get close to others, I feel uneasy about it.
Need for Approval	It's important to me to avoid doing things that others won't like. I worry that I won't measure up to other people. It's important to me that others like me.
Preoccupation with Relationships	I worry a lot about my relationships. I wonder how I would cope without someone to love me. I worry that others won't care about me as much as I care about them.
Relationships as Secondary	Achieving things is more important than building relationships. Doing your best is more important than getting on with others. I am too busy with other activities to put much time into relationships.

tionships as Secondary factor is consistent with Bartholomew's (1990) concept of the dismissing style, in which individuals are seen as protecting themselves against hurt and vulnerability by emphasizing achievement and independence.

In terms of the dimensions underlying Bartholomew's model (positive and negative attitudes to self and others), the item content represented on the Preoccupation with Relationships and Need for Approval scales pertains primarily to attitudes to the self, whereas the Discomfort with Closeness and Relationships as Secondary scales primarily assess attitudes to others. The Confidence scale, on the other hand, assesses attitudes to both self and others.

Relationship between the Three- and Five-Factor Solutions

The five-factor solution involves two factors that were previously part of Anxiety, and two factors that were previously part of Avoidance, plus the Confidence factor. Specifically, Anxiety breaks up into Need for Approval and Preoccupation with Relationships; similarly, Avoidance tends to break up into Discomfort with Closeness and Relationships as Secondary. It should be noted, however, that in the five-factor solution the items pertaining to trust load on the Discomfort with Closeness factor, and the Confidence factor does not deal directly with issues of trust and comfort. After we removed items that were factorially complex and retained items loading above .40, 40 items remained. There were 8 items on the Confidence scale, 10 items on the Discomfort with Closeness scale, 7 items on the Need for Approval scale, 8 items on the Preoccupation with Relationships scale, and 7 on the Relationships as Secondary scale. The resulting 40-item measure is presented in Appendix 5.1; this measure is referred to as the Attachment Style Questionnaire.[1]

RELIABILITY

Two types of reliability data were collected on this 40-item measure: internal consistency, as measured by Cronbach's alpha, and test–retest reliability coefficients. Coefficient alphas for the three factors (Security, Avoidance, and Anxiety) were .83, .83, and .85, respectively. For the factors of Confidence (in self and others), Discomfort with Closeness, Need for Approval, Preoccupation with Relationships, and Relationships as Secondary (to achievement), coefficient alphas were .80, .84, .79, .76, and .76, respectively. These coefficients were calculated on the full sample of 470 subjects, and suggest that the scales have high levels of internal consistency.

Test–retest reliability was calculated on the basis of data collected from the subsample of 295 introductory psychology students. Reliability coefficients for the three scales over a period of approximately 10 weeks were .74 (Security), .75 (Avoidance), and .80 (Anxiety); coefficients for the five scales were .74 (both Confidence and Discomfort with Closeness), .78 (Need for Approval), .72 (Preoccupation with Relationships), and .67 (Relationships as Secondary). These coefficients represent acceptable levels of stability.

VALIDITY

The analyses described in this section are based on data from the 295 introductory psychology students, since the remaining subjects were not asked to complete the original forced-choice attachment measure (Hazan & Shaver, 1987) or to provide Likert ratings of the three descriptions contained in that item.

Correlations between Attachment Scales

Three Attachment Scales

All pairwise correlations between the three scales of the Attachment Style Questionnaire were significant: Security correlated negatively with Avoidance ($r = -.49$) and with Anxiety ($r = -.29$); in addition, Avoidance correlated positively with Anxiety ($r = .35$). It is important to note that these correlations are somewhat different from those obtained from the present sample using the three Likert ratings based on the original forced-choice measure: Secure attachment correlated with avoidant ($r = -.38$) and with anxious/ambivalent ($r = -.24$) attachment; on the other hand, anxious/ambivalent and avoidant attachment were not correlated. These latter correlations are consistent with previous research using the Likert ratings, and hence the correlation between the Avoidance and Anxiety factors in the present analysis appears to reflect characteristics of our new measure, rather than any unusual characteristics of this sample.

We also correlated scales derived from our new measure with the three Likert ratings based on the original forced-choice measure of attachment. Each of the three Likert ratings was moderately to highly correlated with the corresponding scale derived from the new measure (see Table 5.6). These results suggest that the new scales are tapping constructs similar to those assessed by the measure developed by Hazan and Shaver (1987).

Five Attachment Scales

All pairwise correlations between the five scales of the Attachment Style Questionnaire were again significant: Confidence correlated negatively with the other four scales (though most strongly with Discomfort with

TABLE 5.6. Correlations between Likert Ratings and Scales of the Attachment Style Questionnaire

Scales	Secure	Avoidant	Anxious/ambivalent
Security	.43	-.25	-.20
Avoidance	-.43	.44	.16
Anxiety	-.24	.04	.57
Confidence	.34	-.14	-.29
Discomfort with Closeness	-.50	.46	.18
Need for Approval	-.17	.13	.40
Preoccupation	-.24	-.06	.60
Relationships as Secondary	-.24	.27	.06

Closeness); all four scales measuring aspects of insecurity were positively intercorrelated (although the two factors reflecting Anxiety and the two factors reflecting Avoidance were more highly intercorrelated than any other pair of factors). See Table 5.7 for intercorrelations among the five scales.

Again, we correlated the five new attachment scales with the Likert ratings derived from Hazan and Shaver's forced-choice measure. The Likert rating of secure attachment was positively correlated with Confidence, and negatively correlated with the four scales measuring aspects of insecurity. The Likert rating of avoidant attachment was strongly correlated with Discomfort with Closeness, and moderately correlated with Relationships as Secondary. The Likert rating of anxious/ambivalent attachment was strongly correlated with Preoccupation with Relationships and Need for Approval (see Table 5.6 for more detail). Again, these correlations support the validity of the new scales in assessing the constructs proposed by Hazan and Shaver (1987).

Relationship between the Attachment Scales and the Forced-Choice Measure

As a further validity check, we carried out analyses of variance, using as the independent variable the original forced-choice measure of attachment. In other words, subjects were divided into secure, avoidant, and anxious/ambivalent groups, and were compared on both three and five factors of the Attachment Style Questionnaire.

Three Factors

On the Security factor, secure subjects scored significantly higher than either of the other groups, $F (2, 292) = 32.69$, $p < .0001$ (see Table 5.8

TABLE 5.7. **Intercorrelations among the Five Attachment Scales**

Scale	Discomfort with Closeness	Need for Approval	Preoccupation with Relationships	Relationships as Secondary
Confidence	–.52	–.39	–.33	–.18
Discomfort with Closeness		.31	.31	.44
Need for Approval			.57	.16
Preoccupation with Relationships				.17

for group means). On the Anxiety factor, anxious/ambivalent subjects scored higher than either of the other two groups, $F(2, 292) = 33.87$, $p < .0001$. On the Avoidance factor, however, the secure group had significantly lower scores than either of the other groups, $F(2, 292) = 28.24$, $p < .0001$, with no significant difference between the scores of the avoidant and anxious/ambivalent subjects on this measure. These findings underline the ambivalence about relationships of the anxious/ambivalent group.

Five Factors

On the Confidence scale, secure subjects scored significantly higher than either of the other groups, $F(2, 292) = 23.10$, $p < .0001$ (again, see Table 5.8 for group means). For Discomfort with Closeness, the secure group scored significantly lower than either of the other groups, $F(2, 292) = 49.37$, $p < .0001$, a result consistent with the finding for the Avoidance scale from the three-factor solution. Anxious/ambivalent subjects scored significantly higher than either of the other two groups on the Preoccupation with Relationships scale, $F(2, 292) = 41.22$, $p < .0001$, and on the Need for Approval scale, $F(2, 292) = 15.40$, $p < .0001$. For Relationships as Secondary, avoidant subjects scored significantly higher than secure ones, $F(2, 292) = 8.11$, $p < .001$.

For both the three- and five-factor scales, these results provide strong support that the new questionnaire measures attachment styles similar to those originally conceptualized by Hazan and Shaver (1987), although

TABLE 5.8. Means of Attachment Groups (Defined by the Forced-Choice Measure) on Three and Five Scales from the Attachment Style Questionnaire

Scale	Secure	Avoidant	Anxious/ ambivalent
Security	56.00[a]	49.23[b]	50.17[b]
Avoidance	37.25[b]	46.15[a]	43.33[a]
Anxiety	43.08[b]	45.48[b]	54.83[a]
Confidence	36.40[a]	32.81[b]	31.71[b]
Discomfort with Closeness	29.17[b]	37.98[a]	35.56[a]
Need for Approval	21.68[b]	23.35[b]	26.38[a]
Preoccupation with Relationships	26.52[b]	26.78[b]	33.44[a]
Relationships as Secondary	14.84[b]	17.61[a]	16.12[ab]

Note. Scores on Security can range from 12 to 72, Avoidance from 15 to 90, and Anxiety from 14 to 84. Scores on Confidence can range from 8 to 48, Discomfort with Closeness from 10 to 60, Need for Approval from 7 to 42, Preoccupation with Relationships from 8 to 48, and Relationships as Secondary from 7 to 42. Scores with different superscripts are significantly different.

they raise issues about the conceptualization of the insecure attachment styles in particular. With regard to the five scales, the secure subjects, as categorized by the original forced-choice measure, were higher in Confidence and lower in Discomfort with Closeness than either of the other groups. The anxious/ambivalent subjects were higher on Need for Approval and Preoccupation with Relationships than both other groups. The avoidant group scored higher than the secure group on Relationships as Secondary. Whereas the avoidant subjects were higher than the secure ones on Discomfort, they were no higher than the anxious/ambivalent subjects.

An important issue to consider is thus the differentiation of the two insecure groups. Although the anxious/ambivalent group obtained higher scores than the avoidant group on Preoccupation with Relationships and Need for Approval, as would be expected, both insecure groups reported similar levels of Discomfort with Closeness and Confidence, and were equally likely to see Relationships as Secondary. In other words, avoidant subjects were different from the anxious/ambivalent subjects only on the two scales related to Anxiety, but not on the two scales normally associated with Avoidance. As we have already noted, part of the problem with the conceptualization of anxious/ambivalent attachment is the fact that the key feature of this attachment style appears to be an ambivalent attitude to relationships, rather than the desire for extreme closeness, which has sometimes been seen as the defining characteristic. This issue is discussed further later in this chapter. It is also important to note in discussion of this measure that this sample of normal individuals did not obtain scores at the top of the range on the insecure scales. Such a finding suggests that the measure should be appropriate for a clinical sample with very high levels of insecurity.

CLUSTER ANALYSIS

We were interested in determining whether distinct clusters of individuals could be identified using the scales of the Attachment Style Questionnaire, and if so, whether the patterns of scores defining the clusters would be consistent with theoretical conceptualizations of adult attachment. For this reason, cluster analysis using Ward's method and squared Euclidian distance was carried out; the scores on the five attachment scales were used as the clustering variables. In order to assess the replicability of the results, we divided the sample randomly into two groups of equal size (n = 235). Although examination of the amalgamation coefficients supported a four-cluster solution, we also considered the possibility of two-

and three-cluster solutions. For each subsample, the two-cluster solution clearly identified a secure group and an insecure group; the secure group obtained higher scores than the insecure group on Confidence, and lower scores on all other scales. It is important to note that for each sample, the secure group remained stable across all solutions, whereas the insecure group was progressively broken down into finer categorizations. Hence, in terms of the attachment scales, the most fundamental and robust distinction is between secure and insecure.

The three-cluster solution for each sample involved subdividing the insecure group from the two-cluster solution to form a preoccupied group and a fearful group. In the four-cluster solution, a dismissing group was formed (in sample 1, this group resulted from the splitting of the fearful group; in sample 2, it resulted from the splitting of the preoccupied group). The final four groups were quite similar across both samples (see Table 5.9 for group means). Members of the secure group were very high in Confidence, and low on all the other factors (Preoccupation with Relationships, Need for Approval, Discomfort with Closeness, and Relationships as Secondary). In other words, the subjects in the secure group had high self-esteem and were confident about their relationships with other people; they were comfortable with closeness and saw relationships as important, without obsessing about them. Members of the fearful group were very low in Confidence, but high on all other factors. That is, these individuals lacked confidence in themselves and others, were uncomfortable with being close to others, and worried a lot about their relationships and

TABLE 5.9. Means of the Four Clusters on the Five Scales of the Attachment Style Questionnaire

Scale	Sample	Secure	Preoccupied	Dismissing	Fearful
Confidence	Sample 1	39.07[a]	32.29[b]	33.41[b]	26.13[c]
	Sample 2	38.27[a]	30.28[c]	34.03[b]	27.81[d]
Discomfort with Closeness	Sample 1	28.57[d]	31.21[c]	40.14[b]	43.53[a]
	Sample 2	26.70[c]	34.19[b]	36.95[b]	45.62[a]
Need for Approval	Sample 1	18.64[c]	26.50[a,b]	24.00[b]	29.27[a]
	Sample 2	19.02[c]	28.21[a]	23.44[b]	28.08[a]
Preoccupation with Relationships	Sample 1	24.33[c]	30.92[b]	29.34[b]	34.83[a]
	Sample 2	24.16[c]	34.05[a]	27.83[b]	32.23[a]
Relationships as Secondary	Sample 1	14.26[b]	15.77[b]	18.76[a]	18.83[a]
	Sample 2	12.99[c]	14.41[c]	18.10[b]	24.54[a]

Note. See Table 5.8 footnote for score ranges. Scores with different superscripts are significantly different.

whether other people approved of them. The members of the dismissing group were high on Relationships as Secondary; moderately high in Discomfort with Closeness, and moderate in Confidence, Preoccupation with Relationships and Need for Approval. These individuals emphasized achievement to the exclusion of relationships; they were reasonably confident in themselves, but uncomfortable with being close to others and somewhat concerned about the approval of others. The subjects in the preoccupied group were high on Preoccupation with Relationships and Need for Approval, moderate on Discomfort with Closeness, low to moderate in Confidence, and low in Relationships as Secondary. That is, they worried a lot about their relationships and whether others approved of them, and they emphasized the importance of relationships; they tended to be uncomfortable with closeness, however, and to lack confidence in themselves and in others.

In terms of Bartholomew's (1990) model, these results tend to provide strong support for the existence of four rather than three groups, especially given that the three groups obtained from the three-cluster solution did not represent the three discrete styles postulated by Hazan and Shaver. The clusters derived also provide considerable support for the actual groups hypothesized in Bartholomew's model. The profile of the secure group, for example, is consistent with previous conceptualizations of secure attachment: The secure subjects, being high on confidence and low on all four scales related to insecurity, clearly had positive attitudes toward both self and others. The profiles of the remaining three groups raise some important conceptual issues concerning the nature of insecure forms of attachment.

In contrast to the secure subjects, the fearful subjects were low on Confidence and high on all four factors related to insecurity, and thus clearly showed negative attitudes toward both self and others. This result is consistent with Bartholomew's formulation. Moreover, the present results show that this group not only was characterized by all the aspects of insecure attachment, but was distinguishable even from the other insecure groups in terms of their extremely low scores on Confidence and their extremely high scores on Discomfort with Closeness and Relationships as Secondary. Hence this group differed from the others not only in qualitative terms (by endorsing all aspects of insecurity), but also in quantitative terms (compared to the other subjects, they were very insecure).

As expected, the subjects in the dismissing group were high on Discomfort with Closeness and Relationships as Secondary, reflecting their negative attitudes to others. Contrary to previous conceptualizations, however, they also showed moderate levels of Preoccupation with Relationships and Need for Approval—findings suggesting that they did not hold unreservedly positive attitudes toward themselves. Thus it appeared that their attempts to maintain distance in their personal relationships might be, at least in part, anxiety-driven.

Similarly, the preoccupied group conformed to previous conceptualizations, insofar as their high levels of Preoccupation with Relationships and Need for Approval reflected their negative attitudes to self; at the same time, however, their moderate levels of Discomfort with Closeness belied the picture of preoccupied subjects as eager for intimacy, wishing to attain extreme closeness in relationships, and being unreservedly positive in their attitudes toward others. Rather, ambivalence about closeness appeared to be a central feature of this group; for this reason, we would suggest that the name originally given to such individuals, "anxious/ambivalent," more clearly expresses the complexity of their attitudes to relationships. In support of this argument, it should be recalled that on the original forced-choice attachment measure (designed to test Hazan & Shaver's [1987] conceptualization of three attachment styles), avoidant and anxious/ambivalent subjects were not reliably differentiated in terms of avoidance (as assessed by the factor derived from our three-factor solution), or in terms of Discomfort with Closeness or Relationships as Secondary. Perhaps the preoccupation about relationships that characterizes members of this group is driven by ambivalence: Since their attitudes toward relationships are complex and somewhat contradictory (intimacy is desired but at the same time engenders discomfort), they are more likely to think and worry a lot about their close relationships.

The numbers of subjects in the final four groups were very similar across the two samples, supporting the stability of the solution. Specifically, the percentages falling into the various clusters were as follows: secure, 40.4% and 37.4% (samples 1 and 2, respectively); dismissing, 24.7% and 26.8%; preoccupied, 22.1% and 24.7%; and fearful, 12.8% and 11.1%. It should be noted that the percentage of subjects in the secure group is somewhat lower than that generally reported in studies of adult attachment. This result is not really surprising, since in the present procedure we adopted a different approach to attachment classifications. Most of the previous research has relied on subjects' self-reported classifications (which may be fairly strongly influenced by factors such as response bias); in addition, the definition of secure attachment imposed by the clustering procedure was a very stringent one (i.e., high on Confidence and low on all other scales). It should also be noted that in comparison to data reported by Bartholomew and Horowitz (1991), based on interviews designed to measure the four attachment styles, the fearful group in the present research was relatively small. Again, the definition of this attachment group imposed by the clustering procedure was stringent, and as noted previously, this style represents an extreme form of insecure attachment.

Dimensions Underlying Attachment

In order to further explore the attachment dimensions underlying the four-cluster solution, we carried out a discriminant-function analysis (separately for each subsample), with cluster membership as the grouping variable and the five attachment scales as predictors. For each sample, there were two significant discriminant functions. The first function accounted for roughly 80% of the between-groups variability, and was defined by Preoccupation with Relationships, Need for Approval, and Confidence (negative correlation). The second function was defined by Discomfort with Closeness and Relationships as Secondary. Examination of the group centroids revealed that the first function provided maximal discrimination between the secure group on the one hand and the fearful group on the other, with the preoccupied group also obtaining relatively high scores; the second function also provided maximal discrimination between secure and fearful groups, with the dismissing group also scoring relatively high (see Figure 5.1; for convenience, we have plotted the group centroids for the full subject sample). The group centroids clearly illustrate the high degree of insecurity characteristic of the fearful subjects.

These analyses not only provide evidence for four attachment groups, but reveal underlying dimensions that are consistent with those hypothesized by Bartholomew. As noted earlier, Bartholomew's dimensions re-

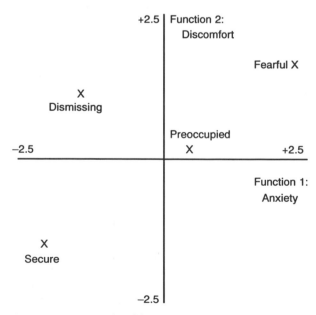

FIGURE 5.1.   Group centroids of four clusters on two discriminant functions.

flect the object of mental models (self or other) and the predominant feeling about that object (positive or negative). Bartholomew sees models of the self as reflecting a social response style of high versus low dependency, and models of others as reflecting the response style of high versus low avoidance. In the present analysis, the first dimension (defined by the first discriminant function) reflects primarily positive versus negative models of self (i.e., dependency); the second dimension reflects positive versus negative models of others (i.e., avoidance). These dimensions bear some resemblance to the two dimensions that we and other researchers have reported, based on adaptations of Hazan and Shaver's original forced-choice measure (Feeney et al., 1994; Simpson, 1990; Strahan, 1991). Specifically, as noted earlier, the dimensions underlying the early measure appear to be Comfort with Closeness (a bipolar factor that contrasts aspects of the original secure and avoidant descriptions) and Anxiety. The present data support both Discomfort and Anxiety as the key dimensions underlying adult attachment, although the Confidence scale of the Attachment Style Questionnaire is contrasted with Anxiety rather than with Comfort. The latter result is consistent with the item content of this scale: As mentioned previously, the Confidence scale measures confidence in relating to others, but does not deal with issues of trust or comfort with intimacy.

Utility of Three and Five Attachment Scales in Delineating Attachment Groups

Recognizing that factor analysis of the Attachment Style Questionnaire had produced a three-factor solution that captured the basic elements of adult attachment, we were interested in comparing the utility of the three- and five-factor solutions in delineating attachment groups. For this reason, we repeated the cluster analysis, using the three attachment scales as clustering variables (again, we split the sample in order to assess the stability of the solution). The results of the clustering were much less clear than those obtained from the five attachment scales. For each sample, the two-cluster solution again produced clear secure and insecure groups. The three- and four-cluster solutions, however, were unstable (in one sample, the three clusters were similar to the three groups proposed by Hazan & Shaver, while the four clusters resembled those discussed by Bartholomew; in the other sample, both three and four clusters simply represented varying degrees of security-insecurity). These results suggest that although the five attachment scales contain similar item content to the three scales, they provide clearer and more stable delineation of the various attachment groups.

APPLICABILITY WITH A YOUNGER SAMPLE

In order to ensure that the measure developed was suitable for a younger sample and for those who had not had much experience of romantic relationships, we also administered the Attachment Style Questionnaire to a sample of 248 eighth-grade students (approximately equal numbers of males and females) from three high schools in a large metropolitan area. The three schools were selected to cover the range of socioeconomic backgrounds. Most of the children were 12 or 13 years of age.

In order to check the internal consistency of the five attachment scales with this sample, coefficient alphas were calculated. These coefficients were .73 (Confidence), .73 (Discomfort with Closeness), .67 (Need for Approval), .73 (Preoccupation with Relationships), and .70 (Relationships as Secondary).

As a further assessment of the validity of the Attachment Style Questionnaire, and particularly of its usefulness with a sample of high school students, subsamples of these students were also administered the ICPS Family Functioning Scales (Intimacy, Conflict, and Parenting Style; Noller, Seth-Smith, Bouma, & Schweitzer, 1992) and/or the Junior Eysenck Personality Questionnaire (EPQ; Eysenck & Eysenck, 1975). Family functioning was assessed because of the strong theoretical link between experiences in the family of origin (notably with parents) and the development of attachment style (e.g., see Bowlby, 1973). Since attachment theory can be regarded as a general theory of personality development (Bowlby, 1980), we also considered it important to assess the link between attachment style and basic aspects of personality.

Attachment Style and Family Functioning

Canonical correlation analysis was used to relate the five attachment scales to the three scales derived from the ICPS Family Functioning Scales: Intimacy, Conflict, and Parenting Style (controlled vs. democratic). This analysis was based on data from 137 subjects. With all pairs of canonical variates included, Wilks's lambda was .67 ($p < .001$). With the first pair of canonical variates removed, subsequent tests of the association between the two sets of measures were not significant. The results showed that a linear combination of all the attachment scales was related to a combination of all the family functioning scales. Specifically, perceptions of high family intimacy, democratic parenting, and low levels of family conflict were associated with high scores on Confidence, and with low scores on all scales measuring aspects of insecure attachment (see Table 5.10). These results are consistent with theory relating attachment style to the quality of parenting.

Attachment Style and Personality Variables

Canonical correlation analysis was also used to relate the five attachment scales to the four personality scales derived from the EPQ: Toughmindedness, Extraversion, Neuroticism, and the Lie scale. This analysis was based on data from 116 students. With all pairs of canonical variates included, Wilks's lambda was .47, ($p < .001$). The dimension reduction analysis indicated that there were two highly significant pairs of canonical variates (see Table 5.10). The first pair of variates related Neuroticism to Preoccupation with Relationships and Need for Approval; the second pair of variates related Extraversion to Confidence (in self and others), and to low levels of Discomfort with Closeness and lack of emphasis on Relationships as Secondary (to achievement). These results support the concurrent validity of the Attachment Style Questionnaire. It is important to note that the Lie scale of the EPQ was uncorrelated with the five attachment scales, suggesting that scores on these scales are relatively unaffected by subjects' desire to portray themselves in a favorable light.

SEX DIFFERENCES AND SIMILARITIES

On two samples, we checked for gender differences on the scales of the Attachment Style Questionnaire. For the sample of 295 first-year university students, there was a significant gender effect only for Relationships

TABLE 5.10. Canonical Correlations with Scales of the Attachment Style Questionnaire

Family functioning (ICPS)			
Confidence	.88	Intimacy	.89
Preoccupation with Relationships	-.67	Conflict	-.86
Discomfort with Closeness	-.64	Parenting Style	.76
Need for Approval	-.60	(democratic)	
Relationships as Secondary	-.54		
Personality (EPQ)			
Dimension 1			
Preoccupation with Relationships	.81	Neuroticism	.97
Need for Approval	.71		
Dimension 2			
Relationships as Secondary	-.86	Extraversion	.73
Confidence	.67		
Discomfort with Closeness	-.57		

as Secondary, $F(1, 293) = 17.36$, $p < .0001$, with males much more likely to view relationships as secondary to achievement than females. On the sample of 248 high school students, there were gender effects on three of the scales. (Note that the number of subjects in these analyses varies slightly because of missing data.) For Discomfort with Closeness, males ($M = 34.43$) scored higher than females ($M = 31.82$), $F(1, 217) = 5.16$, $p < .05$. Males ($M = 32.65$) scored lower than females ($M = 34.50$) on Confidence, $F(1, 224) = 4.81$, $p < .05$. There was also a strong gender difference on Relationships as Secondary, with males ($M = 21.87$) scoring higher than females ($M = 18.53$), $F(1, 224) = 14.70$, $p < .0001$. In the older sample, then, the only attachment scale affected by gender was the Relationships as Secondary scale; this finding was equally strong in the younger sample. In the young sample, there were also differences on two other scales, with males reporting more discomfort with closeness and less confidence than females. Early work on adult attachment using the forced-choice measure revealed no relationship between gender and endorsement of the three attachment styles (Feeney & Noller, 1990; Hazan & Shaver, 1987). With the use of continuous measures, there have been some reports of gender differences on some scales. Collins and Read (1990), for example, using an 18-item scale measuring dependence, anxiety, and comfort with closeness, obtained the counterintuitive finding that males were more comfortable with closeness than were females. This finding contrasts with that of the present analysis, at least for the younger sample, where females reported being more comfortable with closeness and more confident about relating to others.

Where researchers have worked with a four-group model of attachment, the added construct of "dismissingness" (Bartholomew, 1990; Bartholomew & Horowitz, 1991) has been included. It is interesting to note, therefore, that Bartholomew and Horowitz found that men scored significantly higher than women on an interview-based rating of dismissingness. In the present study, using a related measure (the Relationships as Secondary scale), we obtained a similar gender difference across both adolescent and adult samples. This relatively strong and stable finding fits with conceptualizations of gender roles, in terms of the instrumental-expressive dichotomy (Parsons & Bales, 1955).

SUMMARY

The results of our analyses support the utility of the Attachment Style Questionnaire. The scales derived from the Attachment Style Questionnaire show adequate reliability, even with younger subjects who have had little experience of romantic relationships. The validity of the scales is indicated by a number of findings: the pattern of associations with previous measures of attachment style; the predictable patterns of correlations with measures of family functioning and personality; and the lack of correlation with Lie scores (EPQ). In addition, cluster analyses suggested that relatively distinct attachment groups can be identified on the basis of the scales.

The results raise a number of issues concerning the conceptualization of attachment style. First, our findings point to the central distinction as being between secure and insecure attachment. In particular, the strongest group differentiation in the cluster analyses corresponded to this dichotomy: The formation of additional clusters further subdivided the insecure group, with the secure group always remaining intact.

Second, as the pattern of results described above implies, it is nevertheless possible to distinguish different types of insecurely attached individuals (i.e., there is more than one way of being insecure). The results of our cluster analyses lend partial support to the four styles hypothesized by Bartholomew, and we were able to uncover two underlying dimensions reflecting models of the self and models of others. It should be noted that the mental models of some individuals (the fearful group) combine all of the aspects of insecurity.

Third, our insecure groups (whether defined by the clustering procedure based on the scales of the Attachment Style Questionnaire or by the original forced-choice measure) were not as clearly differentiated from one another as theoretical models of attachment would suggest, particularly in terms of Discomfort with Closeness. Our results suggest that the preoccupation with relationships that characterizes the preoccupied group may be driven by their very ambivalence about closeness, and, furthermore, that the approach to relationships adopted by dismissing subjects is anxiety-driven, at least in part. Certainly our results do not fit with the notion that dismissing and preoccupied attachment are clearly and diametrically opposed (Bartholomew & Horowitz, 1991). With regard to the differentiation of insecure groups, it is useful to recall that despite the large degree of overlap between the content of the three and the five attachment scales, the five scales provided clearer delineation of groups (for one sample, three- and four-cluster solutions based on three attachment scales merely divided insecure subjects into groups defined by degrees of insecurity, rather than by discrete profiles of attachment concerns).

Working with such a broad-based measure that clearly contains all of the essential elements of attachment theory has enabled us to address fundamental issues, such as the underlying dimensions of attachment and the nature of attachment styles. Our results tend to suggest that the crucial distinction is between secure and insecure attachment; on the other hand, there is some evidence for different ways of being insecure, and it is also clear that the mental models of some individuals combine all of the aspects of insecurity. Clearly, further work needs to be carried out on the utility of the Attachment Style Questionnaire, but the work reported here supports the value of more fundamental research into the attachment construct.

Appendix 5.1. Attachment Style Questionnaire

Show how much you agree with each of the following items by rating them on this scale: 1 = totally disagree; 2 = strongly disagree; 3 = slightly disagree; 4 = slightly agree; 5 = strongly agree; or 6 = totally agree.

Confidence	1.	Overall, I am a worthwhile person.
Confidence	2.	I am easier to get to know than most people.
Confidence	3.	I feel confident that other people will be there for me when I need them.
Discomfort	4.	I prefer to depend on myself rather than other people.
Discomfort	5.	I prefer to keep to myself.
R as S	6.	To ask for help is to admit that you're a failure.
R as S	7.	People's worth should be judged by what they achieve.
R as S	8.	Achieving things is more important than building relationships.
R as S	9.	Doing your best is more important than getting on with others
R as S	10.	If you've got a job to do, you should do it no matter who gets hurt.
N for A	11.	It's important to me that others like me.
N for A	12.	It's important to me to avoid doing things that others won't like.
N for A	13.	I find it hard to make a decision unless I know what other people think.
R as S	14.	My relationships with others are generally superficial.
N for A	15.	Sometimes I think I am no good at all.
Discomfort	16.	I find it hard to trust other people.
Discomfort	17.	I find it difficult to depend on others.
Preoccupation	18.	I find that others are reluctant to get as close as I would like.
Confidence	19.	I find it relatively easy to get close to other people.
Discomfort	20.	I find it easy to trust others. (R)
Discomfort	21.	I feel comfortable depending on other people. (R)
Preoccupation	22.	I worry that others won't care about me as much as I care about them.
Discomfort	23.	I worry about people getting too close.
N for A	24.	I worry that I won't measure up to other people.
Discomfort	25.	I have mixed feelings about being close to others.
Discomfort	26.	While I want to get close to others, I feel uneasy about it.
N for A	27.	I wonder why people would want to be involved with me.

Preoccupation	28. It's very important to me to have a close relationship.
Preoccupation	29. I worry a lot about my relationships.
Preoccupation	30. I wonder how I would cope without someone to love me.
Confidence	31. I feel confident about relating to others.
Preoccupation	32. I often feel left out or alone.
Confidence	33. I often worry that I do not really fit in with other people. (R)
Discomfort	34. Other people have their own problems, so I don't bother them with mine.
N for A	35. When I talk over my problems with others, I generally feel ashamed or foolish.
R as S	36. I am too busy with other activities to put much time into relationships.
Confidence	37. If something is bothering me, others are generally aware and concerned.
Confidence	38. I am confident that other people will like and respect me.
Preoccupation	39. I get frustrated when others are not available when I need them.
Preoccupation	40. Other people often disappoint me.

Note. Items marked (R) need to be reverse-scored. R as S, Relationships as Secondary; N for A, Need for Approval; Discomfort, Discomfort with Closeness; Preoccupation, Preoccupation with Relationships.

NOTE

1. The matrix of factor loadings and other relevant information is available from us at the Department of Psychology, University of Queensland, Brisbane, Queensland 4072, Australia.

REFERENCES

Ainsworth, M. D. S., Blehar, M. C., Water, E. & Wall, S. (1978). *Patterns of attachment: A psychological study of the Strange Situation.* Hillsdale, NJ: Erlbaum.

Bartholomew, K. (1990). Avoidance of intimacy: An attachment perspective. *Journal of Social and Personal Relationships, 7,* 147–178.

Bartholomew, K., & Horowitz, L. M. (1991). Attachment styles among young adults: A test of a four-category model. *Journal of Personality and Social Psychology, 61,* 226–244.

Bowlby, J. (1973). *Attachment and loss: Vol. 2. Separation: Anxiety and anger.* New York: Basic Books.

Bowlby, J. (1980). *Attachment and loss: Vol. 3: Loss: Sadness and depression.* New York: Basic Books.

Collins, N. L., & Read, S. J. (1990). Adult attachment, working models, and relationship quality in dating couples. *Journal of Personality and Social Psychology, 58,* 644–663.

Eysenck, H. J., & Eysenck, S. B. G. (1975). *Manual of the Eysenck Personality Questionnaire (Junior and Adult)*. Sevenoaks, England: Hodder & Stoughton.

Feeney, J. A. (1991). *The attachment perspective on adult romantic relationships*. Unpublished doctoral dissertation, University of Queensland.

Feeney, J. A., & Noller, P. (1990). Attachment style as a predictor of adult romantic relationships. *Journal of Personality and Social Psychology, 58*, 281-291.

Feeney, J. A., & Noller, P. (1991). Attachment style and verbal descriptions of romantic partners. *Journal of Social and Personal Relationships, 8*, 187-215.

Feeney, J. A., Noller, P., & Callan, V. J. (1994). Attachment style, communication and satisfaction in the early years of marriage. In K. Bartholomew & D. Perlman (Eds.), *Advances in personal relationships: Vol. 5. Adult attachment relationships* (pp. 269-308). London: Jessica Kingsley.

George, C., Kaplan, N., & Main, M. (1984). *Attachment interview for adults*. Unpublished manuscript, University of California at Berkeley.

Hazan, C., & Shaver, P. R. (1987). Romantic love conceptualized as an attachment process. *Journal of Personality and Social Psychology, 52*, 511-524.

Henderson, S., Byrne, D. G., & Duncan-Jones, P. (1981). *Neurosis and the social environment*. Sydney: Academic Press.

Levy, M. B., & Davis, K. D. (1988). Love styles and attachment styles compared: Their relations to each other and to various relationship characteristics. *Journal of Social and Personal Relationships, 5*, 439-471.

Noller, P., Seth-Smith, M. Bouma, R., & Schweitzer, R. (1992). Parent and adolescent perceptions of family functioning: A comparison of clinic and nonclinic families. *Journal of Adolescence, 15*, 101-114.

Parker, G., Tupling, H., & Brown, L. B. (1979). A parental bonding instrument. *British Journal of Medical Psychology, 52*, 1-10.

Parsons, T., & Bales, R. F. (1955). *Family, socialization, and interaction process*. Glencoe, IL: Free Press.

Simpson, J. A. (1990). Influence of attachment styles on romantic relationships. *Journal of Personality and Social Psychology, 59*, 971-980.

Strahan, B. J. (1991). Attachment theory and family functioning: Expectations and congruencies. *Australian Journal of Marriage and Family, 12*, 12-26.

West, M. W., & Sheldon, A. E. (1988). Classification of pathological attachment patterns in adults. *Journal of Personality Disorders, 2*, 153-159.

West, M. W., Sheldon, A. E., & Reiffer, L. (1987). An approach to the delineation of adult attachment: Scale development and reliability. *Journal of Nervous and Mental Disease, 175*, 738-741.

Wilhelm, K., & Parker, G. (1988). The development of a measure of intimate bonds. *Psychological Medicine, 18*, 225-234.

PART III

Life-Span Developmental Perspectives

CHAPTER 6

Parental Attachment, Peer Relations, and Dysphoria in Adolescence

JOANNA BATGOS
BONNIE J. LEADBEATER

Classic views of adolescent–parent relationships include beliefs that adolescents desire independence from their parents and that a primary developmental task of adolescence is to achieve emotional autonomy from them. This point of view was clearly articulated in Freud's (1905/1953) description of what he saw as one of the most painful psychic achievements of adolescence–detachment from parental authority. Following evolutionary theory, he believed that this separation from family was essential for altruistic engagement in extrafamilial relationships and for the progress of civilization. Freud claimed that this detachment was particularly problematic for girls:

> At every stage in the course of development through which all human beings ought by rights to pass, a certain number are held back; so there are some who have never got over their parents' authority and have withdrawn their affection from them either very incompletely or not at all. They are mostly girls, who, to the delight of their parents, have persisted in all their childish love far beyond puberty. (1905/1953, p. 227)

The implications of attachments to parents for extrafamilial relationships in adolescence have not been extensively studied. In this chapter, we argue that mental representations of self and other that are established in and reflective of ongoing relations with parents influence the quality of relations with peers in adolescence. We explore the mental representations of self and other that are involved in secure and insecure attachments and in depressive cognitions. Specifically, we review the theoretical and research literatures that suggest a relationship among secure attachments, protection from dysphoria, and positive relationships with peers. We also review the literature that posits a relationship between insecure attachments and vulnerability to dysphoria. Dysphoric experiences are expected to influence the quality of adolescents' peer relationships.

The view that adolescents must achieve independence from their parents in order to become well-functioning adults has been raised to the point of cultural common knowledge; it appears in our jokes, comic strips, and beliefs about the inevitability of a gap between generations. Adolescence also continues to be seen by psychologists as the phase in which increased physical, cognitive, and social capabilities underlie a growing push toward differentiation, independence, and autonomy from parents (e.g., Erikson, 1963; Hauser, Powers, & Noam, 1991). However, attention to the importance of relationships in adolescents' lives has been heightened recently by criticism by authors from multiple domains of the excessive individualism that has come to dominate our views of the mature self in Western culture. Taylor (1988) traces the development of the modern focus on the differentiated, introspective, moral self from classical Greek beliefs that gave no special status to the first-person perspective. Cushman (1990) situates the Western "empty" self historically and economically in the shift from community-based religious, rural, agricultural communities to scientific, industrial, urban economies that emphasize individual productivity and consumerism. Gilligan (1982; Gilligan, Lyons, & Hanmer, 1989) differentiates two separate moral voices—one focused on justice issues of individual rights and responsibilities, and the other on relational problems of care, concern, and hurt. Miller (1976) argues that psychology has overlooked the importance of relationships in understanding human development, to the detriment of women's mental health; she contends that a model of healthy psychological development must acknowledge attachments and provide an understanding of how the self develops such skills as empathy and responsiveness in relating to others.

Recent empirical research has begun to investigate the quality of adolescents' connections with their parents and the continuing importance of these relationships in adolescence. Youniss and Smollar (1985) characterize changes in adolescent–parent relationships in terms of transformations from relations built on unilateral authority to relationships built on mutuality, which acknowledge the growing autonomy of the adolescent in the context of continued respect for parents. Hauser et al. (1991) also propose that families in which adolescents and parents listen and are emotionally available for each other are important for healthy attachments. Hauser et al. argue that concerns with relationships with both family and peers grow in importance during adolescence:

> We nevertheless see the family as the most important presence during adolescence. The many deep identifications that adolescents have

made with their parents and siblings over the years cause them to incorporate aspects of their families' cognitive and emotional styles, defenses, strengths, vulnerabilities, and cherished beliefs. At another level, children assimilate their family's myths and paradigms for understanding the world. (p. 232)

GENDER DIFFERENCES IN ATTACHMENTS

Infants enter the world as social beings, both dependent on and prepared for relating to others; they experience their initial sense of relatedness in early family relationships. However, several theorists (Chodorow, 1978; Jordan & Surrey, 1986; Miller, 1976; Surrey, 1984) have argued that because of socialization practices that encourage their continuous identification with their mothers, girls develop internal mental representations of the self in relation to another, and they remain more preoccupied with interpersonal connections than boys. The developmental goal for the adolescent girl (and, we would argue, for the adolescent boy as well) is not to "separate" from her parents, but to redefine her relationship to them in ways that affirm her developmental changes and abilities (Gilligan et al., 1989; Miller, 1976).

A "self-in-relation" model that accounts for the continuing importance of relatedness in adult development and describes a "self" that evolves in the context of close relationships and intimate attachments has been suggested by Miller and her colleagues (Miller, 1976; Miller, Jordan, Kaplan, Stiver, & Surrey, 1991; Surrey, 1984, 1987). Theoretical and empirical work has shown that women, in particular, define the self within a context of relationships to others—that is, in terms of their ability to construct and maintain relationships (Jordan & Surrey, 1986; Kaplan, Klein, & Gleason, 1985). This self-in-relation model has much in common with attachment theory; it views the capacity for mutuality or relatedness as a developmental advance in mature relationships, rather than an extension of childhood dependency.

The distinction between "dependency" and "mutuality" is an important one for self-in-relation theory, and one that mirrors the controversy between the terms "dependency" and "attachment" in the attachment literature. "Dependency" and "attachment" are often used interchangeably to refer to behaviors that maintain closeness between a child and another person. However, Bowlby (1969) notes that the term "dependency" should be reserved for contact based upon caretaking of a child by a caregiver, and does not include the myriad of other close interactions and nurturance between parent and child, which he labels "attachments." As Bowlby proposes, a self-reliant person is one who has the ability to rely on others when necessary. Attachments to others are important in male and female adolescent development (Bowlby, 1969, 1980). The self-in-relation theorists label mature forms of relatedness "mutuality," which is more similar to the notion of "secure attachment" than to "dependency" (Gilligan et al., 1989; Jordan, 1986).

Self-in-relation theorists posit a developmental process in which maturation is in the direction of achieving greater mutuality in relationships—that is, an understanding of the self as a separate individual, yet still connected to others. Connections recognize experiences of mastery and empower both individuals in a relationship. In the developmental growth process, the agentic self develops the capacity for relationships with increasing levels of differentiation within the context of human relationships. Providing nurturance to others, skillful communication, and empathic understanding are acts of self-definition and mastery. Women exercise personal power within the context of maintaining and growing in relationships. The growth of a daughter's ability to engage and respond to her mother results in interactions that leave both participants "feeling more aware of self and other, and therefore, more energized to act" (Surrey, 1987, p. 6).

These theorists describe a self that is developed within the context of relationships, and have begun to question the validity of the dichotomies of dependence and independence, autonomy and connectedness (Gilligan, 1990; Miller, 1976; Surrey, 1984, 1987). They believe, rather, that autonomy and relatedness are linked in a dialectical fashion, for to be separate from others and achieve a mature sense of autonomy necessitates an "other" to recognize one's autonomy. Many traditional theories of personality focus on bipolar dimensions of experience. They posit autonomy–relatedness or agency–communion as polar opposites, and give one priority in discussions of psychological development (e.g., Erikson, 1963). But they are intertwined, and indeed the existence of one necessitates the other (Blatt, 1990). Miller and her colleagues believe that traditional models of development do not acknowledge that the self concerned with relationships is an active self. However, within this model, the self is seen as "subject," one who desires and is the author of his or her own experience, not a dependent "object" of others' desires.

Thus, the concept of a self within this theory is not one of a static individual being attended by the other, but of a self inseparable from dynamic interaction. A self-in-relation is not objectified and separate, but a self engaged in an "interactional, ongoing 'process of being' rather than a static structure dedicated to increasing self-sufficient functioning" (Miller et al., 1991, p. 4). The ability to relate to others does not impair the individual's ability to be effective as a self. A more articulated sense of self results from a developmental process that emphasizes an increasing ability to attune to, influence, and be influenced by others. From infancy, the child begins to develop an internal representation of a self as a self-in-relation to others, and begins to develop a sense of others and their feelings. These abilities grow into an ability to empathize with another, and the child develops an internal sense of himself or herself as an agent who can affect interactions with others. However, from the beginning, development of the "self" is "inseparable from dynamic interaction" (Miller, 1990, p. 440). This is a view that acknowledges intrapsychic phenomena, yet sees the relational context between self and other as the primary source of growth. This early interacting sense of self is reinforced particularly for female infants, both by mothers and by fathers. Girls are encouraged to develop empathic skills and to attend to relational issues (Miller, 1990).

This model argues that as a result of socialization for relatedness from infancy through latency and preadolescence, adolescent girls' sense of self-esteem is based in feeling competent and included in relationships. Miller (1990) points out that this is very different from traditional definitions of self-esteem. Indeed, a girl's sense of self-efficacy may be bound up with her emotional connections to others, and with her ability to negotiate and affect those connections. Miller (1976, p. 83) states that "women's sense of self becomes very much organized around being able to make and then to maintain affiliations and relationships."

The relationship differentiation process described by the self-in-relation theorists posits that the motive for connection to others leads to greater authenticity in self, other, and self-with-other. The growing authenticity between mother and daughter does not mean that conflict does not occur. Indeed, resolving misunderstandings and conflicts is viewed as an important growth experience in the development of mutuality between mother and daughter. An authentic relationship is one in which neither participant is self-defeating or egocentric (Miller et al., 1991). Gilligan (1990) views adolescent girls who resist attachment as illustrating the problems that come from a relationship's remaining static, and not developing into a more mature, mutual relationship. A mutual relationship is characterized by each individual's being increasingly able to share feelings, thoughts, and perceptions—to influence the other and be influenced by the other.

Theorists explain this process as developing a sense of a self as a self-in-relation, which is carried to new relationships (Jordan & Surrey, 1986). Adolescent girls report greater intimacy with their mothers than with their fathers (Benson, Harris, & Rogers, 1992; Furman & Buhrmester, 1985; Youniss & Ketterlinus, 1987), rate their mothers as the most important persons in their lives (Kaplan et al., 1985), and desire to have more connection and access to their mothers through late adolescence (Kaplan et al., 1985). These experiences of connections with mothers may be reflected in connections with peers. Consistent with the definition of "self-esteem" as the ability to negotiate connections to others, research has shown that adolescent girls do experience a loss of self-efficacy when relationships fail. Hill and Lynch (1983) report that 12- to 14-year-old girls worry more than boys about what other people think of them, and care more about being well liked. Stern (1989) notes that paradoxically, when adolescent girls are asked to describe themselves, they include a great deal of information about others, particularly about their relationships with others. Adolescent females are socialized to be responsive to others, and thus are more vulnerable to failures in the interpersonal domain.

Empirical work on adolescents' differential vulnerabilities to threats to their personal competence (e.g., achievement or academic failures) and interpersonal relationships (e.g., breakups with boyfriends or girlfriends) also supports hypothesized gender differences in the centrality of relationships for girls' development (see Leadbeater, Blatt, & Quinlan, in press, for a review). Female adolescents are more vulnerable than males to negative events affecting members of their social networks, and females report more family- and peer-related stress than males do (Compas & Wagner, 1991; Siddique & D'Arcy, 1984). In addition, correlations between interpersonal stress and psychological symptoms are stronger for females than for males, suggesting that adolescent girls may be more vulnerable to the negative effects of interpersonal stress (Compas & Wagner, 1991).

Although we might thus expect adolescent females to be more attuned to relationships than adolescent males, recent empirical work also suggests that relationships with parents are still important to adolescent males. Adolescents care about parental opinion and approval because they want acknowledgment of their individuality and new status as they leave childhood and move toward adulthood. Youniss and Ketterlinus (1987) asked 605 adolescents how well they thought their parents knew them, and found that both males and females judged that their mothers knew them fairly well, but females judged that their fathers did not know them very well. Youniss and Smollar (1985) also found that adolescents made distinctions between their mothers and fathers in terms of what they talked about with them, with mothers described by both males and females as more open to listen to problems than fathers. Fathers were found to emphasize achievements and to minimize the importance of adolescents' social skills with peers. Benson et al. (1992) studied the relationship between adolescent identity and attachment to parents in 268 late adolescents. They found that for both males and females, identity achievement was related to attachment to mothers, but unrelated to attachment to fathers. In addition, attachments to mothers were significantly greater than attachments to fathers for both males and females. The authors state that their findings support the assertion that the secure base provided by an attachment to the mother acts as a protective factor against an inability to achieve a sense of identity. In summary, these studies suggest that both male and female adolescents have close bonds with their parents, and that these attachment bonds may be closer for mothers than for fathers.

ATTACHMENT AND ADOLESCENCE

Attachment theory provides a framework for understanding how attachments to parents may be reflected in attachments to peers, and how problems in adolescent attachments reflect disturbances in interpersonal relationships. "Attachment" is defined as an enduring affectional relationship between child and caregiver, the purpose of which is to provide protection and nurturance for the child. Attachment behaviors are abilities that are inborn and form a basic motivational system of behavior that characterizes mother-infant interaction (Bowlby, 1980). The goals of this behavior system are maintaining proximity to a caretaker and thereby ensuring the infant's survival (Bowlby, 1980). Through repeated interaction with the mother (or other primary caretaker), a child develops an "internal working model" of this caregiving relationship. These internal working models can be considered to be mental representations of the self in relation to others (Bretherton, 1992).

Internal working models include affective as well as cognitive components. They also define the self and expectations of others for future interactions, and are used by the individual as a framework for later attachment relationships to others (Bowlby, 1980). Theory and research on internal working models suggest that these models of relationships tend to continue, and are reinforced by the individual's interactions with others. Perhaps because of biases that favor assimilation over accommodation, individuals tend to put themselves into situations that reinforce their early internal working models (Hazan, 1992). Hunter and Youniss (1982) found that adolescents did judge their peers to be similar to their parents on major dimensions of their relationships.

Ainsworth's (Ainsworth, Blehar, Waters, & Wall, 1978) three types of attachments in infants—"secure," "anxious/ambivalent," and "avoidant"— delineate individual differences in the quality of children's early relationships with their mothers. Mother-child attachments have also been found to predict quality of attachments to peers in toddlers (Waters, Wippman, & Sroufe, 1979). Securely attached infants believe that their mothers are accessible and responsive, and thus internalize the belief that they themselves are competent and deserving of empathy. They will seek their attachment figures when distressed. Anxiously/ambivalently attached babies lack confident expectations of their mothers' accessibility and responsiveness. They may have experienced inconsistent, neglectful, or overindulgent behavior from their mothers. They develop a sense of themselves as unworthy of comfort and help, view others as rejecting or unreliable, and are preoccupied with closeness to others. As feelings become part of these infants' internal working models of themselves in relationships, future interactions are disturbed by their sense of themselves as unlovable and of others as unreliable. Avoidantly attached infants actively avoid their mothers on reunion after separation, in what seems to be a defensive maneuver against previous rejection experienced in overly intrusive or noncontingent, insensitive interactions.

Attachment issues become especially salient as children enter adolescence, when increasing involvement with peers challenges self-definitions, as well as intimacy and perspective-taking abilities (Sullivan, 1953). Given the many changes that early adolescents face, positive relationships with parents may serve as "one important sphere of security and comfort in the adolescent's rapidly changing world" (Petersen, Sarigiani, & Kennedy, 1991, p. 267). Secure attachments to mothers provide adolescents with a template for healthy peer relationships and may help the adolescents to negotiate the interpersonal tasks of adolescence, such as maintaining friendships and dating.

This argument is supported by empirical work suggesting that adolescents who perceive secure relationships with their parents exhibit higher self-esteem and emotional well-being (Armsden & Greenberg, 1987; Benson et al., 1992), and less depression and social anxiety (Papini, Roggman, & Anderson, 1991), than adolescents who perceive insecure relationships with their parents. In addition, the attachment-adjustment link has been found to be stronger for mother-child dyads than for father-child dyads (Benson et al., 1992; Larose & Boivin, 1992; Papini et al., 1991). Research exploring life stressors during adolescence has also found that ongoing stress in family relationships is a better predictor of negative psychological symptoms in adolescence than acute life events (Daniels & Moos, 1990).

Indeed, it is *disengagement* from parents that seems to be problematic for adolescents. A series of studies by Ryan and Lynch (1989) with male and female adolescents suggests that emotional autonomy represents emotional detachment in early adolescence. These authors used the Emotional Autonomy Scale (Steinberg & Silverberg, 1986), a 20-item measure of self-reliance and self-regulation, which measures independence from parents as emotional resources. One study explored the relationship between attachment to parents and emotional autonomy. Boys were found to be higher on emotional autonomy than girls, but no sex differences were found on attachment to parents. Avoidantly attached adolescents also had the highest levels of emotional autonomy, compared to securely and anxiously/ambivalently attached adolescents; this effect was more pronounced for avoidantly attached males than for avoidantly attached females. A second study assessed the relationship between adolescents' self-concepts and emotional autonomy. Emotional autonomy was shown to be positively related to perceived parental rejection, and inversely related to family cohesion, parental acceptance, and self-perceived lovability. No gender differences were found in this study. Ryan and Lynch (1989) argue that Steinberg and Silverberg's (1986) measure is assessing detachment, or a reluctance to depend on parents. They believe that their findings reflect the feelings of detachment or alienation experienced by avoidantly attached individuals who cannot experience their parents as emotional resources. These authors believe that autonomy in adolescence is not facilitated by detachment (or emotional autonomy as measured by the Steinberg & Silverberg scale), but rather by attachment to parents. Emotional autonomy may reflect problems of attachment, with highly emotionally autonomous adolescents lacking a sense of their parents' love.

In an interview study of nine adolescent girls with "problematic attachments" to their mothers, Salzman (1989) compared their descriptions of maternal nurturance, dependability, and understanding to insecure attachment classifications. The subgroup of young women labeled as anxiously/ambivalently attached often identified with their mothers' vulnerabilities, and saw themselves as like their mothers (needy, clingy). They had difficulty accepting any dependency needs in themselves, and often compulsively gave to others, while harshly rejecting any personal needs for nurturance. They had trouble feeling justifiably angry at their mothers, and were willing to absorb pain instead of possibly hurting their mothers with angry feelings. For the avoidant group, there was a mixture of admiration, resentment, and apprehension toward their "powerful" mothers. These young women described power struggles with their mothers, whom they viewed as competent, domineering, and ambitious. Their relationships were characterized by unresolved conflicts and avoidance of conflict. Although these girls maintained distance from their mothers, they admitted to longings for connection and guidance. For all of the girls, attachments, even when flawed or painful, remained important.

Given theoretical and empirical work suggesting that adolescent girls may actively seek connections more than adolescent boys, we would expect to find more anxiously/ambivalently attached females than males, because such individuals actively seek connections. We would also expect that males, because of socialization that discourages them from actively seeking relationships, will outnumber females in the avoidantly attached category. These expectations were partially confirmed in a study by Kobak and Sceery (1988), which found that a sample of anxiously/ambivalently attached adolescents was predominantly female (75%).

ATTACHMENT AND INTERPERSONAL COMPETENCE

Substantial research in the area of early adolescent peer relationships has focused on "interpersonal competence"–interpersonal knowledge and skills, and the ability to use those skills (Cauce, 1986). The growth in importance of the peer group during adolescence brings with it new demands for increased ability to negotiate with others. Whereas longitudinal research with infants and toddlers suggests a relationship between attachment and interpersonal competence, research on the relationship between adolescent attachments and interpersonal competence has only begun.

Evidence from cross-sectional studies does suggest that positive parent–child relationships are associated with more intimate peer relationships and greater interpersonal competence. Gold and Yanof (1985) studied adolescent girls' relationships with their mothers and close female friends. Girls' reports of higher levels of affection with their mothers and of maternal democratic parenting styles were associated with more intimate relationships with friends. These findings also suggest that close relationships with parents do not disappear in adolescence in favor of peer relationships. Hauser et al. (1991) studied 14- to 15-year-old adolescents and their parents over a 3-year period, assessing adolescent ego development, self-esteem, and family interaction patterns. They found that adolescent ego development, characterized in part by a greater capacity for supportive relationships, was positively associated with parental acceptance.

Kobak and Sceery (1988) explored the coherence of internal working models of attachment during late adolescence and their relationship to social competence and emotional adjustment. Using the Adult Attachment Interview, these authors classified 53 college students (26 males, 27 females) into groups paralleling the Ainsworth attachment classifications. Students who were securely attached were rated by their peers as more ego-resilient and less anxious than the other groups. They also reported higher levels of social competence and social support than the avoidant group. Students in the avoidant group were rated by their peers as highest on measures of hostility, and reported more loneliness and lower levels of familial support than the other two groups of students. No information on the gender of these students was reported. Students in the anxious/ambivalent group were viewed by their peers as the most anxious and reported high levels of personal and psychological distress (e.g., anxiety, depression, and loneliness). This group rated their families as more supportive than the avoidant group, suggesting that even though these individuals are anxiously/ambivalently attached, they seek connections. Females predominated in this group (75%).

Although adolescents' attachments are expected to be associated with the quality of their attachments to peers, we suggest that this is an indirect relationship, mediated by perceptions of themselves as worthy of attention and of others as available, nurturant supports. A secure attachment to parents may protect an adolescent against dysphoric views of the self as unlovable and worthy of punishment, and of others as unsupportive and punitive. Recent work with conduct-disordered boys supports a theoretical model in which negative parental characteristics (e.g., harsh disciplinary practices) lead to dysphoric experiences, which in turn lead to poor social skills with peers (Bierman & Smoot, 1991; Sroufe & Rutter, 1984). We propose a similar sequence, with poor attachments and their resulting internal working models leaving adolescents at risk for dysphoric experiences and impaired peer relationships.

SUBTYPES OF DYSPHORIA

Insecure attachments result in internal mental representations of the self as unlovable or unworthy of attention and support, and deserving of punishment. Facing the stresses of puberty and adolescence, an adolescent with such a mental representation of the self may be more vulnerable to experiences of dysphoria, or mild depression.

Depressive disorders encompass a wide range of problems, including feelings of sadness (dysphoria), a syndrome or cluster of mild depressive symptoms (dysthymia), or a more severe clinical disorder of depressive symptomatology (e.g., bipolar disorder, major depression). Although the occurrence of dysphoria is not a clinically defined disorder, these subclinical levels of depressive experiences may place individuals at risk for later clinical depression or for problem behaviors such as delinquency and eating disorders (Leadbeater et al., in press).

The reported rates of clinical depression for male and female adolescents range from 5% to 8.6%, but as many as 56% report experiences of dysphoria on self-report assessments (for reviews of this literature, see Leadbeater et al., in press; Petersen, Compas, & Brooks-Gunn, 1991). Negative mental representations of self and other are common to both insecure attachments and experiences of dysphoria, yet the links between the mental representations characteristic of insecure attachments and dysphoria have not been investigated (Cummings & Cicchetti, 1990).

Recent theoretical and empirical work on subtypes of dysphoria suggests how dysphoria may be linked to negative perceptions of self and other. The delineation of two dysphoric subtypes also aids in our under-standing of the relationship among adolescents' attachments to their mothers, resulting predispositions to dysphoria, and the effects of dys-phoria on peer relationships. Investigators from various theoretical per-spectives suggest differentiating subtypes of depression and dysphoria according to the experiences or issues that lead individuals to become depressed (Blatt & Zuroff, 1992). Psychoanalytic, cognitive-developmental, cognitive-behavioral, object relations, and interpersonal theorists all stress the difference between a dysphoria focused on interpersonal issues of dependency and loss of others, and a dysphoria focused on self-critical issues of guilt and punishment by others (Blatt & Maroudas, 1992).

Comparable to descriptions of anxious/ambivalent attachment, inter-personal dysphoria is characterized by feelings of helplessness and fears of being abandoned, and by the wish to be cared for. Individuals with this dysphoric subtype have an intense need to be in contact with others. The self is viewed as unlovable, and others are valued for their ability to pro-vide love and care. These individuals actively seek connections to others, and may resist expressing disagreement with or anger at others for fear of losing connections. Their relationships are idealizing; they defend against stress and separation by denial or by searching for substitutes.

Comparable to descriptions of avoidant attachment, self-critical dys-phoria is characterized by feelings of inferiority and guilt, and by a chronic fear of being criticized. Individuals with this dysphoric subtype have a fear of failing to live up to others' expectations. The self is viewed as unwor-thy, and others are valued for their ability to provide approval. These indi-viduals seek the approval of others, but may withdraw from interactions if they feel rejected. Their relationships are marked by hostility, distrust, and avoidance. They defend against stress and separation by projection (Blatt & Homann, 1992; Blatt & Zuroff, 1992).

Several assessments of these two types of dysphoria have been devel-oped, including the Sociotropy–Autonomy Scale (Beck, Epstein, Harrison, & Emery, 1983), which measures interpersonal issues such as concerns about disapproval and pleasing others, and autonomy issues such as freedom from control and achievement; and a scale developed specifically for adolescents, the Adolescent Depressive Experiences Questionnaire (DEQ-A; Blatt, Schaffer, Bers, & Quinlan, 1990). The DEQ-A provides ado-lescents with Likert-type statements about self-concept (e.g., "I tend to be very critical of myself") and experiences (e.g., "After an argument, I feel very lonely"), which assess fears of loss, dependency, and self-blame. This instrument has been used in a wide variety of settings with both non-clinical and clinical samples, and does appear to differentiate between inter-personal and self-critical dysphorics (Blatt & Zuroff, 1992).

Consistent with the expected gender differences in subtypes of attachment, gender differences have been found for the subtypes of dysphoria: Female adults exhibit higher levels of interpersonal dysphoria, and male adults exhibit higher levels of self-critical dysphoria (Chevron, Quinlan, & Blatt, 1978; Whiffen & Sasseville, 1991). Research with adolescents has found that females appear more vulnerable to interpersonal dysphoria than males, but no gender differences have been found for self-critical dysphoria in adolescents (Baron & Peixoto, 1991; Blatt, Hart, Quinlan, Leadbeater, & Auerbach, 1993).

ATTACHMENT STYLES AND SUBTYPES OF DYSPHORIA

The theoretical link between Ainsworth's attachment classifications and these interpersonal and self-critical subtypes of dysphoria is compelling (see Blatt & Homann, 1992). Shaver (1992) argues that even for adults, "the mind is continually asking the question, is an attachment figure available?" We are arguing that experiences of dysphoria amplify the way in which this question is asked by adolescents. Dysphoric vulnerabilities accentuate attachment styles carried from childhood, and may affect the impact of those styles on later relationships: Adolescents who perceive inconsistency and ambivalence in their relationships with their mothers, and who internalize a sense of others as inconsistently available and of themselves as unworthy of love, may find it difficult to assume that extrafamilial relationships can be maintained in the absence of others. Preoccupation with gaining the attention of others may leave children and adolescents vulnerable to dysphoric states, which are experienced as fears of loneliness and abandonment. Desperately seeking love and care from others, these individuals often idealize their relationships. Difficulties in expressing anger may arise, for fear of losing others.

Similarly, children who experience their mothers as rejecting and critical may internalize a sense of others as hostile and of themselves as unworthy of love—in other words, avoidant attachment, characterized by compulsive self-reliance. They may feel worthless and develop a severely self-critical stance, internalizing the rejecting and restrictive parent. They may fear loss of approval for failing to meet harsh parental expectations. This avoidant attachment may leave adolescents vulnerable to self-critical dysphoria.

Although studies have not been conducted specifically to test the relationship between subtypes of dysphoria and insecure attachments for early adolescents, both retrospective and longitudinal studies of child-parent relationships suggest that a general lack of consistency and nurturance from parents, or experiences of parents as authoritarian, critical, and rejecting, are associated with adult depression. In a study of female college students, McCranie and Bass (1984) found that women with interpersonal dysphoria (as measured by the adult form of the Depressive Experiences Questionnaire) described their mothers as dominating, controlling, and emphasizing conformity, whereas women with self-critical dysphoria described both parents as controlling, inconsistent, and emphasizing achievement. Although theory suggests that inconsistent parental behavior would lead to interpersonal dysphoria, Blatt and Zuroff (1992) suggest that the lack of a significant relationship between parental inconsistency and interpersonal dysphoria in the McCranie and Bass (1984) study may have been attributable to interpersonally dysphoric individuals' inability to recognize and express dissatisfaction with their parents, for fear of losing those relationships.

Other studies also provide support for the link between parental behavior and dysphoria. In studies of nonclinical and hospitalized adults, using both self-report measures of relationships with parents (Parker, Tupling, & Brown, 1979) and investigators' ratings of depressed individuals' parent descriptions (Blatt, Wein, Chevron, & Quinlan, 1979), researchers found negative descriptions of parents to be associated with adult depression.

In a longitudinal study, Gjerde, Block, and Block (1991) found significant prospective correlations between parenting during preschool years and adolescent dysphoria for mother–daughter dyads. Girls whose mothers had received high scores on both authoritarian control and positive engagement (measured when the girls were aged 5) were found to have more dysphoria at age 18 than their male and female peers. This finding is especially interesting, as *positive* engagement with a controlling mother was linked to dysphoria. The authors suggest that the combination of negative control and positive involvement puts girls in a "double bind" and limits their opportunities for self-efficacy. Similar findings were reported in a study of parenting experiences and self-criticism, with parental restrictiveness and rejection when girls were 5 years old related to self-criticism when the girls were aged 12 (Koestner, Zuroff, & Powers, 1991). This relationship held even when mother-reported temperamental differences among children were taken into account. In addition, follow-up analyses at age 31 revealed that this self-critical affect remained stable into adulthood.

Research also suggests that retrospective reports of parental behavior from self-critical individuals accurately reflect the nature of their experiences with their parents and are not merely manifestations of concurrent dysphoria. Brewin, Firth-Cozens, Furnham, and McManus (1992) found a significant relationship between the degree of self-criticism in women and reports of a maternal lack of care, even after possible confounds of social desirability and current mood state were controlled for. Gotlib,

Mount, Cordy, and Whiffen (1988) found that adult women suffering from postpartum depression reported negative parental behaviors from childhood, and that the level of negative behaviors endorsed did not change when depression remitted. Daniels and Moos (1990) found that depressed adolescents reported high levels of stress in family relationships, and also found similar levels reported by their nondepressed siblings, suggesting that the adolescents' experiences of depression were not resulting in a response bias to overreport negative events.

SUBTYPES OF DYSPHORIA AND INTERPERSONAL COMPETENCE

These dysphoric subtypes may also have implications for the continuing development of internal working models of relationships. Studies of these subtypes of dysphoria in undergraduate (generally female) samples show that individuals with interpersonal or self-critical dysphoria interact with friends in different ways. Women with interpersonal dysphoria describe themselves as unassertive with friends, seem concerned with keeping peace in relationships (Zuroff & Fitzpatrick, 1989), and perceive their friends as friendly (Zuroff & Franko, 1986). In contrast, women with self-critical dysphoria describe themselves as unwilling to engage in self-disclosure with close friends, have relationships characterized by unsatisfactory conflict resolution and low levels of trust (Zuroff & Fitzpatrick, 1989), and describe their friends as less supportive (Zuroff & Franko, 1986). In studies of nonclinical samples (Blatt & Zuroff, 1992), interpersonally dysphoric individuals appeared to seek and maintain good interpersonal relationships, whereas self-critical individuals appeared to seek and find interpersonal relationships that were less nurturant and more conflict-ridden. These relationships may confirm both their negative self-appraisals and their appraisals of others as unsupportive or critical. Although these studies have focused on college-aged individuals, they provide hypotheses about the interpersonal environments of these individuals that may be relevant for younger adolescents.

A MODEL OF THE RELATIONSHIPS BETWEEN ATTACHMENT, DYSPHORIA, AND INTERPERSONAL COMPETENCE

Discussions of adolescent attachment could benefit from an understanding of the relationship between attachment styles and vulnerability to self-critical and interpersonal subtypes of dysphoria. Although impaired parent-child relationships have been theoretically linked to subsequent depression in adults (Cummings & Cicchetti, 1990), the distinction between interpersonal and self-critical dysphoria adds to our understanding of the quality of dysphoric experiences for adolescents. Research that explores the link between the thought processes characteristic of insecure attachments and the thought processes characteristic of dysphoria can greatly add to our understanding of the consequences of insecure attachment in early adolescence for later social functioning.

Together, the theory and research cited on attachment, dysphoria, and interpersonal competence in adolescence suggest that insecurely attached adolescents are more vulnerable to self-critical and interpersonal subtypes of dysphoria, and are more likely to exhibit poorer interpersonal competence with peers, than securely attached adolescents. As seen in Figure 6.1, we propose that securely attached adolescents will be protected against dysphoric experiences and will have peer relationships characterized by reciprocity and high levels of perceived social support. Anxiously/ambivalently attached adolescents are expected to show a greater propensity toward interpersonal dysphoria than securely or avoidantly attached adolescents. Their peer relationships are expected to be characterized by ambivalence and an inability to negotiate conflicts. These individuals may be preoccupied with relationships, may idealize others and view them as supportive, and may possess the skills necessary to initiate interactions. However, given their idealized expectations and urgent needs for closeness, they may also exhibit deficits in the interpersonal competence skills required for maintenance of relationships. In contrast, avoidantly attached adolescents are expected to show a greater propensity toward self-critical dysphoria than securely or anxiously/ambivalently attached adolescents. It is expected that their peer relationships will be characterized by higher levels of hostility and conflict, and by lower levels of self-disclosure and perceived social support, than those of securely or anxiously/ambivalently attached adolescents.

Most empirical work exploring the relationships between attachment and dysphoria has focused on the children of depressed mothers (Cummings & Cicchetti, 1990); little research has focused on relationships between attachment and dysphoria in normal adolescents. Given the salience of issues of attachment and autonomy in adolescent development, research involving the relatively unexplored dimensions of interpersonal and self-critical dysphoria may be of particular importance. A study is currently underway to test the model that we propose with 136 adolescent girls (ages 13-16) and their mothers. We are investigating the relations between maternal attachment (assessed both by Hazan & Shaver's [1987] measure of attachment and by Collins & Read's [1990] Attachment Inventory), vulnerability to interpersonal and self-critical dysphoria (assessed by the DEQ-A), and the

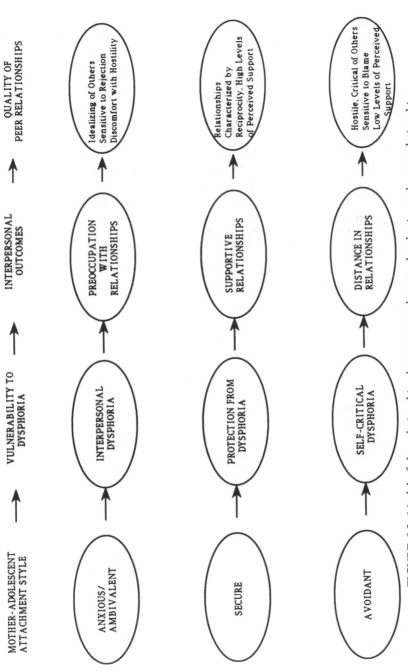

FIGURE 6.1. Model of the relationships between attachment, dysphoria, and peer relationships.

quality of peer relationships (assessed by the Adolescent Interpersonal Competence Questionnaire [AICQ]; Buhrmester, 1990). Pilot data for 110 girls suggest that insecurely attached girls are more likely to report interpersonal and self-critical dysphoric experiences than securely attached girls. In addition, insecurely attached girls are more likely to exhibit impaired peer relationships as assessed by the AICQ.

Specifically, our sample includes 61% ($n = 67$) securely attached, 24% ($n = 27$) avoidantly attached, and 15% ($n = 16$) anxiously/ambivalently attached adolescent girls (according to Hazan & Shaver's [1987] method of attachment classification). This distribution parallels findings from Hazan and Shaver's (1987) study of adults, in which 56% of their sample was classified as secure, 24% as avoidant, and 20% as anxious/ambivalent. A multivariate analysis of variance, used to explore attachment group differences on the DEQ-A subscales (which assess interpersonal dysphoria, self-critical dysphoria, and self-efficacy) was significant, $F(6, 208) = 7.24$, $p < .001$. Follow-up univariate F tests showed, as expected, that anxiously/ambivalently attached girls reported higher levels of interpersonal dysphoria ($\bar{X} = 1.05$, $SD = 0.87$) than securely attached ($\bar{X} = 0.15$, $SD = 0.86$) or avoidantly attached ($\bar{X} = 0.47$, $SD = 0.78$) girls, $F(2, 107) = 7.78$, $p < .001$. Securely attached girls reported lower levels of self-critical dysphoria ($\bar{X} = -0.37$, $SD = 0.98$) than either anxiously/ambivalently attached ($\bar{X} = 0.69$, $SD = 1.33$) or avoidantly attached ($\bar{X} = 0.49$, $SD = 1.09$) girls, $F(2, 107) = 10.42$, $p < .001$. No group differences were found for self-efficacy.

Our findings suggest that anxious/ambivalent attachment is linked to interpersonal dysphoria, but that both anxious/ambivalent and avoidant attachment styles are linked to self-critical dysphoria. This indicates that both types of insecure attachments may leave girls vulnerable to self-criticism, but that anxiously/ambivalently attached girls also express added fears of loneliness and abandonment. It may be that girls in this group, who do not possess the confidence that others will be there for them, also feel unworthy of consistent love and care. Ainsworth et al. (1978) describe a sense of being unlovable and unworthy of comfort and help as a defining feature of anxious/ambivalent attachment. Thus, a punitive and critical stance toward the self is present, along with anxiety about relationships. Avoidantly attached girls, while harboring feelings of worthlessness as well, are less likely to admit their longings for connections.

In addition, our data indicate that anxiously/ambivalently and avoidantly attached girls differ in the quality of their relationships to peers. The AICQ assesses five domains of interpersonal competence with peers: initiation of relationships, negative assertion, self-disclosure, providing emotional support, and conflict management. Multivariate analysis of variance, used to explore attachment group differences on these five subscales, was significant, $F(10, 204) = 3.92$, $p < .001$. Follow-up univariate analyses showed significant differences among the three attachment groups on self-disclosure, $F(2, 107) = 8.45$, $p < .001$, with securely attached girls ($\bar{X} = 3.57$, $SD = 0.64$) more likely to self-disclose to friends than avoidantly attached girls ($\bar{X} = 2.93$, $SD = 0.67$), but not anxiously/ambivalently attached girls ($\bar{X} = 3.26$, $SD = 0.91$). In addition, securely attached girls were more likely to initiate interactions, $F(2, 107) = 6.39$, $p < .002$ ($\bar{X} = 3.61$, $SD = 0.65$) than either anxiously/ambivalently attached ($\bar{X} = 2.97$, $SD = 0.90$) or avoidantly attached ($\bar{X} = 3.20$, $SD = 0.85$) girls. Securely attached girls were also more likely to assert themselves in conflict situations, $F(2, 107) = 11.62$, $p < .001$ ($\bar{X} = 3.49$, $SD = 0.67$) than either anxiously/ambivalently attached ($\bar{X} = 2.81$, $SD = 0.69$) or avoidantly attached ($\bar{X} = 2.91$, $SD = 0.59$) girls. No differences were found among the groups for providing emotional support and conflict management.

The two pathways of insecure attachments we have investigated describe individuals with very different mental representations of relationships and different interpersonal styles. This model also has implications for psychotherapy, as interpersonally and self-critically dysphoric individuals may react differently to specific therapeutic interventions (Blatt, 1992) because of the different ways in which they experience interpersonal interactions. Anxiously/ambivalently attached adolescents with interpersonal and self-critical dysphoria may initially respond more positively to interventions with an interpersonal orientation, which validate their strong desires to be connected to others. They may then be open to exploring issues of self-criticism within the context of an interpersonally oriented therapy. Avoidantly attached adolescents with self-critical dysphoria may initially engage with interventions that are less interpersonally charged, such as cognitive–behavioral interventions. But for both types of individuals, addressing their interpersonal styles is thought to be essential. In summary, it may be that adolescents with secure attachments to their mothers have a strong model for both connection in relationships *and* acceptance of autonomy. As Leadbeater et al. (in press) note, a secure sense of personal competence and a context of supportive, reliably present relationships may be the real protectors of adolescent emotional health.

ACKNOWLEDGMENTS

Preparation of this chapter was supported in part by an American Fellowship from the American Association of University Women Educational Foundation to Joanna Batgos, and by a William T. Grant Faculty Scholars Award to Bonnie J. Leadbeater.

REFERENCES

Ainsworth, M. D. S., Blehar, M. C., Waters, E., & Wall, S. (1978). *Patterns of attachment.* Hillsdale, NJ: Erlbaum.

Armsden, G. C., & Greenberg, M. T. (1987). The Inventory of Parent and Peer Attachment: Individual differences and their relationship to psychological well-being in adolescence. *Journal of Youth and Adolescence, 16,* 427-453.

Baron, P., & Peixoto, N. (1991). Depressive symptoms in adolescents as a function of personality factors. *Journal of Youth and Adolescence, 20,* 493-500.

Beck, A. T., Epstein, N., Harrison, R. P., & Emery, G. (1983). *Development of the Sociotropy-Autonomy Scale: A measure of personality factors in psychopathology.* Unpublished manuscript, University of Pennsylvania.

Benson, M. J., Harris, P. B., & Rogers, C. S. (1992). Identity consequences of attachment to mothers and fathers among late adolescents. *Journal of Research on Adolescence, 2,* 187-204.

Bierman, K. L., & Smoot, D. L. (1991). Linking family characteristics with poor peer relations: The mediating role of conduct problems. *Journal of Abnormal Child Psychology, 19,* 341-356.

Blatt, S. J. (1990). Interpersonal relatedness and self-definition: Two personality configurations and their implications for psychopathology and psychotherapy. In J. Singer (Ed.), *Repression: Defense mechanisms and personality* (pp. 299-335). Chicago: University of Chicago Press.

Blatt, S. J. (1992). The differential effect of psychotherapy and psychoanalysis on anaclitic and introjective patients: The Menninger Psychotherapy Research Project revisited. *Journal of the American Psychoanalytic Association, 40,* 691-724.

Blatt, S. J., Hart, B., Quinlan, D. M., Leadbeater, B. J., & Auerbach, J. (1993). The relationship between dependent and self-critical depression and problem behaviors in adolescents. *Journal of Youth and Adolescence, 22,* 253-269.

Blatt, S. J., & Homann, E. (1992). Parent-child interaction in the etiology of depression. *Clinical Psychology Review, 12,* 47-91.

Blatt, S. J., & Maroudas, C. (1992). Convergence of psychoanalytic and cognitive-behavioral theories of depression. *Psychoanalytic Psychology, 9,* 157-190.

Blatt, S. J., Schaffer, C. E., Bers, S., & Quinlan, D. M. (1990). *The Adolescent Depressive Experiences Questionnaire.* Unpublished research manual, Yale University.

Blatt, S. J., Wein, S. J., Chevron, E. S., & Quinlan, D. M. (1979). Parental representation and depression in normal young adults. *Journal of Abnormal Psychology, 88,* 388-397.

Blatt, S. J., & Zuroff, D. C. (1992). Interpersonal relatedness and self-definition: Two prototypes for depression. *Clinical Psychology Review, 12,* 527-562.

Bowlby, J. (1969). *Attachment and loss: Vol. 1. Attachment.* London: Hogarth Press.

Bowlby, J. (1980). *Attachment and loss: Vol. 3. Loss: Sadness and depression.* New York: Basic Books.

Bretherton, I. (1992, May). *Internal working models of attachment and resilient coping.* Plenary address at the 22nd Annual Symposium of the Jean Piaget Society, Montréal.

Brewin, C. R., Firth-Cozens, J., Furnham, A., & McManus, C. (1992). Self-criticism in adulthood and recalled childhood experience. *Journal of Abnormal Psychology,* *101,* 561-566.

Buhrmester, D. (1990). Intimacy of friendship, interpersonal competence, and adjustment during preadolescence and adolescence. *Child Development, 61,* 1101-1111.

Cauce, A. M. (1986). Social networks and social competence: Exploring the effects of early adolescent friendships. *American Journal of Community Psychology, 14,* 607-628.

Chevron, E. S., Quinlan, D. M., & Blatt, S. J. (1978). Sex roles and gender differences in the experience of depression. *Journal of Abnormal Psychology, 87,* 680-683.

Chodorow, N. (1978). *The reproduction of mothering: Psychoanalysis and the sociology of gender.* Berkeley: University of California Press.

Collins, N. L., & Read, S. J. (1990). Adult attachment, working models, and relationship quality in dating couples. *Journal of Personality and Social Psychology, 58,* 644-663.

Compas, B. E., & Wagner, B. M. (1991). Psychosocial stress during adolescence: Intrapersonal and interpersonal processes. In M. E. Colton & S. Gore (Eds.), *Adolescent stress: Causes and consequences* (pp. 67-85). New York: Aldine/ De Gruyter.

Cummings, E. M., & Cicchetti, D. (1990). Toward a transactional model of relations between attachment and depression. In M. T. Greenberg, D. Cicchetti, & E. M. Cummings (Eds.), *Attachment in the preschool years: Theory, research, and intervention* (pp. 339-372). Chicago: University of Chicago Press.

Cushman, P. (1990). Why the self is empty. *American Psychologist, 45,* 599-611.

Daniels, D., & Moos, R. H. (1990). Assessing life stressors and social resources among adolescents: Applications to depressed youth. *Journal of Adolescent Research, 5,* 268-289.

Erikson, E. (1963). *Childhood and society* (2nd ed.). New York: Norton.

Freud, S. (1953). Three essays on the theory of sexuality. In J. Strachey (Ed. and Trans.), *The standard edition of the complete psychological works of Sigmund Freud* (Vol. 7, pp. 125-243). London: Hogarth Press. (Original work published 1905)

Furman, W., & Buhrmester, D. (1985). Children's perceptions of the personal relationships in their social networks. *Developmental Psychology, 21,* 1016-1024.

Gilligan, C. (1982). *In a different voice.* Cambridge, MA: Harvard University Press.

Gilligan, C. (1990). Remapping the moral domain: New images of the self in relationship. In C. Zanardi (Ed.), *Essential papers on the psychology of women* (pp. 480-495). New York: New York University Press.

Gilligan, C., Lyons, N. P., & Hanmer, T. J. (Eds.). (1989). *Making connections: The relational worlds of adolescent girls at Emma Willard School.* Troy, NY: Emma Willard School.

Gjerde, P. F., Block, J., & Block, J. H. (1991). The preschool family context of 18 year olds with depressive symptoms: A prospective study. *Journal of Research on Adolescence, 1,* 63-91.

Gold, M., & Yanof, D. S. (1985). Mothers, daughters, and girlfriends. *Journal of Personality and Social Psychology, 49,* 654-659.

Gotlib, I. H., Mount, J. H., Cordy, N. I., & Whiffen, N. E. (1988). Depression and perceptions of early parenting: A longitudinal investigation. *British Journal of Psychiatry, 152,* 24-27.

Hauser, S. T., Powers, S. I., & Noam, G. G. (1991). *Adolescents and their families: Paths of ego development.* New York: Free Press.

Hazan, C. (Discussant). (1992, May). *Attachment throughout life: Reworking the working model.* Symposium conducted at the meeting of the 22nd Annual Symposium of the Jean Piaget Society, Montréal.

Hazan, C., & Shaver, P. (1987). Romantic love conceptualized as an attachment process. *Journal of Personality and Social Psychology, 52,* 511-524.

Hill, J. P., & Lynch, M. E. (1983). The intensification of gender-related role expectations during early adolescence. In J. Brooks-Gunn & A. C. Petersen (Eds.), *Girls at puberty: Biological and psychosocial perspectives* (pp. 201-228). New York: Plenum.

Hunter, F. T., & Youniss, J. (1982). Changes in functions in three relations during adolescence. *Developmental Psychology, 18,* 806-811.

Jordan, J. V. (1986). *The meaning of mutuality* (Work in Progress No. 23). Wellesley, MA: Stone Center, Wellesley College.

Jordan, J. V., & Surrey, J. L. (1986). The self-in-relation: Empathy and the mother–daughter relationship. In T. Bernay & D. W. Cantor (Eds.), *The psychology of today's woman* (pp. 81-104). New York: Analytic Press.

Kaplan, A. G., Klein, R., & Gleason, N. (1985). *Women's self-development in late adolescence* (Work in Progress No. 17). Wellesley, MA: Stone Center, Wellesley College.

Kobak, R. R., & Sceery, A. (1988). Attachment in late adolescence: Working models, affect regulation, and representations of self and others. *Child Development, 59,* 135-146.

Koestner, R., Zuroff, D. C., & Powers, T. A. (1991). Family origins of adolescent self-criticism and its continuity into adulthood. *Journal of Abnormal Psychology, 100,* 191-197.

Larose, S., & Boivin, M. (1992). *Quality of parent-adolescent attachment and social adjustment among college students.* Paper presented at the 22nd Annual Symposium of the Jean Piaget Society, Montréal.

Leadbeater, B. J., Blatt, S. J., & Quinlan, D. M. (in press). Depression and problem behaviors in adolescents: Gender-linked pathways in the development of psychopathology. *Journal of Research on Adolescence.*

McCranie, E. W., & Bass, J. D. (1984). Childhood family antecedents of dependency and self-criticism: Implications for depression. *Journal of Abnormal Psychology, 93,* 3-8.

Miller, J. B. (1976). *Toward a new psychology of women.* Boston: Beacon Press.

Miller, J. B. (1990). The development of women's sense of self. In C. Zanardi (Ed.), *Essential papers on the psychology of women* (pp. 437-454). New York: New York University Press.

Miller, J. B., Jordan, J. V., Kaplan, A. G., Stiver, I. P., & Surrey, J. L. (1991). *Some misconceptions and reconceptions of a relational approach* (Work in Progress No. 49). Wellesley, MA: Stone Center, Wellesley College.

Papini, D. R., Roggman, L. A., & Anderson, J. (1991). Early-adolescent perceptions of attachment to mother and father: A test of the emotional-distancing and buffering hypotheses. *Journal of Early Adolescence, 11,* 258-275.

Parker, G., Tupling, H., & Brown, L. B. (1979). A parental bonding instrument. *British Journal of Medical Psychology, 52,* 1-10.

Petersen, A. C., Compas, B. E., & Brooks-Gunn, J. (1991). *Depression in adolescence: Implications of current research for programs and policy.* Washington, DC: Carnegie Council on Adolescent Development.

Petersen, A. C., Sarigiani, P. A., & Kennedy, R. E. (1991). Adolescent depression: Why more girls? *Journal of Youth and Adolescence, 20,* 247-272.

Ryan, R. M., & Lynch, J. H. (1989). Emotional autonomy versus detachment: Revisiting the vicissitudes of adolescence and young adulthood. *Child Development, 60,* 340-356.

Salzman, J. P. (1989). Save the world, save myself. In C. Gilligan, N. P. Lyons, & T. J. Hanmer (Eds.), *Making connections: The relational worlds of adolescent girls at Emma Willard School* (pp. 110-146). Troy, NY: Emma Willard School.

Shaver, P. R. (1992, May). *Forms of adult attachment and their cognitive emotional underpinnings.* Plenary address at the 22nd Annual Symposium of the Jean Piaget Society, Montréal.

Siddique, C. M., & D'Arcy, C. (1984). Adolescence, stress, and psychological well-being. *Journal of Youth and Adolescence, 13,* 459-473.

Sroufe, L. A., & Rutter, M. (1984). The domain of developmental psychopathology. *Child Development, 55,* 17-29.

Steinberg, L., & Silverberg, S. (1986). The vicissitudes of autonomy in adolescence. *Child Development, 57,* 841-851.

Stern, L. (1989). Conceptions of separation and connection in female adolescents. In C. Gilligan, N. P. Lyons, & T. J. Hanmer (Eds.), *Making connections: The relational worlds of adolescent girls at Emma Willard School* (pp. 73-87). Troy, NY: Emma Willard School.

Sullivan, H. S. (1953). *The interpersonal theory of psychiatry.* New York: Norton.

Surrey, J. L. (1984). *The "self-in-relation": A theory of women's development* (Work in Progress No. 2). Wellesley, MA: Stone Center, Wellesley College.

Surrey, J. L. (1987). *Relationship and empowerment* (Work in Progress No. 30). Wellesley, MA: Stone Center, Wellesley College.

Taylor, C. (1988). The moral topography of the self. In S. Messer, L. Sass, & R. Woolfolk (Eds.), *Hermeneutics and psychological theory: Interpretive perspectives on personality, psychotherapy, and psychopathology* (pp. 299-320). New Brunswick, NJ: Rutgers University Press.

Waters, E., Wippman, J., & Sroufe, L. A. (1979). Attachment, positive affect and competence in the peer group: Two studies in construct validation. *Child Development, 50,* 821-829.

Whiffen, V. E., & Sasseville, T. M. (1991). Dependency, self-criticism, and recollections of parenting: Sex-differences and the role of depressive affect. *Journal of Social and Clinical Psychology, 10,* 121-133.

Youniss, J., & Ketterlinus, R. D. (1987). Communication and connectedness in mother- and father-adolescent relationships. *Journal of Youth and Adolescence, 16,* 265-280.

Youniss, J., & Smollar, J. (1985). *Adolescent relations with mothers, fathers, and friends.* Chicago: University of Chicago Press.

Zuroff, D. C., & Fitzpatrick, D. (1989). *Romantic relationships of dependent and self-critical women.* Paper presented at the annual convention of the Eastern Psychological Association, Boston.

Zuroff, D. C., & Franko, D. L. (1986). *Depressed and test anxious students' interactions with friends: Effects of dependency and self-criticism.* Paper presented at the annual convention of the Eastern Psychological Association, New York.

CHAPTER 7

Anxious Romantic Attachment in Adult Relationships

CARL G. HINDY

J. CONRAD SCHWARZ

Our research over the past 10 years has focused on three attachment phenomena that appear to map a domain of experience popularly referred to as "lovesickness" (Hindy & Schwarz, 1984, 1985; Hindy, Schwarz, & Brodsky, 1989). The first of these is "anxious romantic attachment," which can be described as insecurity, emotional dependency, and "clinging" in love relationships. This has been of primary interest to us, and required the development of an assessment instrument. The second, "sexual jealousy," can be broadly defined as the matrix of thoughts, feelings, and behaviors occurring when one perceives a valued sexual attachment to be threatened by an interloper. The third, "postrelationship depression," involves the reaction to the loss of a valued sexual or potentially sexual relationship. We have regarded these three variables as akin to barometers placed at three key points in a romantic relationship: They have been used to measure the character of the attachment at the beginning or early phases of a relationship, when one faces the unknown reactions of a potential partner; later, when the existing relationship is threatened or stressed; and finally, when the relationship ends and the object of attachment is lost.

This research has uncovered some of the situational and interpersonal relationship determinants of these "lovesickness" reactions. However, more importantly, it has demonstrated the heuristic value of an attachment perspective, in which they are viewed as adult manifestations of an underlying attachment system rooted in familial childhood experiences. By focusing on individual differences in people's proneness to these reactions, it has shown how they can be viewed as interrelated at a deeper level, with trait-like qualities understandable in light of early developmental experiences. Only selected aspects centering around the construct of anxious romantic attachment are presented in this chapter, to demonstrate the potential yield of continued research from this attachment theory perspective. Focusing upon this construct also accentuates the considerable overlap with other research cited in this volume. For example, it overlaps considerably with the largest category of recent attachment research, which postulates "anxious/ambivalent attachment" as an adult relationship style carried forth from early, insecure mother-infant attachment (e.g., Bartholomew, 1990; Bartholomew & Horowitz, 1991; Brennan, Shaver, & Tobey, 1991; Feeney & Noller, 1990, 1991; Hazan & Shaver, 1987, 1990; Kobak & Hazan, 1991; Pistole, 1989; Shaver & Hazan, 1988). It also points to a convergence with the constructs of "desperate love" and "fusional relations," which are derived from psychoanalytic theory and relevant to increasingly popular object relations theories (e.g., Sperling, 1985, 1988, 1989; Sperling & Berman, 1991).

The Anxious Romantic Attachment Scale (see Appendix 7.1) was developed through rational, item-analytic, and construct-validational approaches to scale development. With several different samples of college students and young adults, the scale has demonstrated high internal consistency for both males and females. It is not correlated with the Marlowe-Crowne Social Desirability Scale, and, as evidenced by its pattern of discriminant validity, appears to be free from acquiesence response set. Item statistics show that respondents make good use of the long, Likert-type scales, with item responses and total scale scores well centered and normally distributed. Scale scores range quite broadly, with no sex differences found.

In the first investigation to be described here, male college students completed the scale on their "two most typical or most representative past relationships." In the second, main investigation, older participants of both sexes were asked to complete it about their "four most important past relationships." It is important to note that we have not relied on just one completion, because we want to get at people's tendency to have a pattern of such relationships. By prompting participants to report on salient relationships, and taking an average across multiple completions, we believe that we are getting at something that better represents their dating or romantic relationships as a whole. This average across relationships is what we have referred to as "tendency toward anxious romantic attachments" (TTARAT; Hindy & Schwarz, 1984).

THE FIRST INVESTIGATION

A total of 133 unmarried undergraduate males volunteered for the first study, which was presented as "an investigation of the getting-acquainted process." They attended a questionnaire session and, several months later, an experimental session. In the first session, participants spent approximately 2 hours completing reports of their parents' child-rearing behaviors, as well as several measures of personality variables converging on the concept of self-esteem. In addition to general information about their dating histories, they provided more detailed information on each of their "two most typical or representative past relationships," including a measure of romantic love, the Anxious Romantic Attachment Scale, and depression inventories to assess the magnitude of their depression when each relationship ended.

Of these 133 men, 124 returned later in the college semester to participate in the experimental session. In this "getting-acquainted" segment, each was presented with a clipboard at the top of which was a Polaroid photo of a woman the subject would be getting to know. Subjects were led to believe that the woman was also a research volunteer and that her picture had just been taken upon her arrival. They completed measures of their mood and their expectations in anticipation of meeting the woman. Then each subject was brought to an interviewing room where, in order to get acquainted, he was left alone with her for 10 minutes. Afterward each subject completed the measures of moods and expectations again, which allowed us to assess changes resulting from the encounter. Unbeknownst to the men, the attractive women with whom they had met were experimental accomplices who previously had been instructed to act in a warm and interested manner toward the men or, alternatively, in a cool and indifferent manner. The men were randomly assigned to one or the other condition and the accomplices were also rotated between the two roles on a random schedule.

Experiential and Relationship Correlates, and Family Antecedents

Looking first at correlations of TTARAT with other variables from the questionnaire session, we found the following. On the general dating variables, participants scoring higher on TTARAT did not differ in their frequency of dating in the past year, or in their rating of overall dating enjoyment. However, during the same year they dated more different women, more frequently believed that they were "in love," experienced this love earlier in the relationships, felt it more intensely, and declared their love ("said 'I love you'") to more of their dating partners. Looking at their "two most typical past relationships," on which we had obtained more focused data, we found that they had spent more time on the telephone with these partners, but that they had not actually spent more time with them face to face. They reported stronger feelings for their partners, both at the time of the first date and at the strongest point (the emotional zenith) of each relationship. However, at these two points the strength of their feelings was not correlated with their estimates of how strongly their partners felt about them. During these relationships, compared with men scoring lower on TTARAT, men who scored higher on TTARAT experienced far more intense positive states (such as euphoria and heightened sense of personal worth) *and also* negative states (such as depression and anxiety, agitation and restlessness, and emotional instability). The higher a man's score on TTARAT, the greater the likelihood that a relationship ultimately was terminated by the woman, and the stronger the postrelationship depression.

In sum, these data seem consistent with the clinical impression of the anxiously romantically attached person as one who overly invests his or her emotions in a relationship. He or she attempts to secure reciprocation and to stabilize relationships by extensive contact and with declarations of affection. More than others, anxiously attached individuals experience relationships as more imbalanced or unrequited, and throughout their relationships have roller-coaster-like mood swings. Ultimately, and despite their wishes, the relationships end, and they have a very difficult time coping with the loss.

Next, we looked at the general self-esteem measures (generalized expectations for affection, generalized expectations for success in life, social distress and fears of negative evaluation, and overall dating anxiety). We found that chronically low or chronically high expectations for love and affection, or chronically high or low self-evaluations, were not the keys to understanding anxious romantic attachment. We hypothesized that it would be *unpredictable* parental affection in childhood and the resulting lack of stable expectations—the lack of a clear "internal working model"—that would render these men prone to emotional vicissitudes and fluctuating self-esteem in their later love lives. Nonetheless, these same men might feel quite confident about themselves in other areas. Consistent with this hypothesis, men high on TTARAT did not distinguish themselves on the global, static (i.e., one-time) attributes such as those assessed with these measures. Standard deviations were consistently higher on these measures for such men, but there were no significant correlations with TTARAT. This was a notable finding also in further establishing the discriminant validity of our TTARAT measure and its relative freedom from response sets.

Looking next at information that subjects higher on TTARAT provided on their parents' earlier child-rearing behaviors, we found that they perceived their mothers and fathers as more love-inconsistent. When all of the parenting measures were used in a post hoc attempt to construct the best statistical model to predict later TTARAT, the best multiple-regression models were ones in which one parent (either mother or father) was highly possessive of the child, while the other parent was love-inconsistent.

In the experimental session premeasures of emotions, men scoring high on TTARAT distinguished themselves from men scoring low. Overall, as they awaited meeting the attractive woman, their emotions were more negative, suggesting that they found the uncertainty (i.e., the fear of rejection) to be especially stressful. They were higher on measures of concentration, surgency, anxiety, and especially aggression: A fight-or-flight emotional pattern seemed to exist for these men. Although TTARAT was not correlated with positive versus negative expectations prior to meeting the woman, these expectation scores did have a greater standard deviation for high-TTARAT men, indicating that their expectations were spread more widely in anticipation of what for them was apparently a greater unknown.

Warm versus cold treatment by a woman had a notably different impact on men who were prone to anxious romantic attachments. After warm treatment by a woman, men scoring higher on TTARAT had a greater surge of positive mood and a greater increase in their expectations. However, after being treated coolly by a woman, the high-TTARAT men decreased their expectations but reported the same mood that they reported prior to meeting the woman. By contrast, subjects lower on TTARAT reported what would "normally" be expected: worsened mood *and* decreased expectations following cool treatment. In fact, for these men, the decrease following the cool treatment was quite similar in magnitude to the increase following the warm treatment. Thus, it seems that subjects prone to anxious romantic attachments were aware cognitively that they had not been well received since they lowered their expectations; however, they protected themselves emotionally. This is interesting because it jibes with clinical descriptions of anxiously romantically attached individuals: They ratchet their emotions upward with each sign of affection received, and they are very difficult for unwilling partners to discourage. If the high-TTARAT men in this study took signs of affection strongly to heart, while ignoring rebuffs, one can begin to understand how they might start down the path toward another anxious romantic attachment.

THE SECOND INVESTIGATION

These encouraging results from the first study left us wishing for both more extensive and intensive data, to assess more variables with increased reliability, in order to further articulate situational and personality correlates as well as childhood antecedents of TTARAT. This wish was grandly fulfilled by linking this project to the ongoing study of family dynamics and late adolescent psychopathology being conducted by Schwarz at the University of Connecticut. The Family Dynamics Study, then nearing completion, provided an enviable data base in which 369 students of both sexes in their freshman year of college had already completed an exhaustive set of questionnaires and psychological tests. In addition, each student's mother, father, a sister or brother, and a college roommate or best friend had filled out many parallel measures about their observations of the student and the student's family. All family respondents had contributed their perspectives on such issues as mother's and father's child-rearing behaviors and personalities, the parents' marital adjustment, and the degree to which either parent exerted a dominant influence over the child. The student and the sister or brother also rated the closeness of the student's relationship with each parent, and the two parents rated their own and each other's personalities. The student's college roommate or best friend provided still another, independent source of data about various attributes of the student, once again on many of the same instruments. (A listing of the major instruments, and raters/informants for each, can be found in Appendix 7.2.) Aggregating these multiple reports across informants, and combining variables into more robust factors, made it possible to obtain more reliable, generalizable indices of family background and personality. By conducting a follow-up study of the same students, we could bring these data, less clouded by the problems of single scales and isolated self-reports, to bear on the attachment variables of interest to us. (For readers interested in this aggregation strategy, there is a body of literature that discusses and demonstrates its significance and potential yield, while underscoring the limitations of traditional single-source measurements [e.g., Rushton, Brainerd, & Pressley, 1983; Schwarz, Barton-Henry, & Pruzinsky, 1985; Schwarz & Mearns, 1989; Wachs, 1987]. Especially relevant are the papers coauthored by Schwarz, which use the same data base to dramatically demonstrate the incremental gains obtained in assessing parental child-rearing behavior as the number of raters/informants is increased.)

We were successful in following up 66% of the former participants in the Family Dynamics Study. A total of 244 young adults, who by then were college seniors or recent college graduates, agreed to complete additional attachment measures. Because they were now older and had had more dating experience, it was possible to expand on the strategy of data collection on multiple relationships, pioneered in the first investigation. Hence the subjects were asked to provide data on their "four most important past romantic relationships." For each relationship they answered the 33 questions of the Anxious Romantic Attachment Scale, which were averaged to give a score on TTARAT. Other questions included how long each relationship lasted, whether or not it was exclusive, how intensely the partners felt about each other, and how much time they spent together. Each participant was asked to rate his or her romantic partners on certain key characteristics, and to report on a wide range of emotions that he or she might have experienced in the course of each relationship. With regard to each relationship, a subject also completed a measure of romantic jealousy and a depression inventory modified to retrospectively assess depression at the time the relationship ended.

Although the Anxious Romantic Attachment Scale once again showed high internal consistency (alpha coefficients > .90), orthogonal factor rotation allowed us to tease out two clear factors. Therefore, we decided to decompose TTARAT into two subscores in this study. With unit weighting, we summed the items loading highest on each factor to create separate subscales, which we labeled Romantic Anxiety and Romantic Obsession. The items comprising each subscale are indicated in Appendix 7.1, and their differing nature is evident. The Romantic Anxiety factor seems to tap feelings of anxiety and fear, indicated by the underlying lack of confidence and repeated questioning of the partner's affections and continued availability. The Romantic Obsession factor captures the consuming preoccupation with the partner and the relationship, to the neglect of other people, interests, and responsibilities in the person's life. It is statistically evident, but also quite obvious, that these overlap and generally occur together. But the distinction seemed interesting on practical grounds, since people who score high on TTARAT, as well as those presenting for counseling, sometimes experience obsession more strongly than anxiety or vice versa. It seemed interesting on theoretical grounds as well, because it overlaps in interesting ways with Bartholomew's more recent distinction between "fearful" and "preoccupied" styles of adult attachment (Bartholomew, 1990; Bartholemew & Horowitz, 1991). Hence we decided to aggregate these variables across relationships to gauge participants' tendencies toward each, and carry them forward into our statistical analyses. As it turned out, they showed similar patterns of correlations with other variables, but some illuminating differences encourage further pursuit along these lines.

Experiential and Relationship Correlates

First to be noted among the findings was the expected interrelationship among the "barometers" of the attachment system—namely, that people high on TTARAT were clearly more prone to sexual jealousy and postrelationship depression. The strong correlation of TTARAT with postrelationship depression replicated a finding of the first study. Separating TTARAT into the two factors revealed that the Romantic Obsession factor was especially predictive of depression when the relationships ended. It makes sense that a more consuming attachment, in which a person's outer and inner lives are more highly interwoven with the partner, would predict greater depression upon severance of the tie. Romantic Anxiety was less predictive of postrelationship depression than was Romantic Obsession, especially for women. The lesser impact of Romantic Anxiety may be attributable to a partially compensating sense of relief that the emotional roller-coaster ride had come to an end, or perhaps the Romantic Anxiety component was less indicative of the strength of attachment; both these factors may affect the sexes differentially. The compensating sense of relief may be less for men than for women. A man's failure to "win" a woman's commitment and the loss of "control," even in the face of a lesser attachment, may be more ego-threatening or unearthing of earlier narcissistic injuries in a way that seems more characteristic of male development. Men may suffer a greater loss of masculine self-worth, pride, and the like, which is less a function of the magnitude of the foregone attachment, whereas for women the loss of the attachment itself may be more important. In our book (Hindy et al., 1989) we discuss this at greater length, along with other data supporting two types of postrelationship depression: grieving depression and self-punishing depression.

The findings for sexual jealousy seemed to parallel those for depression. Jealousy, while correlated with TTARAT, was more strongly correlated with the Romantic Obsession component than with the Romantic Anxiety component, especially for women. Overall, for both men and women, jealousy was experienced more intensely by those who expressed stronger attachment to highly valued partners (i.e., Romantic Obsession) than those who felt more anxious about their partners. But for men the distinction was somewhat less. This is consistent with what clinicians more typically hear from men who are suddenly alarmed at the possibility of interlopers, yet previously did not seem obsessed with their partners. Often to their partners' dismay, these men may seem more concerned with securing or controlling relationships than with fully embracing them or enjoying them; when faced with the threat, they state, "I didn't know what I had until now, when I might lose it!" Though it is beyond the scope of the present chapter, in our book (Hindy et al., 1989) we have theorized a typology of jealousy that parallels our typology of depression. The jealousy typology is supported by data suggesting that romantic relationships fulfill different patterns of needs for different people, and therefore give rise to different patterns of emotions when those relationships are threatened in jealousy situations.

Returning to our examination of the correlates of TTARAT, we found that both men and women high on TTARAT experienced a wide range of emotions with significantly greater intensity. They had more intense positive emotions of joy, interest, and sexual arousal, but also more extreme negative emotions of distress, fear, shame, anger, contempt, and disgust. Most strongly correlated with TTARAT was the measure of distress—assessed with the rating scale adjectives of "downhearted," "sad," "miserable," and "discouraged"—indicating the negative side of greater passion. The positive emotions of joy, interest, and sexual arousal were more strongly associated with the Romantic Obsession aspect of TTARAT, whereas anger and shame were more strongly associated with the Romantic Anxiety factor. There were some differences between the men and women that are consistent with clinical observations and cultural stereotypes. For example, among men there was a stronger link between TTARAT scores (especially the Romantic Anxiety factor) and outer-directed emotions, with the more insecure men expressing greater anger, contempt, and disgust toward their partners. Women seemed more inclined to turn the insecurities inward; more insecure women had stronger experiences of fear and guilt. The correlations with feelings of sexual arousal were stronger for women than for men. Sexual arousal was more strongly correlated with Romantic Obsession for women than for men, and was correlated with Romantic Anxiety only for women. Participants' reports of the extent of sexual activity with their partners followed the same pattern. The young women who were more sexually involved in relationships in which they ultimately were disappointed experienced considerably more shame. These data are consistent with the general observation that sexuality is not so closely tied to love for young men in our culture, whereas for women it requires and constitutes a greater investment in a relationship, and therefore is more strongly linked to the strength of the attachment and the fear of losing it.

The frequency of contact between partners, the length of the relationship, and relationship intensity (frequency of contact × length of relationship) all had strong positive correlations with Romantic Obsession, but were uncorrelated with Romantic Anxiety. By contrast, imbalances in expectations about relationship parameters, and imbalances of affection, were the strongest predictors of Romantic Anxiety. For example, if the subject was dating the partner exclusively but the partner was seeing others, the Romantic Anxiety score ran very high. Of all the relationship variables assessed, by far the strongest predictor of Romantic Anxiety was a variable labeled "love inequity": the greater the subject's own love than the partner's love, then the greater the magnitude of Romantic Anxiety.

Recall that we asked participants to rate each of their four romantic partners on 10 personal characteristics. Factor analysis of these 10 characteristics resulted in three very clear factors: Prospects for Success, Social Appeal, and Emotional Responsiveness. Prospects for Success included socioeconomic status, prospects for success in life, and intelligence. Physical attractiveness, popularity with peers, and self-assurance loaded most highly on Social Appeal. The third factor, Emotional Responsiveness, was comprised of the characteristics of emotional consistency, trustworthiness, generosity, and warmth.

We found that a subject's Romantic Obsession score correlated most strongly with the partner's Social Appeal score, and that among items on that factor, physical attractiveness was the most important. Perhaps in addition to the physiologically arousing aspects of a physically attractive partner, the social appeal of a partner indexed the self-esteem reward value of the partner to the subject. The correlations between Romantic Obsession and partner's attractiveness were slightly stronger for men than for women. For women, but not for men, the Romantic Obsession score had a low but significant correlation with the partner's score on Prospects for Success. These sex differences are consistent with the widely held beliefs that partners' physical attractiveness is more important to men, and that partners' achievement potential is more important to women because of its impact on lifestyle and family security. We found that a subject's Romantic Anxiety score was more strongly correlated than the Romantic Obsession score with the partner's Emotional Responsiveness score. This was a very strong negative correlation: The lower the partner's Emotional Responsiveness, the greater the participant's Romantic Anxiety. It comes as no surprise, then, that the highest levels of TTARAT occurred when a vulnerable person became attached to a partner who was outwardly very attractive but emotionally fickle.

Childhood and Family Antecedents

We now turn our attention to the person source of variance—the attachment system and our findings about childhood antecedents. Our data suggest several different family background patterns related to later insecurity in romantic love relationships. The most commonly occurring configurations are presented and discussed here. Although there were different modal patterns for sons versus daughters, each was likely to be found among both sexes. The patterns were also somewhat different for Romantic Anxiety versus Romantic Obsession, giving a little more insight into this distinction. Common to all of these configurations was the impact upon a child's emerging mental representation of love relationships. It can be seen how children growing up within such family systems would fail to develop stable expectations for love and affection. Lacking this internalized ballast, they became prone to the emotional buffeting, ego inflation and deflation, fear, and defensive patterns that we found to exist in their later love relationships.

The "family portraits" described below may seem like clinical case histories—the familiar unstructured accounts given by patients to their therapists during the troubling upheavels for which the patients are seeking help. They are not, and therefore avoid some sources of bias well known to exist in the case history approach. Instead, we have reconstructed them from the convergence in our multiple-respondent data base, using multivariate statistical techniques to discern commonalities amidst the large amount of quantitative, retrospective data. Although they may sound like those depicted in the burgeoning popular psychology of dysfunctional families, there is another important distinction. In that popular literature, one typically reads of very troubled individuals who are coming to terms with family backgrounds of severe discord, including alcoholism, marital violence, child abuse and neglect, divorce, stepfamilies, and various traumatic family circumstances. In those more extreme cases, readers may easily conclude, "Of course these kids are going to have problems when they grow up." Indeed, in the most deviant cases one would expect numerous variables, both relevant and irrelevant, to deviate from the norm. Our data, by contrast, show that even comparatively subtle developmental forces, such as parents' attitudes and disciplinary behaviors toward children, the degree of the parents' marital happiness, and coalitions within an intact family, can have an important impact on the later love relationships of the offspring. Even people from outwardly "normal" families, who seem to be functioning well in other regards, can experience insecurity in love relationships which is correlated with earlier family factors. (For example, a prerequisite for participation in the Family Dynamics Study was that each family had to have remained intact at least until a participant's 16th birthday, and that both parents and a sibling could be contacted and would agree to cooperate with participation. The participants themselves were college seniors or recent college graduates, implying that they and their families had certain means and competence to attain this status at a state university.) Therefore we speak in terms of developmental forces rather than "traumas," and of personality and relationship patterns rather than frank psychopathology; we encourage other researchers to pursue similarly reliable and robust means of retrospective data collection that permit these to be studied coherently. Finally, the family systems nature of our findings, which include the important but often neglected role of fathers (e.g., Phares, 1992), underscores the urgent need for researchers to look beyond the impact of "bad mothering."

The Origins of Insecure Love: Daughters

Overall, for women who scored high on TTARAT, it appears that their childhood homes were below average in providing emotional security, stability, and caring warmth and concern. Their fathers were experienced as more hostile–either in a controlling and fault-finding manner, which could cause these young women to doubt their ability to secure the affections of men, or in a rejecting and neglecting way, which might result in an emotional void and strong need for compensatory relationships with men. Their parents' marital relationships were significantly more troubled than average, which probably had direct effects on their personality development, as well as indirect effects through the distortion of family alliances and boundaries. Their mothers were more lax in exerting parental control, structure, and guidance. Some of these mothers were notably passive and incapable of sheltering the girls from the fathers' hostility, while others overcompensated in an emotionally overinvolved, pampering-to-please way that magnified the rift between daughters and their fathers, and can be viewed as a model of the enmeshed, dependent relationships that these girls would later establish with men. The best predictors of a daughter's later emotional security in a love relationship were found to be a warm and satisfactory parental relationship, a close emotional bond with the father, and a combination of parental firmness and nurturance. However, a daughter scoring high on TTARAT experienced the opposite pattern: disengagement and dissatisfaction in the parents' marriage, a chasm between daughter and father, excessive discipline and control from one parent, and a blurring of the parent–child role distinctions and lack of guidance from the mother. Somewhat different family types were found for women scoring high in Romantic Anxiety versus Romantic Obsession.

High Romantic Anxiety. In Table 7.1 are summary variables describing the type of family background found most frequently for a woman scoring high on Romantic Anxiety. There was a high level of conflict between the parents; while the father might sublimate his discontent into work and other pursuits, the mother was especially dissatisfied with the marriage. The father was seen as hostile, and his negativity pervaded the family life. He did not maintain an emotional bond with the daughter; meanwhile, the mother, much more lax and yielding, formed a coalition with her daughter against the father.

In this type of family, both the mother and the daughter were unhappy with the father and seemed to form one side of a divided family. Although the mother and daughter found themselves on the same "side," their degree of emotional bonding, and the mutuality of their alliance, were less clear. For the most romantically anxious women and their mothers, the coalition seemed to be less of an emotional bond than a mutually self-protective alliance against the fathers. Often such a daughter was parentified, and was bolstering and protecting a mother who could not hold her ground with the father. Alternatively, the mother might be too weak and passive to oppose the father, and too fearful to form an alliance with

TABLE 7.1. Summary Variables Characterizing the Family
Background of a Daughter Who as an Adult Scored High on
Proneness to Romantic Anxiety

Parents' personality and child-rearing traits:
Father hostile and controlling
Mother lax in disciplining daughter

Parents' marital relationship:
Marital conflict and dissatisfaction (mother especially dissatisfied)
Father dissatisfied with mother's communication style

Daughter's relationships with parents:
Daughter not emotionally attached to father
Daughter in coalition with mother

the daughter that might bring about greater repercussions later on. Regardless, the unfortunate net result was that the daughter failed to establish with either parent the necessary relationship of firm guidance and nurturance.

Considering how daughters generally see less of their fathers than their mothers, it is notable how these fathers' characteristics had such a great impact. It suggests that the father–daughter relationship is in some ways prototypical of later heterosexual relationships. It may shape a girl's mental representations of men and relationships, especially her initial expectations of warmth and reliable attachment or rejection and inconsistency from men. In the type of family that caused a daughter to score high later on Romantic Anxiety, these expectations were shaped by a father who enforced unrealistically high standards with punitive criticism. Yet, as even the most rejecting father attempted at times to "make it up to the daughter"—whether as a function of his guilt feelings or his vacillating moods—confusing inconsistency was the likely end result. Not surprisingly, such a father also scored high on the measure of love inconsistency. Anxiety may have been instilled in the daughter through this combination of uncertainty and painful consequences, much as early laboratory studies with animals created "experimental neurosis." Transported into the daughter's adult romantic relationships, this could result in pervasive insecurity about her ability to please men, and to obtain and maintain affection. A young woman's mental representation of men and relationships might be envisioned as a photographic plate that has developed a sharp image through consistent and steady exposure during a broad critical period of childhood. In this type of family, the shifts and fluctuations in the images projected back to the daughter might cause a blurring of the image, which, once set, would be difficult to change.

High Romantic Obsession. In Table 7.2, the summary variables are listed that characterized the type of family most often leading to a high score on Romantic Obsession for a daughter. Because high Romantic Obsession was generally found along with high Romantic Anxiety, the similarities with Table 7.1 are not surprising. However, the subtle differences make intuitive sense. In regard to instilling high Romantic Obsession, the father's overt rejection seems to have been more important. The daughter was cut off from a relationship with the father. The mother was also cut off, as indicated by the marital relationship variables, which indicated low marital adjustment but not much marital conflict or concern for communication. Neither mother nor daughter had much sense of relationship or connectedness with the father. This was different from the family prototype for high Romantic Anxiety, where the father was very controlling yet still very involved. There the mother maintained a "conflict-habituated" relationship, with the resulting anger, tension, and anxiety, rather than face a relationship void; the daughter likewise tried repeatedly to win over the father, while acquiring expectancies for emotional punishment in relationships with men. In the family prototype for high Romantic Obsession, the parents had emotionally disengaged, and the daughter had already lost her hopes for the relationship and sense of connectedness with her father. The coalition with the mother was more of a consolation or substitute gratification, rather than an alliance in struggling with the father. (Whereas relationships and connectedness are very important for the establishment of self-esteem in female adolescents, instrumental achievement and masculine adequacy seem to be the counterparts for adolescent males. Consistent with this, it can be seen below that frustrations and losses in regard to achievement recognition and respect were central in the family prototype for sons' high Romantic Anxiety and Romantic Obsession.)

TABLE 7.2. Summary Variables
Characterizing the Family Background of
a Daughter Who as an Adult Scored High
on Proneness to Romantic Obsession

Parents' personality and child-rearing traits:
    Father hostile and rejecting
    Mother lax in disciplining daughter

Parents' marital relationship:
    Low marital adjustment

Daughter's relationships with parents:
    Daughter not emotionally attached to father
    Daughter in coalition with mother

To the extent that a daughter lacked this important sense of relationship with her father, she might bring to adult romantic relationships the needy, wish-fulfilling, "in love with love" qualities that characterize the romantically obsessed. Although she might yearn to have a man's love, her first-hand experience during her critical developmental years was limited. She experienced her mother's love, but might assume that a man's love would magnificently transcend it. Her "photographic plate" might see the light only of her fantasies—romantic imagery constructed from fairy tales and other idealized observations.

The Origins of Insecure Love: Sons

Some men who scored high on TTARAT had parents with high expectations, especially when it came to achieving outward success, status, and recognition. Yet these parents were described as cold and domineering, and not providing the emotional support—the encouragement, acceptance, warmth, and affection—necessary for these sons to develop the self-confidence to pursue such lofty goals comfortably, or to feel secure and take pleasure in their accomplishments. One can imagine them kept in a state of perpetual anxiety because of unfulfilled parental expectations, developing a pattern of self-doubt, and emerging unable to assert their worthiness.

Other men scoring high on TTARAT had parents who appeared to be at the opposite extreme: very warm and loving, easy-going, lavishing acceptance and approval upon their sons, and allowing them relatively free rein and self-direction. However, the impact of these indiscriminately approving parents may not have been so different from that of parents who were uncompromising and nonsupportive. Indiscriminate approval connotes a lack of concern for standards, as well as a failure to provide adequate criteria for performance. It may have denied the sons the opportunity to obtain the meaningful feedback, genuinely validating approval, and realistic internalized standards necessary for self-confidence. Both parenting styles were deficient in what we found to be crucial for the sons' later emotional security: firmness and love, challenge and support.

A general sex difference previously noted was that family factors for daughters tended to focus on interpersonal relationships, whereas for men they hinged more upon achievement and self-confidence. Consistent with this observation, it can be seen that the parents' marital adjustment did not emerge as a significant determinant of insecurity in sons, whereas it was tremendously important for daughters.

High Romantic Anxiety. Table 7.3 lists parental characteristics that were found to contribute in a cumulative way to a high score on Romantic Anxiety in a son. Such parents were rated as demanding and control-

TABLE 7.3.   Summary Variables Characterizing the Family Background of a Son Who as an Adult Scored High on Proneness to Romantic Anxiety

Father		
Achievement-controlling, non-nurturant, and/or hostile, rejecting	*combined with*	Dominant, nonpermissive

Mother		
Intellectually stimulating, autonomous, non-nurturant, and/or rejecting, critical	*combined with*	Assertive, nonpermissive

ling, and portrayed as pressuring their sons to surpass others in achievements, especially those of an intellectual nature. Both mothers and fathers apparently shared a narcissistic need to project images of ambition and successful outward appearances, and seemed to expect the same of their sons. Fathers were likely to enforce this with punitive means, and neither mothers nor fathers extended warmth, affection, empathy, or nurturance.

Sons were found to have higher levels of Romantic Anxiety if their fathers were dominant in combination with achievement-controlling, and the mothers were autonomous and assertive. "Dominant" in this usage means that the fathers were especially likely to use psychological means of control (such as instilling guilt and anxiety), to press for achievement, to punish failure, and to maintain the high level of orderliness that they expected. In doing so, it seems that they transmitted their own self-punitive styles, inferiority complexes, and defensiveness to their sons. For example, the personality indices showed these fathers to be cool, controlled, and rational so long as things were proceeding according to their own wishes, but prone to aggressive and seemingly irrational outbursts if they were challenged or if control was usurped. When their sons challenged their authority, they would ventilate their frustations upon the sons in an attempt to regain control. Because sons were more likely to be romantically anxious if their mothers were autonomous and assertive, it is likely that these sons witnessed their fathers going through greater control struggles with their wives as well. The sons may have learned through direct modeling some of the controlling behaviors later evident in their romantic relationships. The panic and rage of an anxiously attached man when his romantic partner asserted her autonomy in a threatening way, or in the extreme case tried to withdraw from him, resulted in the son's "instant replay" of Dad's behavior.

The highest levels of Romantic Anxiety were seen when parents, in addition to the above-described characteristics, would go so far as to act in rejecting ways toward their sons. Most troubling was the configuration in which a father was hostile and detached from a son, while the mother was highly critical and love-inconsistent, or rejecting of him.

In sum, we can envision the romantically anxious man as coming from a family that traded fiercely in the commodity of approval. At times the parents may have glorified him and basked in his accomplishments, but only so long as he continued to meet their exacting standards. Although high levels of achievement often may have resulted, the son was motivated by fear of failure and punishment, rather than by concrete rewards, praise, and the inherent pleasure of mastery. This negative motivation, and the need to prove himself repeatedly or risk failure and humiliation, could become an ongoing theme in the son's life. His mental representations of love relationships might take on the same coloration, as yet another class of psychological situations involving achievement versus failure, love/approval versus shame/humiliation. Thus, the romantically anxious man worried about whether he would pass or fail the courting test, for rejection, to him, was a mark of failure. For the son who experienced repeated rejection by his parents, the loss of a love partner might be tantamount to the feared irretrievable loss of his acceptability, dignity, and sense of self-worth.

High Romantic Obsession. The parental characteristics summarized in Table 7.4 represent one of two family patterns found to correlate with a high score on Romantic Obsession in a son. Many of these are the same characteristics described above as causing high Romantic Anxiety in a son; this is to be expected, because this type of young man (unlike the second type described below) was also high on Romantic Anxiety. The father was achievement-oriented and controlling, whereas the mother emphasized the intellectual development of the son and was strict, critical, and rejecting. Both parents were low on both nurturance and permissiveness.

These findings give the impression that deficiencies of love and affection caused these sons to crave emotional acceptance, while acquired fears

TABLE 7.4. Summary Variables Characterizing One Possible Family Background of a Son Who as an Adult Scored High on Proneness to Romantic Obsession

	Father	
Achievement-controlling, non-nurturant	*combined with*	Firm, nonpermissive
	Mother	
Intellectually stimulating non-nurturant, and/or rejecting, critical, strict	*combined with*	Firm, nonpermissive

of disapproval and rejection left them prone to high Romantic Obsession and Romantic Anxiety. Furthermore, the criticisms and rejections of their youth seem to have caused a negative self-concept and a dependency upon the feedback of others in order to feel good about themselves. The strength of their Romantic Obsession therefore reflected their need, or wish, for a woman who would love them abundantly. In their relationships with women, they acted as if the women should somehow provide compensation for their earlier deprivations, prove them lovable, and keep inflated their sagging self-esteem.

Table 7.5 presents the summary characteristics of the second type of family that led to a high Romantic Obsession score in a son. It is striking that these characteristics are diametrically opposite to those in the first type. These were exceedingly nurturant and permissive parents, who scored very low on the negative attributes of being demanding, controlling, or rejecting. Although the sons emerging from these families scored very high on Romantic Obsession, they did not score high on Romantic Anxiety. Also, they differed in other notable ways from those of the first family type. These men were highly conforming, scored among the lowest on drug and alcohol use, and appeared to be very inhibited and socially isolated. They were heterosexually avoidant and had very little dating or sexual experience; when they did have romantic liaisons, these tended to be brief.

One gets the impression that these families esconced their sons in a cocoon of love and support. In so doing, they may have insulated their sons from the challenges and stressors from which self-confidence develops, failed to provide needed criteria for success or failure, and instead provided such ease and comfort that the separation/individuation process was impeded. These families seem to have been socially insular or peripheral, and unable to provide the sons with an accurate working model for life outside of the home. They were apparently deficient in their ability to convey the social knowledge and skills needed for success outside the home, and did not provide role models of self-confident assertiveness. Therefore the sons, lacking the skills and courage to venture

TABLE 7.5. Summary Variables Characterizing Another Possible Family Background of a Son Who as an Adult Scored High on Proneness to Romantic Obsession

	Father	
Nurturant	*combined with*	Permissive
	Mother	
Nurturant and/or nonrejecting, noncritical	*combined with*	Permissive

outside of the home and to pursue romantic relationships appropriately, might resort to romantic fantasies as wish fulfillment. Their brief forays with women were heavily colored by fantasy; hence their high Romantic Obsession.

Other Findings and Future Directions

Because of space limitations, we cannot discuss several additional research findings and methodological issues that have emerged. For example, what about the people who scored among the lowest on the Anxious Romantic Attachment Scale, virtually denying any and all experiences that could be classified as Romantic Anxiety or Romantic Obsession? We found similar family patterns associated with this, suggesting that at a deeper level these individuals might be quite similar to those at the other extreme. By avoidance and emotional distancing, they may have found another (albeit limiting) means of coping with their deficient or distorted mental representations of attachment relationships. The low-scoring pattern was far more prevalent for men than for women. We have conjectured that they manifest the adult counterpart of "avoidance," the other category of insecure attachment described by Ainsworth and her collegues in studying mother–infant attachment. Similarly, we found family patterns that seemed to predispose individuals to greater experiences of jealousy when relationships were threatened, and to greater depression when attachments were broken. Although long-term follow-up and longitudinal studies will ultimately be needed to fully exploit the implications of attachment theory for adult relationships, our data seem to coalesce in encouraging ways with the now substantial body of research that has emerged since the mid-1980s.

Appendix 7.1. Anxious Romantic Attachment Scale

0_____1_____2_____3_____4_____5_____6_____7_____8
Not a   Definitely
all true;   true; agree
disagree   completely
completely

o   (1)   I felt that if ____ rejected me, I might never get over it.
o   (2)   I spent much time analyzing my relationship with ____, weighing it in my mind.
o   (3)   While I was dating ____, I had little desire to see other women (men).
o   (4)   From the beginning, I was eager to see ____ almost every day.

(continued)

Appendix 7.1. (*continued*)

0____1____2____3____4____5____6____7____8

Not at	Definitely
all true;	true; agree
disagree	completely
completely	

o	(5)	I would often lie awake at night thinking about being with ____.
a	(6)	"She (he) loves me, she (he) loves me not": It seemed that ____'s feelings for me changed very frequently and unpredictably.
a	(7)	I often wished that ____'s feelings for me were as strong as my feelings for her (him).
a	(8)	____ seemed very capable of *both* hurting *and* comforting me.
a	(9)	Sometimes I felt that I was forcing ____ to show more feeling, more commitment.
o	(10)	After just a few dates, I felt that I might be in love with ____.
o	(11)	I spent a lot of time daydreaming about love, romance, and sex with ____.
o	(12)	The ending of my relationship with ____ was long and drawn-out, rather than sudden.
	(13)	I made a bold attempt to win ____'s favor.
a	(14)	As a girlfriend (boyfriend), ____ was certainly temperamental.
o	(15)	When my relationship with ____ was definitely over, I felt that I had "hung on" too long.
a	(16)	"Uncertain" is a word that well captures the nature of my relationship with ____.
o	(17)	During my relationship with ____, my friends and school work got much less attention.
	(18)	My feelings for ____ seemed to grow strong when she (he) expressed her (his) uncertainty about our relationship.
o	(19)	"Exciting" is a word that captures the nature of my relationship with ____.
o	(20)	I wanted to spend more and more time with ____, feeling that I just couldn't see her (him) often enough.
	(21)	I am not usually as "moody" as I was during my relationship with ____.
	(22)	I was afraid that ____ would stop loving me.
a	(23)	I often felt that I was giving more than I was receiving in my relationship with ____.
a	(24)	____ made me *both* very happy *and* very sad.
	(25)	I saw "warning signs" of trouble in my relationship with ____ but tried to ignore them.
a	(26)	It annoyed me when ____ seemed unsure of her (his) feelings for me.
a	(27)	I knew that ____ didn't care for me as much as I had hoped she (he) would, but I couldn't accept it.

a	(28)	Things might have worked out better if ____'s feelings were as strong as mine were.
o	(29)	I felt preoccupied with feelings about ____.
o	(30)	____ and I talked very frequently about our relationship.
a	(31)	____ said or implied that she (he) felt "suffocated" or "smothered" by the attention and affection given her (him).
	(32)	I felt an aching of the "heart" (a region in the front center of the chest) when I wasn't sure how ____ felt about me.
a	(33)	I was unable really to believe in ____'s feelings for me.

Note: Items marked "a" were scored on the Romantic Anxiety factor. Items marked "o" were scored on the Romantic Obsession factor. All items were used in computing total scores on "tendency toward anxious romantic attachment" (TTARAT). Each was scored in an additive manner, so that high scores indicated a greater magnitude of the variable.

Appendix 7.2. Major Instruments Aggregated across Multiple Completions (Raters) from the Schwarz Family Dynamics Study Data Base

	Rater				
Target and instruments	Student	Friend	Sibling	Mother	Father
I. *Mother's child-rearing behaviors and personality*					
Children's Report of Parental Behavior Inventory (CRPBI; Schaefer, 1965; Schwarz, Barton-Henry, & Pruzinsky, 1985; Schwarz & Mearns, 1989)	×		×	×	×
Parent Behavior Form (PBF; Worell & Worell, 1974; Schwarz & Mearns, 1989)	×		×	×	×
Relationship with Mother and Father Scale (Schwarz, 1991)	×	×			
Love Inconsistency Scale (Schwarz & Zuroff, 1979, 1990)	×		×	×	×
Competence Scale of the Clarke Parent-Child Relations Questionnaire (Paitich & Langevin, 1976; modified by Schwarz, 1979a)	×		×	×	×
Adjective Checklist (ACL; Gough & Heilbrun, 1983; Schwarz, Wheeler, & Rausch, 1992)				×	×

(*continued*)

Appendix 7.2. (*continued*)

Target and instruments	Rater				
	Student	Friend	Sibling	Mother	Father
II. *Father's child-rearing behaviors and personality* [Instruments and raters identical to those on mother, above]					
III. *Parents' marital adjustment*					
Marital Adjustment Test (MAT; Locke & Wallace, 1959)	×		×	×	×
Inter-Parental Conflict Scale (IPC; Schwarz, 1990a)	×		×	×	×
Inter-Parental Influence Scale (IPI; Schwarz, 1990)	×		×	×	×
Marital Communication Inventory (Bienvenu, 1970)				×	×
Marital Status Inventory (Weiss & Cerreto, 1980)				×	×
IV. *Student's personality*					
Adjective Checklist (ACL; Gough & Heilbrun, 1983; Schwarz, Wheeler, & Rausch, 1992)	×	×	×	×	×
Personal Attributes Rating Scale (PARS; Schwarz, 1979b)	×	×	×	×	×
Millon Clinical Multiaxial Inventory (MCMI; Millon, 1983; Wheeler & Schwarz, 1989)	×	×			
Psychological Screening Inventory (PSI; Lanyon, 1973)	×	×			
Extended Personal Attributes Questionnaire (EPAQ; Spence, Helmreich, & Holahan, 1979)	×	×	×		
Various self-report measures of sexual behavior and fantasies, substance use/abuse, and delinquent behavior (Schwarz, 1986)	×				

REFERENCES

Bartholomew, K. (1990). Avoidance of intimacy: An attachment perspective. *Journal of Social and Personal Relationships, 7,* 147-178.

Bartholomew, K., & Horowitz, L. M. (1991). Attachment styles among young adults: A test of a four-category model. *Journal of Personality and Social Psychology, 61*(2), 226-244.

Bienvenu, M. (1970). Measurement of marital communication. *The Family Coordinator, 81,* 506-520.

Brennan, K. A., Shaver, P. R., & Tobey, A. E. (1991). Attachment styles, gender and parental problem drinking. *Journal of Social and Personal Relationships, 8,* 451-466.

Feeney, J. A., & Noller, P. (1990). Attachment styles as a predictor of adult romantic relationships. *Journal of Personality and Social Psychology, 58*(2), 281-291.

Feeney, J. A., & Noller, P. (1991). Attachment style and verbal descriptions of romantic partners. *Journal of Social and Personal Relationships, 8,* 187-215.

Gough, H. G., & Heilbrun, A. B. (1983). *The Adjective Checklist manual.* Palo Alto, CA: Consulting Psychologists Press.

Hazan, C., & Shaver, P. R. (1987). Romantic love conceptualized as an attachment process. *Journal of Personality and Social Psychology, 52*(3), 511-524.

Hazan, C., & Shaver, P. R. (1990). Love and work: An attachment-theoretical perspective. *Journal of Personality and Social Psychology, 59*(2), 270-280.

Hindy, C. G., & Schwarz, J. C. (1984). *Individual differences in the tendency toward anxious romantic attachments.* Paper presented at the Second International Conference on Personal Relationships, Madison, WI.

Hindy, C. G., & Schwarz, J. C. (1985). *"Lovesickness" in dating relationships: An attachment perspective.* Paper presented at the 93rd Annual Convention of the American Psychological Association, Los Angeles.

Hindy, C. G., Schwarz, J. C., & Brodsky, A. (1989). *If this is love, why do I feel so insecure?* New York: Atlantic Monthly Press.

Kobak, R. R., & Hazan, C. (1991). Attachment in marriage: Effects of security and acuracy of working models. *Journal of Personality and Social Psychology, 60*(6), 861-869.

Lanyon, R. I. (1973). *Psychological Screening Inventory: manual.* Goshen, NY: Research Psychologists Press.

Locke, H., & Wallace, K. (1959). Short marital-adjustment and prediction tests: Their reliability and validity. *Marriage and Family Living, 21,* 251-255.

Millon, T. (1983). *Millon Clinical Multiaxial Inventory manual* (3rd ed.). Minneapolis: National Computer Systems.

Paitich, D., & Langevin, R. (1976). The Clarke Parent–Child Relations Questionnaire: A clinically useful test for adults. *Journal of Consulting and Clinical Psychology, 44,* 428-436.

Phares, V. (1992). Where's Poppa? The relative lack of attention to the role of fathers in child and adolescent psychopathology. *American Psychologist, 47,* 656-664.

Pistole, M. C. (1989). Attachment in adult romantic relationships: Style of conflict resolution and relationship satisfaction. *Journal of Social and Personal Relationships, 6,* 505-510.

Rushton, P., Brainerd, C., & Pressley, M. (1983). Behavioral development and construct validity: The principle of aggregation. *Psychological Bulletin, 94,* 18-38.

Schaefer, E. S. (1965). Children's report of parental behavior: An inventory. *Child Development, 36,* 355-369.

Schwarz, J. C. (1979a). *The Parental Competency Scale.* (Available from Dr. J. Conrad Schwarz, Department of Psychology U-20, University of Connecticut, 406 Babbidge Road, Storrs, CT 06269-1020)

Schwarz, J. C. (1979b). *The Personal Attributes Rating Scale (PARS).* (Available from Dr. J. Conrad Schwarz, Department of Psychology U-20, University of Connecticut, 406 Babbidge Road, Storrs, CT 06269-1020)

Schwarz, J. C. (1986). *Description of the Family Dynamics Study data base.* (Available from Dr. J. Conrad Schwarz, Department of Psychology U-20, University of Connecticut, 406 Babbidge Road, Storrs, CT 06269-1020)

Schwarz, J. C. (1990a). *The development and validation of the Schwarz Inter-Parental Conflict Scale (IPC).* (Available from Dr. J. Conrad Schwarz, Department of Psychology U-20, University of Connecticut, 406 Babbidge Road, Storrs, CT 06269-1020)

Schwarz, J. C. (1990b). *Development and validation of the Schwarz Inter-Parental Influence Scale (IPI).* (Available from Dr. J. Conrad Schwarz, Department of Psychology U-20, University of Connecticut, 406 Babbidge Road, Storrs, CT 06269-1020)

Schwarz, J. C. (1991). *The development and validation of measures of emotional attachment and coalition with mother and father.* (Available from Dr. J. Conrad Schwarz, Department of Psychology U-20, University of Connecticut, 406 Babbidge Road, Storrs, CT 06269-1020)

Schwarz, J. C., Barton-Henry, M. L., & Pruzinsky, T. (1985). Assessing childrearing behaviors with the CRPBI: A comparison of ratings by mother, father, student, and sibling. *Child Development, 56,* 462-479.

Schwarz, J. C., & Mearns, J. (1989). Assessing parental childrearing behaviors: A comparison of parent, child, and aggregate ratings from two instruments. *Journal of Research in Personality, 23,* 450-468.

Schwarz, J. C., Wheeler, D. S., & Rausch, S. P. (1992). *The validity of personality factor scores based on self, other, and aggregated ratings from the Adjective Checklist (ACL).* Unpublished manuscript.

Schwarz, J. C., & Zuroff, D. (1979). Family structure and depression in college students: Effects of parental conflict, decision-making power, and inconsistency of love. *Journal of Abnormal Psychology, 88,* 398-406.

Schwarz, J. C., & Zuroff, D. (1990). *Development and validation of the Schwarz/Zuroff Love Inconsistency Scale (LI).* (Available from Dr. J. Conrad Schwarz, Department of Psychology U-20, University of Connecticut, 406 Babbidge Road, Storrs, CT 06269-1020)

Shaver, P. R., & Hazan, C. (1988). A biased overview of the study of love. *Journal of Social and Personal Relationships, 5,* 473-501.

Spence, J. T., Helmreich, R. L., & Holahan, C. K. (1979). Negative and positive components of psychological masculinity and femininity and their relationship to self-report of neurotic and acting-out behavior. *Journal of Personality and Social Psychology, 37,* 1673-1682.

Sperling, M. B. (1985). Discriminant measures for desperate love. *Journal of Personality Assessment, 49*(3), 324-328.

Sperling, M. B. (1988). Phenomenology and developmental origins of desperate love. *Psychoanalysis and Contemporary Thought, 11*(4), 741-761.

Sperling, M. B. (1989). Fusional relations in the borderline and normative realm: Desperate love. In R. Fine (Ed.), *Current and historical perspectives on the borderline patient.* New York: Brunner/Mazel.

Sperling, M. B., & Berman, W. H. (1991). An attachment classification of desperate love. *Journal of Personality Assessment, 56*(1), 45-55.

Wachs, T. D. (1987). Short-term stability of aggregated and nonaggregated measures of parental behavior. *Child Development, 58,* 796-797.

Weiss, R. L., & Cerreto, M. C. (1980). The Marital Status Inventory: Development of a measure of dissolution potential. *American Journal of Family Therapy, 8,* 80-85.

Wheeler, D. S., & Schwarz, J. C. (1989). Millon Clinical Multiaxial Inventory (MCMI) scores with a collegiate sample: Long-term stability and self-other agreement. *Journal of Psychopathology and Behavioral Assessment, 11,* 339-352.

Worell, L., & Worell, J. P. (1974). *The Parent Behavior Form.* (Available from Dr. Judith P. Worell, Department of Education and Counseling Psychology, 235 Dickey Hall, University of Kentucky, Lexington, KY 40506)

CHAPTER 8

Attachment in Marital Relations

WILLIAM H. BERMAN
LAUREN MARCUS
ELLEN RAYNES BERMAN

Intimate relationships have a significant impact on people's health, well-being, and survival (Antonucci, Chapter 10, this volume; Bloom, Asher, & White, 1978). Theories of intimate relationships in general and marital relationships in particular, however, have been emerging slowly in psychology. Sociological and anthropological theories of marriage (Fincham & Bradbury, 1990) address a sociocultural level of understanding, rather than an exploration of the structure and process of marital interaction itself. Recent efforts to develop psychological theories of marriage (e.g., Fincham, Bradbury, & Scott, 1990; Jacobson & Margolin, 1979) have begun to pursue this latter goal, but are only exploring limited aspects of marriage. The purpose of this chapter is to outline the potential contribution of attachment theory to an understanding of marital interaction and marital disruption, and to review research related to attachment in the marital relationship.

PSYCHOLOGICAL THEORIES OF MARRIAGE

Within the field of psychology, theories of marriage can be divided into three basic domains: the social theories involving social exchange and social learning principles, drawing on the work of Thibaut and Kelley (1959); the psychodynamic theories involving psychoanalytic (Kernberg, 1976), object relations (Dicks, 1967), and contract theories (Sager, 1976); and the general systems theories that draw on Von Bertalanffy's (1968) work.

Social exchange theory was developed by and applied to marital relationships by the pioneering work of Thibaut and Kelley (1959). It addresses the formation, maintenance, and dissolution of relationships through a quasi-economic model of reinforcements. Rewards and punishments are controlled by the partners and by social approval or sanction. In a close relationship, one individual evaluates the quality of the reinforcers provided by the other person, as well as the availability of these reinforcers in the current relationship compared to their perceived availability in alternative relationships. The individual then seeks to maximize reinforcement, which determines whether (at the bottom line) he or she remains in the relationship or not (Levinger, 1983).

Social learning researchers have identified different patterns of reinforcement in happy versus distressed couples; the latter exhibit significantly more negative responses than the former, for example (Wills, Weiss, & Patterson, 1974). In particular, negative behaviors such as nagging, whining, and withdrawal are related to later marital dissolution (Gottman & Krokoff, 1989). Negative coercive patterns such as the demand-withdrawal cycle, in which an individual inadvertently reinforces negative behavior and is reinforced by the withdrawal of an aversive stimulus, are also more common in distressed couples (Patterson, 1982).

Cognitive processes in marriage have only recently been studied within academic psychology (Baucom & Epstein, 1990; Fincham et al., 1990). Most current research and theory address the impact of an individual's beliefs and attributions about the self, the spouse, and the marriage on the marital relationship. Results indicate that one's beliefs affect how one responds in a given situation, and that some of these beliefs may lead to dysfunction in the marriage. Incongruence between partners is especially damaging—for example, when the wife holds traditional beliefs about her role in the marriage, while the husband believes in a more egalitarian distribution of roles. In addition, attributions for behavior significantly influence satisfaction: The more one attributes negative behavior in the spouse to internal, global, and stable characteristics, the greater the dissatisfaction will be. In contrast, the more one attributes negative behavior to external, specific, or unstable characteristics, the more satisfied one will be in the marriage (Fincham et al., 1990).

A number of psychodynamically oriented theories of marriage have been proposed, most of which tend to be extensions of individual psychoanalytic and object relations theories. Among the most well articulated of the dynamically oriented theories are those of Sager (1976), related to marital contracts; Dicks (1967), drawing on the British object relations school as a basis; and Meissner (1978), who has synthesized ego-psychological and object relations theories.

Sager's (1976) theory of marital contracts posits that each person brings to the marriage a set of conscious and unconscious expectations, beliefs, and demands, which he or she hopes and believes will be fulfilled. This "contract" reflects not only what the partner will do, but also what the individual will do in exchange for the partner's compliance. When two people marry, they form an interactional contract which synthesizes the two individual contracts by defining the processes by which the individual contracts are met. In other words, the interactional contract defines the rules of the marital relationship.

One of the first of the psychoanalytic marital theories was presented by Dicks (1967) while at the Tavistock Clinic. Dicks proposed a complex theory of marital conflict that draws extensively on object relations theory. Each individual maintains fantasized object relationships as well as the real relationship, and each person casts the marital partner, in part or whole, to implement that fantasy relationship. Marital distress arises when the partner does not fulfill that fantasy relationship. Dicks is careful to note that these fantasies are not simply displacements of earlier object relations, but may present contrasts to them, or may otherwise be different from earlier relations. He also proposes that one person may be attracted to another because the partner exhibits characteristics of the self that he or she has repressed. However, over time, the partner becomes hated or persecuted for just that reason: He or she exhibits undesired characteristics of the self that are split off, unconscious, and hated. In addition, some couples interact as if each person were a part of the self.

Meissner (1978) has also addressed marital relationships from an ego-psychological/object relations viewpoint. He emphasizes the interrelationship between the introjective and projective processes of each individual's object-representational structures, and the real interactions between two people found in marriages. He uses the psychoanalytic concept of transference as a model for the process found in marriage, noting that the process is occurring *in situ* rather than in the constructed environment of psychoanalysis. As in Kernberg's (1976) discussions of love from an object relations perspective, the degree of integration of good and bad internal objects has a significant impact on one's ability both to participate in and to gain pleasure from the intimate relationship.

General systems theory is a theory of complex open systems proposed by Von Bertalanffy (1968). Extrapolations of this theory have had a dramatic impact on theories of family relationships, particularly in the field of family therapy. The effect is so significant that some have referred to it as a "paradigm shift" (Hoffman, 1981). Like attachment theory, systems theory draws on principles of cybernetics, including reciprocal causality, positive and negative feedback loops, and homeostasis. However, there is no clearly articulated theory of marriage from a systems perspective (Steinglass, 1978), although recent efforts have been made to use systems theory to understand marital dysfunction (Coyne, 1988). In essence, marital distress is the manifestation of a dysfunctional system. The interactions themselves are not producing the desired result, but because of an organizational system's tendency to maintain homeostasis, the system is unable to change. A central component of systems theory is the concept of triangular relationships, in which the imbalance within a triangle of people creates tension.

These three theoretical fields have largely defined the issues involved in marriage and marital satisfaction. As seen in these theories, two central forces play on the nature of marriage: aspects of the interaction between the two partners, and aspects of each person's internal rules, beliefs, attributions, models, and fantasies about the relationship, known as the "internal working model" (IWM) or "mental representation."[1] One of the most significant distinctions among these theories is their attention to the actual interaction versus internal mental representations of the relationship. The psychoanalytic (Dicks, 1967) and cognitive (Fincham et al., 1990) models of marriage attend primarily to internal mental processes as they affect the marriage. Behavioral models (Jacobson & Margolin, 1979) and social exchange models (Levinger, 1983) address some aspects of cognitive processes, such as the valence of a particular behavior, but they attend more to reinforcements and to observable costs and benefits. Systems-oriented theories (Watzlawick, Weakland, & Fisch, 1974) attend almost exclusively to interactional processes within the couple, and minimize or ignore the mental processes involved. The dialectical tension between internal mental processes and external interactional behaviors presents a significant challenge for researchers desiring a more comprehensive theory of marriage. We believe that attachment theory as defined by Bowlby, Ainsworth, Main, and others provides a vehicle to explore the interface between representational and interactional aspects of marital relations.

The study of marriage from an attachment theory perspective began with examinations of disruptions of the marital bond. Since the attachment drive is only active at times of threat, stress, or perceived unavailability, initial efforts to understand adult attachment examined points of threat or unavailability, through bereavement (e.g., Parkes, 1972), divorce (e.g., Weiss, 1975), and prolonged separation (McCubbin, Dahl, Lester, Benson, & Robertson, 1976). In fact, many researchers have argued that the intensity of a bond can only be measured by the reaction to disruptions of that bond (Berscheid, 1983; Reite & Boccia, Chapter 4, this volume).

More recent perspectives on adult attachment have been based on studying attachment within an existing marital relationship (Cohn, Silver, Cowan, Cowan, & Pearson, 1992; Kobak & Hazan, 1991; and our own research, described later in this chapter). These studies have emphasized the systems aspects of Bowlby's theory, in which the IWMs of attachment both affect and are modified by current relationships (Bowlby, 1982). As noted by Kobak and Hazan (1991), "working models are the product of the reciprocal interaction between individuals and their partners. Thus it is important to consider how spouses' behavior is associated with their partners' attachment security" (p. 865). The study of infant attachment in ongoing relationships is relatively easy, since activators in infants and toddlers are common, triggered by parents' leaving the room, going out for an evening, or going to work. Among adults, however, there are few predictable situations in which spouses are inaccessible. Adults' greater memory capacities, cognitive abilities (including abstraction and anticipation), and the stability of IWMs of relationships all prevent attachment from being activated during most common brief separations. Activators of attachment may be common among adult couples, but tend to be idiosyncratic and to some degree changeable, and are hence difficult to identify and track in naturalistic research. The following is an example of attachment activation in one couple.

> *Case Example*
>   A middle-aged man had been traveling internationally for years as a salesman. He rarely experienced any distress about his long absences, but always arranged to have contact with his wife at a specific day and time. On the few occasions that she did not call, or the call was disrupted, he became extremely anxious, fearful, and angry —feelings that would not abate until she called. After several years, he realized that she could no longer tolerate his traveling, and within a few months he changed jobs to one that did not require travel. However, he became much more overtly insecure in his relationship to her, and much more insistent on regular contact. Now, if she was later than expected, the same anger and anxiety (that she might die) could be activated.

In this case, physical separation and inaccessibility did not initially disrupt the couple unless the anticipated contact was disrupted. At a later point in their relationship, however, activation of attachment was much more common, possibly because expectations for availability were much greater. In neither case would a researcher be able to use these experiences to generalize to situations that elicit attachment. Recent studies of marital attachment have examined the behavior in marriages as it relates to marital satisfaction, communication, and problem solving (Kobak & Hazan, 1991; Cohn et al., 1992).

Attachment research conducted by W. H. Berman has also progressed from attachment in disruption to attachment in interaction. The first set of studies examined the attachment bond of women to their ex-husbands shortly after a divorce. The goal of this study was to use an experimental research design to examine attachment distress in divorced women, and to develop a measure of attachment distress that did not rely directly on self-report. The second set of studies, currently in progress, examines the attachment bond in existing nonpathological marital relationships. Consistent with the divorce research, this research is using an experimental research design to elicit attachment responses, and a non-self-report method of measuring attachment has been developed.

In the next section, we first briefly review the research on attachment in divorce and bereavement, with particular attention to our research methods and findings. Then we discuss the theoretical implications of attachment theory for marital interaction and marital satisfaction. We begin with a discussion of the activation of attachment in close relationships and within a given attachment relationship. We then explore the nature of the IWM in order to understand the role it plays in relationships, and how it is affected by interactions. Next, we return to the joint contributions of interaction and representation, with particular emphasis on the reciprocal activation processes found in marital dyads. Finally, we present our current research design for studying attachment in marriage, and describe early pilot data obtained with our observational procedure.

RESEARCH ON ATTACHMENT
IN MARITAL DISRUPTION

The first extrapolations of attachment theory to adults were made by Parkes (1972) in his studies of loneliness and bereavement. In his landmark study of bereaved spouses, Parkes (1972) observed many behaviors comparable to those seen in infant–mother separations, such as initial shock and distress, followed by a period of "mitigation." In this period, the surviving spouse experiences continuing preoccupation with thoughts of the spouse; attempts to look for or seek out the spouse; attempts to contact the spouse; focuses attention on parts of the environment associated with the lost spouse; and calls for and cries about the lost spouse. Parkes asserted that these are symptoms of adult separation anxiety, isomorphic with those seen in infants separated from their primary attachment figures.

Following on Parkes' research, Weiss (1975) cogently described the role of attachment in divorced people. He noted that it can persist for many months after the separation, and that it is present in both partners, regardless of who initiated the separation. The symptoms he viewed as separation distress included recurrent thoughts and images of the ex-spouse, and positive feelings expressed about the ex-spouse. He argued that these behaviors could be understood as the "response to the intolerable inaccessibility of the attachment figure" (Weiss, 1975, p. 131).

Several empirical studies have examined the attachment following marital separation using interview or questionnaire data. Hetherington, Cox, and Cox (1976) interviewed many divorced couples over a 2-year period, and suggested that much of the continued conflict and rancor in divorces could be understood as manifestations of continued attachment. Separation distress has been found to be inversely related to adjustment, and was correlated with several variables suggesting a continued connection to the ex-spouse (Berman, 1988b; Brown, Felton, Whiteman, & Manela, 1980; Kitson, 1982). Those with significant attachment distress also reported more difficulties with loneliness and parenting, whereas those with low attachment distress experienced problems in practical and financial areas. Not all research has indicated attachment as a central component of postdivorce adjustment. Spanier and Casto (1979) found no correlation between attachment to the spouse and adjustment, and did not find a high level of continued attachment in their sample.

Extrapolating parent-infant attachment to adult-adult attachment presents problems, however, including the defensive processes available to adults and the multiple internal models that are active in adult relationships (Ainsworth, 1989). In an effort to address these problems, as well as to evaluate the role of attachment in postdivorce adjustment, Berman (1988a) used an experimental design to assess attachment to the spouse following divorce, employing a thought-sampling procedure as the dependent measure. The thought-sampling procedure taps into an individual's stream of consciousness by asking the subject to report whatever thoughts are in his or her mind at the time of the probe question. Since many of the symptoms of separation distress include preoccupation with the lost spouse (Parkes, 1972) or with thoughts or images of the lost spouse (Kitson, 1982; Weiss, 1975), it was assumed that the assessment of cognitive activity would provide a useful method of assessing "spontaneous" or intrusive thoughts about the ex-spouse (Cohen, 1974).

The experimental design was developed to control for the possibility that factors other than attachment could account for behaviors appearing to be attachment-based, such as conflict with the ex-spouse. If continued attachment to the ex-spouse (preoccupation, concern, longing, etc.) has a direct affect on adjustment, a memory of the ex-spouse as a loving, protective attachment figure would be significantly more distressing than other (e.g., conflictual) types of memories, because of the unavailability of this attachment figure. If the attachment-adjustment link is mediated by the amount of conflict (i.e., the more conflict one has, the more one feels distressed by the ex-spouse), then a conflictual memory of the ex-spouse would be more distressing.

Recently divorced women were identified through court records. All women who had been married at least 2 years, had at least one child from the marriage, and were between the ages of 22 and 65 were recruited. Sixty subjects who agreed to participate were asked to recall either (1) a positive or (2) a conflictual memory of the ex-spouse, or (3) a positive memory of a friend. Each subject was asked to describe the memory in detail, and was probed about her feelings both at the time of the memory and currently. She then engaged in a thought-sampling procedure, in which the subject sat in a quiet room by herself and let her thoughts wander. She was interrupted and asked to report on her thoughts at 1-minute intervals; these thoughts were recorded and transcribed. The number of thoughts about the ex-spouse during the thought-sampling task was counted. The frequency of these thoughts was used as a cognitive measure of continued attachment.

Subjects in the positive-spouse memory condition exhibited a higher frequency of thoughts of the ex-spouse than those in the other two conditions, even when desire for divorce and feelings of love for the ex-spouse were controlled for. In other words, the positive memory elicited significantly more spontaneous thoughts about the ex-spouse than either the conflictual or the positive-friend condition. The frequency of thoughts about the ex-spouse following the positive memory was also correlated with questionnaire measures of attachment, with psychological distress, and with the highest level of distress experienced during the divorce. Thoughts of the ex-spouse following the other two conditions were not correlated with these measures. Consistent with attachment theory, thoughts about the ex-spouse following the positive memory were uncorrelated with trait measures of dependency or affiliation.

These results were interpreted to mean that the experience of recently divorced women was significantly affected by memories of their ex-spouse as positive, loving figures. This was consistent with their personal descriptions of the divorce. Many described the onset of distressed feelings, depression, or anxiety at times when they felt particularly close to their ex-spouses, or when they recalled their ex-spouses as good persons whom they had loved. There did not appear to be any relationship between the experience of continued attachment and aspects of the current relationship; the attachment appeared to be related more to the spouse a subject had internalized during the marriage than to the spouse who had left, or whom the subject had left.

The experience of divorced people provides much insight into the process of psychological and emotional separation. However, the attachment bond in this case is inextricably intertwined with anger, conflict, hurt, and realistic traumas associated with divorce. It has become evident that the only way to understand the attachment bond in adults is to explore it in the context of existing attachment relationships.

A THEORETICAL MODEL
OF ATTACHMENT IN MARRIAGE

Bowlby (1988) argued that current relational experiences can affect the nature of the IWM, "updating" it or accommodating it in both beneficial and detrimental ways. It is as yet unclear how the IWMs of two individuals in a close relationship affect their interaction so as to accommodate or assimilate information. We are proposing the following as a theoretical model of how attachment functions interactively in a close adult relationship.

As with children, the attachment drive in adults is activated and terminated by two types of environmental stimuli: those that indicate danger or threat, and those that relate to the accessibility and responsiveness of the attachment figure. Once attachment is activated, the behavioral system severely constrains the types of behaviors an individual can exhibit to those that will increase or maintain proximity to the attachment figure. These behaviors (crying, calling, reaching out, or [in the case of insecure attachment] hostility and/or withdrawal) are significantly likely to convey information regarding danger or the availability of the attachment figure to the other person in the dyad. As a result, the activation and/or termination of one person's attachment system is determined in large part by the activation and termination of the other's. The activation of an adult's attachment system is also significantly affected by his or her IWM, which serves to organize and filter incoming information. Thus both the behavior exhibited by the partner and the schema through which that information is filtered activate and terminate the attachment system. In simple terms, both one's own IWM of attachment and one's spouse's behavior (which draws in part on his or her IWM of attachment) determine the activation–deactivation of the attachment system in any given interaction. This perspective is in contrast to object relations theory and cognitive theory, in which only the individual's IWM determines the meaning of environmental events, and hence his or her emotional response. It is also in contrast to systems models, in which only the interaction determines the response. We describe below how representation and interaction are synthesized. Before we elaborate on this theory, however, a few points of clarification are necessary.

Distinction between Parent–Infant and Adult–Adult Attachment

There are numerous differences between the affectional bonds of a parent to his or her infant and of two adults to each other. Perhaps the most important, however, are the relationship between the two figures, and the relationship between the attachment figure and the IWM. The attachment system in an infant emerges as a genetic process, but develops as an experiential process based on repeated interactions between attachment figure and infant. As the interactions between the child and attachment figure proceed, the child begins to develop an IWM, which exists in some rudimentary form by the end of the first year. Bowlby (1982) made it clear that the attachment-caregiving system is interactive, with bidirectional reinforcement and reciprocal interactions between the primary attachment figure and the infant. Yet the principal dynamic within the parent-infant attachment system is that the availability and responsiveness of the parent determine the nature of the child's IWM of attachment. Consistent with this latter dynamic, most research examining childhood attachment presumes a basically linear model:

Maternal caregiving behavior $\rightarrow$ Child's attachment IWM

In adults, however, intimate relationships such as marriage require a more reciprocal process that encompasses both care-seeking (attachment) and caregiving functions. Reciprocity of caregiving and attachment functions is essential for a healthy marriage. Each member of the couple needs to act in ways that are protective and nurturant, and to be able to accept protection and nurturance. Adult relationships in which one person is predominantly or exclusively serving one function are invariably problematic. In sum, the parent-infant dynamic is largely unidirectional, with the parent providing the caregiving, and the infant exhibiting attachment (care-seeking) behavior. In adults, both partners exhibit both caregiving and care seeking, and the meanings of these behaviors are determined by both partners in the relationship.

The Function of Adult Attachment

The attachment drive provides one of the major motivations for the adult dyad. Bowlby (1982) consistently argued that the "set goal" of attachment for the individual is felt security, with the "function" of protecting the infant from predators. In adults, attachment has been suggested to have the function of emotion regulation (Kobak & Hazan, 1991), particularly negative affect (Howes & Markman, 1989). We disagree that affect regulation is the function of adult attachment as defined by Bowlby (1982), for two reasons.

First, Bowlby (1982) devoted substantial time to the distinction among "function," "cause," and "predictable outcome" of a behavioral system. The distinction among these terms is unfamiliar in most behavioral sciences, and may need clarification. In Bowlby's language, "the causes of any behavior are those factors that activate that particular behavioral system; whereas the function of that behavior derives from the structure of the system, which is such that, when it is in action in its environment of evolutionary adaptedness, a consequence that promotes survival [of the species] commonly results" (Bowlby, 1982, p. 126). In other words, the function is the value of the genetic trait *for the species*. The distinction between function and predictable outcome is that of the distinction between an individual and a population. The predictable outcome is the result that can be observed from the activation–deactivation of the behavioral system in an individual instance. The function is the prevailing result of a population in its environment of evolutionary adaptedness. As such, it is unlikely that the "function" of adult attachment is affect regulation, since the link between the development of an attachment style and affect regulation does not have a clear species value. Rather, these theorists probably mean that the predictable outcome of attachment is affect regulation.

The second reason for disagreement on this point is that it is unlikely that attachment regulates all affect, or even all negative affect, any more than attachment accounts for all behavior in the parent–child dyad. There are many IWMs and behavioral systems, all of which may regulate some emotions to greater or lesser degrees. It may be that the predictable outcome of IWMs or mental representations is affect regulation—a point addressed extensively in object relations theory (see Kernberg, 1976).

Rather, we propose that the regulation of anxiety and some forms of anger is the "predictable outcome" of attachment (Bowlby, 1982, p. 128). We propose that the function of attachment in adults is preservation of a dyadic family unit, which increases species survival. The set goal of adult attachment is regulation of an optimal level of continued and stable proximity–distance with an intimate, which usually leads to the function as defined above. The regulation of proximity, in turn, regulates anxiety–security. The particular IWM determines what is experienced as optimal proximity, which may change if the IWM changes, and determines whether the outcome is related to the function of attachment. In other words, within an individual couple the regulation of relatedness or proximity also regulates emotion, which then either facilitates or hinders dyadic communication, emotional expression, frustration tolerance, and (inevitably) preservation of the species through the ability of the couple to produce and raise children.

Activation of Adult Attachment

We propose that there are two distinct types of activators of attachment: "primary activators," which are the unchanging components of similar interactions that associate a given individual with the attachment IWM; and "secondary activators," which are behaviors and emotions that engage the attachment system within an attachment relationship at a given time. Primary activators are the stimuli that form the basis of and identify an individual with the attachment IWM. Bowlby (1982) identified a wide range of attachment-associated stimuli, which become increasingly restricted in range as the infant develops. These behaviors include visual contact (particularly with the attachment figure's face and eyes), auditory stimulation, and tactile/olfactory contact (sucking, grasping, and clinging). Harlow and Harlow's (1965) studies comparing infant monkeys' responses to cloth and mesh mother surrogates suggests that comforting physical contact is an important primary activator as well. For a young infant, the feel and smell of the attachment figure, and the eye contact made in the early months, may be the most important defining characteristics of that figure, particularly as the attachment is developing. This is consistent with developmental theory, which assumes that sensorimotor representations of self and others are formed during the early months of life (Piaget & Inhelder, 1969; Stern, 1985; Blatt, 1974). Sensations such as smell, feel, and position (clinging) would, by their nature, be activators for a representation that focuses on motoric and sensory input.

Since we are assuming that the attachment system in adults is the same as the attachment system in children, then the primary activators of attachment should be the same for adults and for children. Early interactions between adults in a close relationship that include touching, stroking, and grasping, or eye contact and auditory stimulation, may activate the attachment system by providing each individual with the potential for physical security and comfort. These sensorimotor interactions provide the basis for identifying and experiencing another individual as an attachment figure—someone who offers the possibility of comfort and security. When the attachment drive, including the behavioral system and the IWM, becomes associated with another adult, primary activation has occurred, and the dyad then holds the potential for using the attachment IWM to interpret the meaning of the partner's behavior.

Secondary attachment activators are the stimuli within a given interaction that evoke the attachment behavioral system, resulting in information being processed through the attachment IWM. As such, primary activation occurs only once per relationship, whereas secondary activation occurs countless times within a given attachment relationship. Within a complex adult relationship such as marriage, what determines that a given interaction is experienced as an attachment interaction? Once a relationship is identified as an attachment relationship, with the set goal of an optimal level of proximity, attachment is activated by behaviors that convey threat and/or unavailability, or the primary "attachment" emotions of anxiety or anger (see Figure 8.1). Although distancing behaviors are most likely to convey threat and/or unavailability, we assume that proximity-seeking behaviors can also activate attachment. Any behavior *can* be interpreted as an attachment activator if it alters the psychological proximity or distance within the dyad, hence altering anxiety–security. As

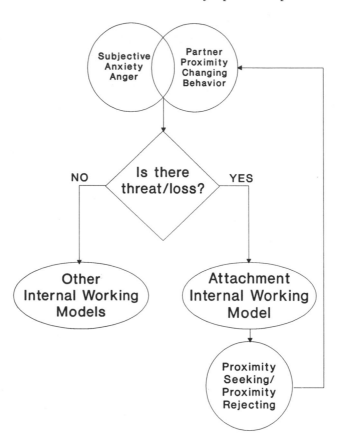

FIGURE 8.1. Secondary activation and deactivation of the attachment system.

such, a simple hug can activate attachment, as can turning away or leaving for work. Once the attachment behavioral system is activated, it is terminated only through re-equilibration of proximity–security (Bowlby, 1982).[2] Secondary activation of attachment engages the individual's attachment IWM, which then determines the meaning of the partner's behavior and prescribes the range of one's behavioral responses. In the next section, we describe the IWM in more detail.

The Attachment Internal Working Model

As we have described above, the attachment IWM is a mental representation of the self and other in interaction. This representational model contributes to the expectations, beliefs, and attributions each person has about himself or herself and the partner. The cognitive theory of marriage places these processes at the center of marital adjustment and satisfaction (Fincham et al., 1990). The attachment IWM establishes the person's belief in the availability and consistency of the attachment figure, and in the person's own worthiness as the receiver of security and comfort (Bowlby, 1982; Kobak & Hazan, 1991; Main, Kaplan, & Cassidy, 1985). In an adult, it also establishes the person's attitudes and beliefs about his or her availability to another. In part, the attachment IWM affects the person's self-worth and self-esteem in the context of an attachment relationship.

We assume that the IWM of attachment described here is consistent with the developmental theories of Stern (1985), Blatt (1974; Behrends & Blatt, 1985), Kernberg (1976), and Main et al. (1985), and with the representational theories of Schank and Abelson (1976) and Lazarus (1992). To summarize briefly, the IWM is constructed of repeated parallel experiences between the self and another, and is a reasonably accurate (but not identical) representation of the child's experience over time. Each IWM is organized around a particular affect state (Lazarus, 1991), and possibly a particular relationship (e.g., mother, father). Each experience is added to the comparable IWM, with differences and similarities integrated in an unspecified quasi-mathematical fashion. That is, the IWM is a function of the child's experiences, probably weighted for the intensity of the emotional experience. As an example, when a child has experienced a parent's leaving the room and returning once, all aspects of the experience are encoded in episodic memory. Stern (1985) argues that each additional experience is combined with the prior episodic memory, with the invariant aspects remaining and the unstable aspects eliminated. To continue the example, the amount of time of the parent's absence may be quite relevant the first time. However, after many such brief encounters in which the time absent varies a great deal, the child will have a model in which a brief absence and return are integral, but the amount of time absent is not.

The organizing principles in the attachment IWM, as in all mental schemata, are the invariant attributes of the interaction (Stern, 1985; Schank & Abelson, 1977). These organizing principles are also the activators and deactivators of the IWM. In general, these may include certain physical characteristics of the attachment figure (Blatt, Brenneis, & Schimek, 1976); actions of both the self and the attachment figure (Blatt et al., 1976; Stern, 1985); and, most importantly, the affects that connect the self and attachment figure (Kernberg, 1976; Lazarus, 1991). Because attachment develops critically during the second half of the first year, at the end of the sensorimotor period (Bretherton, 1991), we suggest that sensorimotor components are central organizing principles of the attachment IWM. These include actions that affect proximity and distance, and the emotions experienced by infants going through separation experiences: security/safety, anxiety, anger/rejection, and detachment/withdrawal. In other words, feelings of anxiety may elicit attachment even if they are not attended by physical distancing. Situations that include both anxiety and distancing will strongly activate the attachment IWM.

The IWM of the attachment relationship is an accumulation of the experiences within that relationship, especially during the second half of the first year. The IWM at this point consists of representations of the child and attachment figure in interaction; they are defined by their behavior, as in Stern's (1985) stage of core self, and Blatt's (1974) sensorimotor stage. Over the next few years, the IWM proceeds through several stages, incorporating and advancing over prior stages—integrating object permanence, conservation, intersubjective experience, and verbally mediated characteristics of self and other. Despite these additions and elaborations of the IWM, we suggest that the original organizing components (proximity-altering behaviors and the affects of anxiety, anger, and detachment) remain as the principal activators and deactivators of attachment.

The nature or style of the attachment IWM is affected by the child's experience with the attachment figure, particularly with regard to the affect that connects the child and attachment figure in the IWM. When the recurrent experiences of the child and attachment figure are fairly consistent over time with respect to distancing behaviors and emotional experience, the IWM develops in an integrated, differentiated interaction pattern (the secure or autonomous style). Distancing leads to anxiety, which activates attachment, followed by proximity-seeking behaviors, physical contact, psychological comfort, and then finally deactivation. If this is the general case, then occasional variations in any one component can become assimilated into the overall schema. As the IWM becomes more differentiated over time, the attributes of the attachment IWM become more specific and detailed and are less likely to become activated, because there is an insufficient match between the real experience and the attachment IWM. More specific, complex activators of the attachment IWM are needed as the child's cognitive complexity increases.

When there are significant fluctuations in the parent–infant interactions that form the IWM (particularly the organizing affect state), there are fewer invariants, and the attributes of the IWM are less differentiated and integrated (Blatt, 1974). In addition, more behaviors such as rejection, parental anger, or detachment may become an integral part of the IWM (as in the avoidant or dismissing, and anxious/ambivalent or preoccupied styles). Under these conditions, we think it is possible that the representation of the attachment relationship may split into separate IWMs that include different patterns of anxiety reduction involving anger, detachment, and dismissal; or that the representation may become a single, poorly differentiated IWM organized primarily by rejection, a lack of anxiety reduction, and/or intense anger that is unresolved by reunion. In either case, the attachment IWM can be evoked much more easily, because the range of behaviors that signal threat/loss is broader. This results in both the tendency to form attachment bonds quickly, and the tendency for them either to be a source of excessive anxiety given the duration and intensity of the relationship, or to be rejected or trivialized. The following is a case in which excessive fluctuations in the attachment relationship resulted in poorly differentiated attachment representation and in hyperactivation of the attachment bond with little capacity to deactivate it.

Case Example
    S, a woman in her early 20s, was raised by a mother given to violent rages; those were often followed by excessive self-recrimination, withdrawal, and occasional suicide gestures. In both S's childhood and adulthood, her experience with her mother included extremely variable reactions to S's anxiety, ranging from excessive attention to cold dismissal to the mother's intentional prolongation of S's distress "because it made her feel loved." In one childhood memory of an event that happened repeatedly, her mother would withdraw into her bedroom following a rage episode, locking the door and leaving S banging on the door crying, "I'm sorry, Mommy, I'm sorry." In psychotherapy, S's normal interactional style was extremely deferential, quiet, and timid. At times, however, if she became anxious about being abandoned by the therapist, she would immediately become defensively angry and at times provocative or withdrawn, as if saying to the therapist, "Go ahead, leave, I dare you." These episodes would end only when the therapist made significant efforts to demonstrate his availability and responsiveness, such as prolonging sessions, talking on the telephone with her, or overtly declaring his commitment to her. On other occasions, only angry limit setting about what was tolerable behavior in psychotherapy, with the threat of termination, ended the ambivalent attachment interaction. At these times the interactions were quite compelling; the therapist's anger provoked insecurity in both the patient and therapist, and promoted a continued attachment-focused interaction between patient and therapist in attempts to re-establish a sense of security about the relationship.

Once the attachment IWM is activated in a particular interaction, it can be deactivated when the affect state changes, or when other attributes of the IWM change. Again, when the IWM is poorly differentiated, or the invariants are less well articulated and differentiated, the IWM may be more difficult to deactivate.

The attachment IWM is crucial to understanding some aspects of marital interaction. The spouse is likely to become an attachment figure because of the primary activation through consistent physical contact. Moreover, the constant movement into and out of intimacy in a marriage provides an important source of secondary activators (distancing actions). The attachment IWM functions as a cognitive filter, determining whether the distancing actions convey a threat/loss, and whether the attachment sequence remains active or is deactivated. Since the IWM includes aspects of the self and the spouse, it also determines important characteristics of the spouse, and determines expectations about future behavior. The next section elaborates on the interface between interactional behaviors and the IWM.

The Internal Working Model and Interaction in Marriage

The concept of the attachment IWM is central to understanding marriage. It explains consistency across relationships, and indicates why individuals selectively attend to some behaviors of the spouse and not others. However, although Bowlby (1988) has allowed for "updating" of the IWM, he has not clearly explained the process of change in the nature of the IWM; nor does the concept of the IWM explain why the same person can have very different experiences in different relationships. Many clinicians have observed individuals who exhibit all the characteristics of an insecure attachment in one relationship, but no longer manifest those characteristics when they enter into another relationship with a psychologically different partner. As such, the IWM is insufficient as an explanatory construct. Our clinical and experimental observations suggest that interactional components must play a significant role in activating and maintaining attachment-based interactions within close relationships.

We suggest that activation of attachment in marriage occurs in a two-stage process involving both the behavior of the attachment figure and the self's IWM of attachment (see Figure 8.2). The attachment figure behaves in ways that alter the proximity–distance between the self and the attachment figure. From the attachment figure's viewpoint, these behaviors may or may not be meaningful. That is, they may or may not convey the same meaning as attachment activators in infants–physical inaccessibility (such as the wife's not calling her traveling husband in the case example described earlier), or unresponsiveness through interpersonal distancing behaviors, such as withdrawal, avoidance of gaze, or avoidance of contact. The first stage of the process is the behavior of the attachment figure. Activation can occur in a variety of contexts in response to behaviors that change the physical/psychological proximity of the attachment figure.

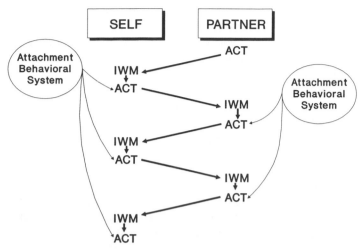

FIGURE 8.2. Internal working models of IWM and interactional behavior (ACT).

The second stage involves each individual's processing the behavior of the other via his or her IWM of attachment. The IWM is activated by the subjective experience of danger or threat, or by the unavailability/unresponsiveness of the attachment figure. The attachment IWM appraises the *meaning* of partner behavior—that is, whether it is separation-related or not, and what the meaning of the separation is (Main et al., 1985). This appraisal then determines the type of response that is given by the self. When the attachment IWM (and hence the attachment system) is activated, the attachment behavioral system severely limits the behavioral repertoire at that point: The self must do those things that will re-establish optimal proximity and security, and reduce or eliminate anxiety.

In adult couples, the attachment process does not stop at this point. Since both self and partner have attachment IWMs, the behavioral response of the self is subsequently filtered by the partner's IWM—first to determine whether the partner's IWM is activated, and then to determine the meaning of the self's behavior. This then determines the partner's behavior. For example, the partner engages in some behavior that potentially implies unavailability or interpersonal distancing. The IWM of the self then determines the meaning of that behavior. If the meaning of the behavior is "unavailability/unresponsiveness," then the attachment behavioral system of the self is activated. The self then responds with attachment-mediated behaviors—actions that either solicit proximity or reject it (in individuals with insecure attachment styles). By their very nature, these behaviors are likely to elicit the attachment system in the partner, as they are overtly either proximity-seeking or proximity-rejecting. Once both partners' attachment systems are activated, they will continue in cycles of behavior-interpretation-response-interpretation until one or both determine that the meaning is *not* "unavailability/unresponsiveness." Each person's attachment system is deactivated only when proximity and/or security is restored. In the following example, the effect of each person's attachment style on the other is illustrated. In the first relationship, the partners repeatedly activated each other's attachment systems, and neither allowed deactivation to take place. In the second relationship, activation was much less frequent for one partner, making it less frequent for both.

Case Example

A young woman with a strongly anxious/ambivalent attachment style became extremely depressed while dating a man with an avoidant style. On many occasions, she would feel anxious and insecure when he would make plans to go home or go to work. She stated that she experienced his behaviors as rejection, confirming her sense that she was unworthy of having a close relationship, and resulting in her seeking contact and reassurance from him. He responded to her contact seeking with more withdrawal and depreciation of her, in efforts to minimize any significance to his separation behaviors. Thus the two would become embroiled in an interaction dominated by their recurrent proximity-seeking and distancing behaviors: she compulsively seeking support and caring, and he rejecting her efforts defensively. Eventually, and with great pain, that relationship ended. The young man confirmed his avoidant attachment by becoming quite depressed after the separation, and repeatedly seeking contact with her after the breakup. She then had a second relationship with a man with a secure attachment style. This resulted in significantly less anxiety, since he did not react to her insecurity with rejection, but rather with caregiving (responsiveness). Frequently he spontaneously offered reassurance to her. As a result, her insecure attachment IWM would be deactivated much more quickly. In fact, when the second relationship ended, she was less distraught and felt less inadequate than after the first breakup.

The secondary activators of attachment—proximity-altering behaviors and/or anxiety—function to initiate attachment, regardless of the nature of the IWM of attachment. The dyadic interactions within a marriage that involve change in the interpersonal distance will potentially initiate attachment. Activation of the attachment behavioral system through distancing behavior engages the attachment IWM, which functions as a filter by which the individual assesses the meaning of the spouse's proximity-seeking or distancing behavior. The attributions, expectations, and beliefs about both the self and the spouse that are inherent in the IWM provide feedback, which will maintain activation of attachment if the overt behavior matches the invariants of the IWM. If it is inconsistent with the IWM, the person attributes the partner's behavior to nonattachment systems and deactivates the attachment system.

If the feedback to the first person sustains attachment, the person's behavioral response will be determined by his or her IWM. Since activation of attachment limits the range of behaviors the person can exhibit to those that will regain optimal proximity, the behavior is then much more likely to activate the partner's attachment system; how he or she responds is then also determined by his or her IWM. Within an interactional framework, the activation of one person's IWM (and his or her resultant behavior) limits the interpretations possible by the partner. This partner's behavior then limits the interpretations (i.e., deactivation of attachment) possible by the first one.

A stylized example may be helpful. A wife with an avoidant attachment style decides to go to bed early one night. This activates the husband's attachment system, since her movement away from him increases their interpersonal distance. Let us assume that he has an anxious/ambivalent style, thus increasing the likelihood that the answer to the question "Is there threat/loss?" is "Yes," since rejection and inconsistency are more likely to be invariants of the anxious/ambivalent IWM. He responds with irritation, stating, "Why are you going to bed so early?" This hostility activates her attachment system, in which hostility and rejection are invariants of an avoidant IWM. She then responds by distancing more—for example, by saying nothing or reacting with hostility. Her response now is determined by the nature of her IWM, which will then determine the nature of his response, and maintain a cycle of attachment-based interaction over an (objectively) minor event. If her IWM is not activated (e.g., anger is not an organizing affect, and the environment and model do not match), she may respond with a neutral response, or perhaps a caregiving response. Either may then deactivate his attachment IWM, as these are typically the deactivators. However, if her IWM is activated by his anger, she will respond from the limited repertoire of behaviors provided by the IWM. Typically, her options are to increase the hostility, or to withdraw and ignore the attachment figure.

In any marital interaction like the example above, two factors will determine whether the attachment IWM is engaged and an attachment interaction is initiated: vulnerability to experiencing threat/anxiety because of withdrawal of the attachment figure, and the extent to which there is real hostility/rejection intended in the proximity change. In any relationship, a covertly angry withdrawal will elicit anxiety, and hence trigger attachment. As noted before, proximity seeking can also evoke the attachment IWM if it generates anxiety. When proximity seeking takes place because of anxiety in one person, the other may respond to the anxiety as well as the proximity, and hence activate attachment.

In general, the more consistent the partner's behavior is with the person's attachment activators, the more likely the person is to maintain the attachment system. When the individual's behavior is inconsistent with expectations for distancing, he or she is less likely to engage or maintain activation of the attachment system. Obviously, then, the more differentiated and articulated the attachment IWM, the more difficult it will be to have concordance between behavior and IWM; conversely, the more global, diffuse, and general the IWM, the easier it will be to have concordance between behavior and IWM. In addition, when spouses have more consistent attachment IWMs, the easier it will be for them to deactivate the system, because of their common deactivators. When the IWMs are inconsistent, each person is less likely to deactivate his or her own attachment IWM because the partner's possible behaviors are not the same as those that are invariant within the person's IWM.

Case Example
    A husband and wife married for more than 20 years both appeared to have avoidant attachment styles. Exploration of how they handled conflict suggested that both were comfortable withdrawing from hostility. During a session, when the wife became angry at her husband, he stated that he had to use the bathroom and left the room. She visibly detached and continued to talk, ignoring him when he returned. In a later session, he expressed some anger, to which she responded by noticing a bird outside the window. He immediately changed the subject, and spoke to the therapist about a completely different topic.

We are considering a number of hypotheses about interactions in marriages, based on the theoretical model we have described up to this point. First, we predict that given the same external stimulus, there will be a greater number of attachment behaviors in people with insecure attachments, and marital distress will be increased for these subjects. Second, in couples with inconsistent attachment styles, attachment behaviors will persist longer and marital adjustment will be worse, particularly for the person with the insecure style. In the remainder of this chapter, we describe research designed to examine these questions, and present pilot data obtained through the use of a standardized procedure.

EMPIRICAL RESEARCH

To explore the role of attachment in marriage and marital satisfaction, we conducted a pilot project designed to assess both the attachment styles of married people, and the presence of attachment behaviors within their interactions. The development of the interactional procedure is described in detail elsewhere (White & Berman, 1991); it is based on the principles that guided the development of the Strange Situation (Ainsworth, Blehar, Waters, & Wall, 1978). In brief, the procedure assesses dyadic behavior not during a marital interaction per se, but rather upon reunion after two different affectively salient interactions. The first of these interactions involves identification of a loving, vulnerable, or affectionate memory, and a request that the spouses discuss the memory with each other in private for 5 minutes. The individuals are then placed in separate rooms for a brief period, and then reunited with instructions to "Relax, talk, do whatever you like" for 5 minutes. After the reunion period, the spouses repeat this sequence of discussion–separation–reunion, but they are asked to discuss an area of conflict in the relationship. In our pilot study, we expected that the first interaction would make all the couples feel closer, but would only elicit attachment for spouses who were insecurely attached. The securely attached would not experience anxiety, and would attribute the proximity-altering behavior to the research context. The conflictual interaction, however, when followed by a physical separation, would universally elicit mild feelings of threat or abandonment; in other words, the conflict–separation situation would be an attachment activator for all the couples.

We then rated videotapes of each person's behavior during the unstructured reunion period for behaviors that we identified as potential adult extrapolations of attachment behaviors in infants and children. A comprehensive review of the literature on the assessment of attachment (White & Berman, 1991) suggested a limited set of nonverbal and verbal behaviors. Adult nonverbal behaviors in the context of a laboratory interaction included changes in proximity to the attachment figure, changes in the amount of physical contact, and changes in the amount of "proximity-seeking and proximity-maintaining" behaviors (e.g., eye contact or smiling). Verbal behaviors included discussion of the period of time the couple was separated, or the discussion period prior to separation; affect tone of the verbalizations was also scored. Interrater reliability (using intraclass correlation coefficients) for the nonverbal behaviors ranged from .50 to .93, all of which were highly statistically significant (White & Berman, 1991).

Eighteen couples were solicited from several sources, including mailings to Fordham University staff and faculty, and couples married at the university chapel. The sample was a predominantly Caucasian, Roman Catholic, college-educated sample. The average age was 31.2 ($SD = 7.7$). No couple was in marital or family counseling, and no individual was in treatment for any major psychiatric disorder. Length of marriage ranged from 4 months to 24 years ($M = 4.5$ years), and 53% of the couples had children. When couples agreed to participate, they gave informed consent, and were then introduced to the interaction procedure as described above. A number of other measures were collected on these subjects as well. Of relevance to the issues discussed here are the following:

1. *The Attachment Style Inventory* (ASI; Sperling & Berman, 1989). The ASI uses a procedure similar to the "Love Quiz" of Hazan and Shaver (1987), but examines four attachment styles, rather than three, in four different categories of close relationships: mother, father, friendship, and sexual. It consists of four brief self-rated paragraphs, one each describing the "dependent" (secure), "hostile," "avoidant," and "resistant/ambivalent" styles, and an item assessing the security-insecurity of the relationship in question. For each type of relationship, the subject rates the degree of his or her agreement with each description on 9-point Likert scales, and also indicates which of the four styles best characterizes his or her attachment style in that relationship. For the pilot study, the scores for the sexual relationship style constituted the primary attachment measure.

2. *The Dyadic Adjustment Scale* (DAS; Spanier, 1976). The DAS was used to examine the quality of marital adjustment in these couples. It has 40 items rating several aspects of marriage, including criticism, joint activities, agreement, and interpersonal attachment. A simple summary score was used for our analyses. The DAS has been used extensively in studies of marital relationships.

Preliminary analyses of the pilot data suggest that attachment style is significantly related to the amount of attachment behavior exhibited. Results are presented here only for the nonverbal behaviors, compared across the dependent ($n = 26$), avoidant ($n = 4$), and resistant/ambivalent ($n = 6$) attachment styles. To examine the relationship of attachment style to attachment behaviors, we conducted a two-factor analysis of variance for attachment style and for condition (positive vs. conflict). In this analysis, the avoidant subjects leaned toward their spouses significantly less than the dependent subjects, $F(1, 33) = 3.3$, $p < .05$, and turned away from their spouses more than the dependent subjects, $F(1, 33) = 3.15$, $p = .05$. They also tended to avert their eyes more often than the dependent subjects following the positive condition, $F(2, 31) = 8.67$, $p < .01$. In each case, the resistant/ambivalent subjects fell midway between the other two groups.

Nine couples in which both members had secure (dependent) attachment styles were compared to nine couples in which one ($n = 8$) or both ($n = 1$) of the members had an insecure attachment style. When comparing those people in matched/secure couples to those in mismatched couples, we found that the spouses in mismatched couples leaned toward each other more often, $F(1, 34) = 4.75$, $p < .05$. In addition, the couples with matched attachment styles ($M = 117.2$) had significantly higher marital satisfaction than those with mismatched attachment styles ($M = 101.5$), $F(1, 34) = 18.69$, $p < .0001$.

These data suggest that attachment behavior plays a significant role in marriage, particularly with reference to changes in proximity in brief interactions. We found that the subjects with nondependent attachment styles reacted differentially to the positive and conflictual interactions for one of the nonverbal measures. The lack of findings regarding other differences in the positive and conflict conditions may be attributable in part to the small sample sizes in each group. It may be, however, that both the positive and conflictual interactions elicited the attachment drive for all subjects because of the separation period in both conditions. Attachment behaviors were present more for the avoidant subjects than for the dependent subjects, as we predicted: Deactivation is less effective for insecure attachment styles. We were unable to test whether a couple with one avoidant spouse and one resistant/ambivalent spouse would have the most prolonged attachment interactions. Attachment appears to be related to marital adjustment as well as specific behaviors: Individuals in marriages with insecure spouses were more unhappy than those with secure spouses. Similar results have been reported by Kobak and Hazan (1991) and by Cohn et al. (1992). Further analyses of these data will provide clarification of the relationship between attachment style and attachment behavior in marriage when the attachment styles of the two people are incompatible.

SUMMARY

Attachment in adults has typically been viewed as a characterological variable that individuals bring from one relationship to the next relatively unmodified. We suggest that although attachment style is a component of individual personality, it is significantly affected both by the individual's sensitivity to attachment activators, and by the behaviors and attachment style of the person's significant life figures (attachment figures). The IWM of attachment mediates the marital relationship for both individuals. For any couple, the nature of the attachment IWM of each member of the couple both shapes and responds to the behaviors of the partner, in a complex interplay between overt behaviors and the meaning each person ascribes to these behaviors. Activators of the attachment system in adults are responsible for engaging each person's attachment behavioral system. Once one member of a couple has activated his or her attachment system, the individual's range of behaviors is constrained to those that most people would interpret as attachment behaviors, thus activating the partner's attachment system. On the basis of this theory, we have proposed that the presence of an insecure attachment in one spouse will significantly affect the marital adjustment and the attachment behavior not only of the insecure spouse, but of the other partner as well.

ACKNOWLEDGMENTS

Preparation of this chapter was supported in part by a Faculty Research Grant and a Faculty Fellowship to William H. Berman. We would like to thank Nick Radcliffe, Joe Ruggiero, and Valerie White for assistance in the research; Alexandra Barsdorf for assistance in preparing the manuscript; and Michael Sperling for substantial comments on an earlier version of this chapter.

NOTES

1. Within the various fields of psychology, numerous labels have been given to the structures in the mind that represent the self, other, relationships, and models of the world. Bowlby (1982) and his followers have used the term "internal working model." In psychoanalytic theory, the concepts of "object relations" (e.g., Kernberg, 1976) and "object representations" (Blatt, 1974; Behrends & Blatt, 1985) have predominated, with "schemata" introduced recently (Safran, 1990). In cognitive psychology, the concept of "schemata" was emphasized by Piaget and Inhelder (1969) to describe the mental models of objects and the world. More recently, "scripts," "plans," and "goals" (Schank & Abelson, 1977), "representations of interactions that have been generalized" (Stern, 1985), and Lazarus's (1991, 1992) "cognitive-motivational-relational models" describe different levels of organization of these mental models of the external world. Although there are important differences among these terms, we use them somewhat interchangeably in this chapter to refer to mental models of relationships.

2. As noted before, people have multiple IWMs of relationships, which overlap to varying degrees. The activators of IWMs in adults also overlap; this is particularly notable in the activation of sexual and attachment IWMs. Physical contact and gazing are the primary activators for both, although the secondary activators may be different. For example, the secondary activators for attachment are changes in proximity and anxiety/anger, whereas the secondary activators for sexual IWMs are arousal and increased proximity. However, if an individual is unable to discriminate the secondary activators effectively, there may be extensive confusion between attachment and sexuality.

This may provide some insight into why individuals with so-called histrionic personality disorder may move rapidly into a sexual relationship, and then feel enormously insecure and betrayed. These people are often said to be seeking nurturance through sexual contact. It may be that the individual experiences confusion of the adult sexual drive and attachment, because they both involve physical contact. Although histrionic patients may be seeking warmth and nurturance, they often receive sexual contact, and then respond with activation of the attachment drive.

It also may go some distance in explaining why, in our culture, women appear both to have more intimate friendships and to benefit more from their close friends. Western society generally discourages physical contact between males, aside from the handshake (which is behaviorally fairly distant from stroking or holding). In contrast, women are much more likely to hug, touch, or stroke each other in friendship. It is possible that these behaviors stimulate the attachment system in female–female relationships, which is discouraged in male-male relationships. This could be tested by examining the intensity and closeness of male-male friendships in cultures that endorse physical contact between males.

REFERENCES

Ainsworth, M. D. S. (1989). Attachments beyond infancy. *American Psychologist, 44,* 709-716.

Ainsworth, M. D. S., Blehar, M. C., Waters, E., & Wall, S. (1978). *Patterns of attachment: A psychological study of the Strange Situation.* Hillsdale, NJ: Erlbaum.

Baucom, D. H., & Epstein, N. (1990). *Cognitive-behavioral marital therapy.* New York: Brunner/Mazel.

Behrends, R. S., & Blatt, S. J. (1985). Internalization and psychological development throughout the life cycle. *Psychoanalytic Study of the Child, 40,* 11-39.

Berman, W. H. (1988a). The role of attachment in the post-divorce experience. *Journal of Personality and Social Psychology, 54*(3), 496-503.

Berman, W. H. (1988b). The relationship of ex-spouse attachment and adjustment following divorce. *Journal of Family Psychology, 1*(3), 312-328.

Berscheid, E. (1983). Emotion. In H. H. Kelley, E. Berscheid, A. Christensen, J. Harvey, T. Huston, G. Levinger, E. McClintock, A. Peplau, & D. Peterson, *Close relationships* (pp. 110-168). New York: W. H. Freeman.

Blatt, S. J. (1974). Levels of object representation in anaclitic and introjective depression. *Psychoanalytic Study of the Child, 29,* 107-157.

Blatt, S. J., Brenneis, C. B., & Schimek, J. G. (1976). *A developmental analysis of the concept of the object on the Rorschach.* Unpublished manual, Yale University School of Medicine.

Bloom, B. L., Asher, S. J., & White, S. W. (1978). Marital disruption as a stressor: A review and analysis. *Psychological Bulletin, 85,* 867-894.

Bowlby, J. (1982). *Attachment and loss: Vol. 1. Attachment* (2nd ed.). New York: Basic Books.

Bowlby, J. (1988). Developmental psychiatry comes of age. *American Journal of Psychiatry, 145,* 1-10.

Bretherton, I. (1991). Pouring new wine into old bottles: The social self as internal working model. In M. R. Gunnar & L. A. Sroufe (Eds.), *Minnesota Symposia on Child Development: Vol. 23. Self processes and development* (pp. 1-41). Hillsdale, NJ: Erlbaum.

Brown, P., Felton, B. J., Whiteman, V., & Manela, R. (1980). Attachment and distress following marital separation. *Journal of Divorce, 3*(4), 303-317.

Cohen, L. J. (1974). The operational definition of human attachment. *Psychological Bulletin, 81*(4), 207-217.

Cohn, D. A., Silver, D. H., Cowan, C. P., Cowan, P. A., & Pearson, J. (1992). Working models of childhood attachment and couple relationships. *Journal of Social Issues, 13,* 432-449.

Coyne, J. (1988). Strategic therapy. In J. F. Clarkin, G. L. Haas, & I. D. Glick (Eds.), *Affective disorders and the family* (pp. 89-113). New York: Guilford Press.

Dicks, H. V. (1967). *Marital tensions: Clinical studies toward a psychological theory of interaction.* London: Routledge & Kegan Paul.

Fincham, F. D., & Bradbury, T. N. (Eds.). (1990). *The psychology of marriage.* New York: Guilford Press.

Fincham, F. D., Bradbury, T. N., & Scott, C. K. (1990). Cognition in marriage. In F. D. Fincham & T. N. Bradbury (Eds.), *The psychology of marriage* (pp. 118-149). New York: Guilford Press.

Gottman, J. M., & Krokoff, L. J. (1989). Marital interaction and marital satisfaction: A longitudinal view. *Journal of Consulting and Clinical Psychology, 57,* 47-52.

Harlow, H. F., & Harlow, M. K. (1965). The affectional systems. In A. M. Schrier, H. F. Harlow, & F. Stollnitz (Eds.), *Behavior of nonhuman primates* (Vol. 2, pp. 287-334). New York: Academic Press.

Hazan, C., & Shaver, P. (1987). Romantic love conceptualized as an attachment process. *Journal of Personality and Social Psychology, 52,* 511-524.

Hetherington, E. M., Cox, M., & Cox, R. (1976). Divorced fathers. *Family Coordinator, 25,* 417-428.

Hoffman, L. (1981). *Foundations of family therapy.* New York: Basic Books.

Howes, P., & Markman, H. J. (1989). Marital quality and child functioning: A longitudinal investigation. *Child Development, 60,* 1044-1051.

Jacobson, N. S., & Margolin, G. (1979). *Marital therapy: Strategies based on social learning and behavior exchange principles.* New York: Brunner/Mazel.

Kernberg, O. (1976). *Object relations theory and clinical psychoanalysis.* New York: Jason Aronson.

Kitson, G. C. (1982). Attachment to the spouse in divorce: A scale and its application. *Journal of Marriage and the Family, 44,* 379-393.

Kobak, R., & Hazan, C. (1991). Attachment in marriage: Effects of security and accuracy of working models. *Journal of Personality and Social Psychology, 60*(6), 861-869.

Lazarus, R. S. (1991). Progress on a cognitive-motivational-relational theory of emotion. *American Psychologist, 46,* 819-834.

Lazarus, R. S. (1992). *Emotion and adaptation.* New York: Basic Books.

Levinger, G. A. (1983). Development and change. In H. H. Kelley, E. Berscheid, A. Christensen, J. Harvey, T. Huston, G. Levinger, E. McClintock, A. Peplau, & D. Peterson, *Close relationships* (pp. 315-359). New York: W. H. Freeman.

Main, M., Kaplan, N., & Cassidy, J. (1985). Security in infancy, childhood, and adulthood: A move to the level of representation. In I. Bretherton & E. Waters (Eds.), Growing points of attachment theory and research. *Monographs of the Society for Research in Child Development, 50*(1-2, Serial No. 209), 66-104.

McCubbin, H. I., Dahl, B., Lester, G. R., Benson, D., & Robertson, M. L. (1976). Coping repertoires of families adapting to prolonged war-induced separations. *Journal of Marriage and the Family, 38,* 461-472.

Meissner, W. W. (1978). The conceptualization of marriage and family dynamics from a psychoanalytic perspective. In T. J. Paolino & B. S. McCrady (Eds.), *Marriage and marital therapy* (pp. 25-88). New York: Brunner/Mazel.

Parkes, C. M. (1972). *Bereavement.* New York: International Universities Press.

Patterson, G. R. (1982). *Coercive family process.* Eugene, OR: Castalia.

Piaget, J., & Inhelder, B. (1969). *The psychology of the child.* London: Routledge & Kegan Paul.

Schank, R., & Abelson, R. (1977). *Scripts, plans, goals and understanding.* Hillsdale, NJ: Erlbaum.

Safran, J. D. (1990). Towards a refinement of cognitive therapy in light of interpersonal theory: I. Theory. *Clinical Psychology Review, 10,* 87-106.

Sager, C. (1976). *Marriage contracts and couple therapy: Hidden forces in intimate relationships.* New York: Brunner/Mazel.

Spanier, G. B. (1976). Measuring dyadic adjustment: New scales for assessing the quality of marriage and similar dyads. *Journal of Marriage and Family Therapy, 38,* 15-28.

Spanier, G. B., & Casto, R. (1979). Adjustment to separation and divorce: A qualitative analysis. In G. Levinger & O. C. Moles (Eds.), *Separation and divorce: Context, causes, and consequences* (pp. 211-227). New York: Basic Books.

Sperling, M. B., & Berman, W. H. (1989, April). *An attachment classification of desperate love: Preliminary findings.* Paper presented at the midwinter meeting of the Division of Psychoanalysis of the American Psychological Association, New York, NY.

Steinglass, P. (1978). The conceptualization of marriage from a systems theory perspective. In T. J. Paolino & B. S. McCrady (Eds.), *Marriage and marital therapy* (pp. 298-365). New York: Brunner/Mazel.

Stern, D. (1985). *The interpersonal world of the infant.* New York: Basic Books.

Thibaut, J. W., & Kelley, H. H. (1959). *The social psychology of groups.* New York: Wiley.

Von Bertalanffy, L. (1968). *General systems theory,* New York: George Braziller.

Watzlawick, P., Weakland, J., & Fisch, R. (1974). *Change.* New York: Norton.

Weiss, R. S. (1975). *Marital separation.* New York: Basic Books.

White, V., & Berman, W. H. (1991). *Manual for the behavioral assessment of attachment in intimate couples.* Unpublished manuscript, Fordham University.

Wills, T. A., Weiss, R. L., & Patterson, G. R. (1974). A behavioral analysis of the determinants of marital satisfaction. *Journal of Consulting and Clinical Psychology, 47,* 802-811.

CHAPTER 9

Attachment Relationships and Life Transitions
An Expectancy Model

MARY J. LEVITT
SHERRILYN COFFMAN
NATHALIE GUACCI-FRANCO
STEPHEN C. LOVELESS

The importance of social relationships to personal well-being across the life span has been documented extensively (Cohen & Wills, 1985; Hinde & Stevenson-Hinde, 1987; Kahn & Antonucci, 1980), but work in this area has been fragmented. Child developmentalists have focused on infant attachment relations, with an emphasis on individual differences in the security of infant-caretaker relationships as precursors of social-developmental outcomes (Ainsworth, Blehar, Waters, & Wall, 1978). The heuristic and clinical value of this approach has been widely recognized, but basic research on normative processes of attachment formation, maintenance, and dissolution, and on the developmental trajectory of social attachments, has been minimal (McCall, 1990). Research with adult populations has been focused on the concept of social support, and there is an expansive literature demonstrating a link between support and well-being (Antonucci, 1990; Cohen & Wills, 1985). However, research on social support has been hampered by a proliferation of measures and a lack of theoretical integration. In a third area of research, social psychologists have recently intensified efforts to study the processes involved in close interpersonal relationships (Holmes & Boon, 1990), but these relationships are rarely considered within the context of the broader social milieu in which they are embedded.

Fortunately, these disparate lines of inquiry have begun to converge. For example, research on individual differences in attachment security has been extended to consider the intergenerational transmission of mothers' early attachment relations to their relations with their own children (Van

IJzendoorn, 1992). In another extension of the work on infant attachment security, researchers have developed measures of adult attachment styles and have reported studies linking a secure adult attachment style to relationship and well-being outcomes (e.g., Shaver & Hazan, 1988). Others have explored the association of attachment relations with outcomes following divorce (Berman, 1988a, 1988b) or the normative leave taking of adolescents from the parental home (Berman & Sperling, 1991). Social support researchers have noted the significance of close relationships with regard to the provision of support, and have suggested equivalency between the security function of attachment relations in childhood and the supportive function of close relations later in life (Antonucci, 1976; Boyce, 1985; Levitt, 1991; Takahashi, 1990).

Thus, the study of close relationships has gathered considerable force in recent years, emerging at the boundary of social and developmental psychology (Masters & Yarkin-Levin, 1984), and driven by a rich body of empirical research across disciplinary lines. At this juncture, integrative efforts to link the proliferation of studies on this topic into a comprehensive theoretical model are needed. Drawing from research on attachment, social support, and close relationships, we attempt in this chapter to specify how supportive relationships are formed, maintained and dissolved across the life span, within the context of the social network. This effort is grounded in the "convoy model" articulated by Kahn and Antonucci (1980).

THE CONVOY MODEL
OF SOCIAL NETWORK RELATIONS

Basic Premises

From the perspective of the convoy model, the individual is surrounded from the beginning of life by a network of social relations that moves with the individual through time. This network serves a protective function by affording the exchange of support between the individual and members of the convoy. In this way, the model is related to the Bowlby-Ainsworth theory of attachment, in which attachment figures are viewed as providers of a "secure base" from which infants develop basic competencies (Ainsworth et al., 1978). However, the convoy model is broader in scope, and attachment relations are considered within the context of the network of relations affecting the individual. The "convoy" is conceptualized as a dynamic hierarchical structure, defined empirically as a series of concentric circles surrounding the individual (Antonucci, 1986), which represent increased levels of intimacy and importance as the circle approaches the individual. Inner-circle relations are defined as persons to whom the individual feels "so close that it's hard to imagine life without them" (Antonucci, 1986, p. 10). According to Kahn and Antonucci (1980), these are likely to be persons who are bound to the individual through both affective and role-related ties, such as close family members. Outer-circle relations are those who are "less close, but still important" to the individual (Antonucci, 1986, p. 11). Attachment relations are viewed as an important subset of the individual's social relations—specifically, those occupying the inner circle of the individual's convoy. Changes in the relations comprising the convoy are hypothesized to occur as a result of individual developmental processes, normative life transitions, or non-normative crises.

Cross-sectional research consistent with the convoy model has been reported. Across age, the inner circle of the convoy has been found to consist primarily but not exclusively of close family members, with more distant relatives, friends, and others occupying the outer circles. Social support is provided largely by inner-circle relations across the life span (Antonucci & Akiyama, 1987; Levitt, 1991). Life-stage differences have been observed (Antonucci & Akiyama, 1987; Levitt, Guacci-Franco, & Levitt, 1993; Levitt, Weber, & Guacci, 1993) primarily in the peripheral circles of the convoy, with shifts in the balance of extended family and friendship relations occurring from early childhood through adulthood. (Friends are more prevalent and provide more support in adolescence and young adulthood.) Of particular interest to us are the processes by which changes in convoy relations occur.

Change and Continuity in Convoy Relations

At one level, understanding convoy change seems relatively simple. Persons are likely to enter or leave the individual's social orbit through such fundamental life changes as birth, death, and geographic relocation. However, when persons are asked to map their networks, they occasionally include deceased individuals, often fail to include newborn family members, and very often include persons who are not in geographic proximity. Conceptualizing the convoy as a personal network of figures who are "close and important" from the perspective of the individual acknowledges the validity of such reports. In this way, the model departs from those that specify contact frequency, interactive dependency, support provision, or role status as determinants of social network structure (Kelley et al., 1983; Furman & Buhrmester, 1985), and emphasizes the affective nature of convoy relationships. Thus, to acquire an understanding of convoy change, it is essential to study the processes leading to alterations in the affective quality of the dyadic relations comprising the convoy.

RELATIONSHIP CHANGE PROCESSES

The Social Expectations Model

A developmental model of normative relationship processes has been proposed by Levitt (1991). The model is depicted in Figure 9.1. In brief, relationships are thought to be initiated through interactions that familiarize relationship partners with each other and foster each partner's expectations regarding support from the other. Interactions with specific relations influence subsequent expectations of similar partners in related contexts. Social expectations are also influenced by life-stage-related social norms. Expectations serve to stabilize relationships until they are tested and disconfirmed. Disconfirmation of expectations destabilizes a relationship, potentially leading to changes in relationship quality, and in extreme cases to dissolution of the relationship. The development of social expectations, the relation of the proposed model to comparable models, the role of normative influences, and the proposed effects of expectations on relationship continuity and change across the life span are discussed in the following sections. Research designed to test aspects of the proposed model by focusing on relationship change across the transition to childbirth is then described.

Development of Social Expectations

Relationships are thought to be initiated through processes of familiarization and mutual responsiveness that occur in social interactions from infancy (Levitt, 1980; Cairns, 1977) through adulthood (Altman & Taylor, 1973; Zajonc, 1968). These interactions engender expectations regarding future encounters with relationship partners. Social expectations emerge in infancy, in the course of interactions with caregivers and others in the social milieu. That infants form such expectancies can be inferred from the active distress they exhibit when their mothers present still, nonreactive faces to them (Tronick, 1989) or when stimulation is withdrawn in experimental extinction paradigms (Lewis, Alessandri, & Sullivan, 1990).

As infants mature cognitively, they recognize specific persons as sources of contingent feedback, providing a basis for early social preferences (Levitt & Clark, 1982). Caregivers may be typically the most preferred, because they are most frequently available and responsive to the infants, but the infants may develop ties to others in their families' social networks through the same processes (Levitt, Guacci, & Coffman, 1993). Cognitive maturation also increases infants' capacity to link contingent events across extended time periods. In early infancy, only responses that occur within a few seconds of the infants' actions will be perceived as contingent (Watson, 1979). For older children and adults, marked in-

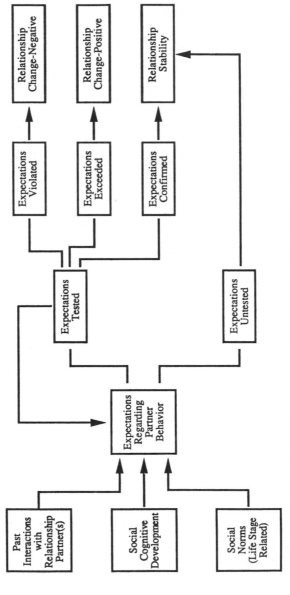

FIGURE 9.1. Hypothesized expectancy model of relationship stability and change. From Levitt (1991). Copyright 1991 by Lawrence Erlbaum Associates, Inc. Reprinted by permission.

creases in memory and communicative capacities allow events that are separated by extended time periods to be perceived as contingent (Weisz, 1986). For example, one might send a gift to a friend in gratitude for a favor granted weeks earlier, and the recipient would be likely to perceive it as contingent on the initial favor, particularly if the rationale for the gift is specified in an accompanying note. Even more extended scenarios can be envisioned, as when one provides considerable support to another in a time of crisis. The recipient may reciprocate years later in response to the needs of the initial provider, and most persons would have little difficulty comprehending the contingency of the second act on the first.

In traditional social exchange models, reciprocity of exchange is viewed as essential to the maintenance of relationships (Mutran & Reitzes, 1984). However, close relationships are not typically characterized by observable reciprocity (Clark, 1984), although individuals tend to perceive these relations as reciprocal (Antonucci & Israel, 1986). From the standpoint of the proposed model, the cognitive capacity to sustain expectations and associate contingent events over prolonged periods of time precludes the need for immediate reciprocity of exchange between close relationship partners. Perceptions of equity or reciprocity depend not on objective exchanges between partners, but rather on expectations that support will be provided as needed (i.e., contingent on each individual's requirements).

In our view, expectations that develop within earlier relationships are generalized to subsequent relationships; they are moderated both by interactions with new relationship partners, and by social norms governing the role of each partner within given cultural contexts and historical time periods.

The Role of Early Experience: Comparable Models

The notion that new relations are mediated by expectancies engendered in past relationship encounters is not new. Within social psychology, the current trend toward viewing person perception (including self-perception) as an outgrowth of attributions based on past interactions can be dated back to the symbolic interactionist views of Cooley and Mead (Schellenberg, 1990) and to the naive psychology of Fritz Heider (Fiske & Taylor, 1991). More recent views have been based on cognitive schema theory, which specifies that individuals categorize incoming information and build a schematic prototype that represents the particular category (Fiske & Taylor, 1991).

Similar views have been expressed by attachment theorists following the lead of John Bowlby and Mary Ainsworth. Initial encounters with a responsive or nonresponsive primary caregiver in infancy are said to engender expectations of future relationships, in the form of a "working model" of others in relation to the self (Bretherton, 1990). The working model is viewed as resistant to change, particularly if interactions with the caregiver were negative, as defensive processes are instituted to maintain the view that the relationship with the caregiver was adequate. In support of this view, Bretherton (1990) cites data indicating that poor relations with mothers are transmitted intergenerationally to affect the relations of daughters with their own offspring. Presumably, negative working models can be altered through therapy or a positive relationship experience, but the conditions under which such changes are likely to occur have not been specified.

Although allowing for the possibility of multiple attachment relations, the concept of the working model is weighted toward the monotropic view that infant relations with a primary caregiver form a dominant prototypic schema. Alternate attachments are viewed as secondary (Ainsworth, 1989), and theorists have been vague regarding the specific influence of multiple attachments on the working model. In keeping with the monotropic emphasis of the theory, empirical work on the concept has been focused on mother-child relations.

From a social network perspective, the construct of the working model, as currently conceptualized, is somewhat limited. First, the monotropic emphasis of the Ainsworth–Bowlby perspective has been questioned. An early critique of the concept was formulated by Margaret Mead (1962), who noted that multiple caretaking is the norm in many cultures. Contemporary researchers have expressed similar concerns regarding the universality of monotropic attachments (Lewis, 1987; Tronick, Morelli, & Ivey, 1992; Van IJzendoorn & Tavecchio, 1987). Even within our own culture, with its emphasis on the nuclear family, infants have been observed to exhibit attachment behavior toward a variety of nonparental relations (Levitt, Guacci, & Coffman, 1993).

Monotropic attachment theory is consistent with cognitive schema theories that emphasize the establishment of a single prototypic representation of the schema. However, prototype models are currently under challenge from alternative models suggesting that categories of information are represented not by a single prototype, but by varying exemplars of the category (Fiske & Taylor, 1991; Smith & Zarate, 1992). From an exemplar model perspective, social expectations would be based not on a specific prototype relationship, but on the degree of similarity between the new relation and one or more of several relations with whom the individual has interacted in the past in related contexts. In this case, mothers' past experiences with their mothers may be salient with regard to their own mothering behavior, but intergenerational transmission of troubled mother-child relations would not necessarily extend to other relationships.

Cognitive exemplar models are consonant with a social network perspective that stresses the importance of examining the totality of an individual's experience with significant network relations in projecting developmental consequences. Measures that are focused exclusively on the parent–child relationship are not likely to capture the full range of experience that will ultimately determine future relationship and well-being outcomes. Exemplar-based social network models can account readily for the existence of simultaneous multiple attachment relations, for positive outcomes that ensue despite poor attachment relations with parental figures, and for anecdotal and clinical evidence that a good relationship (with a grandparent, aunt, neighbor, peer, etc.) can compensate for an insecure attachment to a parent. Thus, in our model, relationship expectations are viewed as based on previous experience with a variety of social network figures.

Normative Influences on Social Expectations

Within the proposed model, social expectations are viewed as determined partly by past and present interactive experiences, and partly by life-stage-related norms governing the roles of relationship partners. For example, imbalances that exist between parents and children with regard to exchanges of support are reinforced through social norms, such as those specifying parents as providers and preadult children as recipients of support; reversals of this arrangement, as when a parent becomes dependent on a young child, are viewed as anomalous. At a later stage in the family life cycle, the norm is reversed, and middle-aged individuals are expected to tend to their elderly parents. The norm-governed nature of this arrangement is reflected in research demonstrating that caregiving to an elderly parent is not particularly contingent on the quality of the individual's relationship with the parent, or on the extent to which the parent provided support to the child in the past (Rossi & Rossi, 1990).

Social norms vary across relations (parent, spouse, child, etc.) and across cultures and time periods, so that what one expects from one's relations depends to some extent on one's cultural milieu and generational cohort. A cross-sectional study of marital satisfaction from young to old adulthood, by Reedy, Birren, and Schaie (1981), illustrates this point. Consistent with attachment theory, couples in the study, regardless of age, viewed emotional security as the most important aspect of their relationship; however, younger couples were more likely to value intimacy and less likely to value loyalty in their relationships than were older couples.

Relationship Continuity and Change

In the foregoing discussion, we have proposed that close relationships are maintained through expectations of support that emerge through interactions with specific relationship partners and are governed to some extent by culturally shared values. As affirmed in current research on social cognition (Fiske & Taylor, 1991), once expectations regarding other persons are solidified, they are quite resistant to alteration. Thus, it is proposed within our model that relationships are maintained through expectations regarding partner support, and that these expectations serve to stabilize the relationship until they are tested in some way. Expectations may be tested at any time, but are particularly likely to be challenged when an individual encounters a life event that precipitates an acute need for support from the partner. To the extent that such events are normative, changes in relationships would be expected to occur regularly across the life span. Periods of normative life transition provide fertile ground for the testing of support expectations. Violations of expectations during these times of heightened need destabilize relationships, potentially resulting in changes in the quality of the relationship. Whether such violations lead to long-term relationship disruption will depend on both the nature of the relationship and the extent of the violation. As specified in the convoy model, relationships with persons in the inner circle, who tend to be linked to the individual through strong affective and role-related ties, are resistant to change. Thus, these relations should be relatively resilient with regard to minor violations of social expectations, and are likely to be severed only if expectancy violation is extreme or recurrent. Outer-circle relations are more vulnerable to disruption.

Our initial attempts to assess the feasibility of the proposed model have been focused on the childbirth transition. From a social network perspective, the addition of a child to an existing network structure is bound to lead to some reorganization of the relations within that structure. A number of researchers have observed changes in the quality of marital relationships across this transition (Belsky, Spanier, & Rovine, 1983; Cowan & Cowan, 1988). Others have focused on the supportive aspect of social relations as a moderator of stress during this period. In general, previous research affirms that childbirth is a major life transition that has important implications for both interpersonal relationships and personal well-being.

The Childbirth Transition

Stress, Social Support, and Postpartum Well-Being

The childbirth transition has been widely recognized as a stressful period for parents (Coffman, Levitt, Deets, & Quigley, 1991; Coffman, Levitt, & Guacci-Franco, 1993; Hopkins, Marcus, & Campbell, 1984; Tietjen & Bradley, 1985), and the stress of this transition places women at a higher-than-normal risk for developing depression and other signs of diminished well-being (Crnic, Greenberg, Ragozin, Robinson, & Basham, 1983; Hopkins et al., 1984). Social support is thought to play an important role in alleviating the stresses of this period (Crnic & Greenberg, 1987), and lack of support has been correlated with multiple outcomes in new mothers (Boukydis, Lester, & Hoffman, 1987). Postpartum depression, for example, has been associated with lack of confidant relationships, lack of close family members nearby, having few close friends that provide support, and conflict in relations with husbands or parents (Cutrona, 1984).

Professional support has been found to have little impact on postpartum well-being (Coffman, Levitt, & Deets, 1991), but the importance of intimate support from spouses or other close persons has been documented repeatedly (Crnic et al., 1983; Tietjen & Bradley, 1985; Levitt, Weber, & Clark, 1986). Lack of a supportive spousal relationship has been the social support factor most commonly associated with postpartum affect (Gotlib, Whiffen, & Wallace, 1991; Levitt et al., 1986). Focusing on mothers of both preterm and full-term infants, Crnic et al. (1983) found evidence that spousal support predicted mothers' life satisfaction and satisfaction with parenting, maternal sensitivity to infants' cues, and infant responsiveness. With a similar sample, Coffman, Levitt, Deets, and Quigley (1991) found significant associations of support from husbands, mothers, and other close relations with postpartum well-being.

Overall, then, research on social support and the childbirth transition suggests that well-being in the postbirth period is dependent on support derived from close attachment relations. However, the magnitude of direct relations between support and well-being indicators tends to be relatively modest in most studies (Cohen & Wills, 1985). Our model specifies that postbirth outcomes depend more on the extent to which expectations for support are confirmed or disconfirmed following birth than on the actual level of support provided by the mother's close relations. Although prior research has not been addressed directly to support expectations, there is evidence to suggest that expectancies are important contributors to postbirth adjustment.

Expectations and Postbirth Outcomes

Research on expectations and postbirth adjustment has been focused primarily on the marital relationship. Belsky (1985), for example, found that when expectations regarding the impact of the infant on the marriage were less realistic, the spousal relationship was more likely to undergo a negative change in the postbirth period. Similarly, Kach and McGhee (1982) reported that women with less realistic expectations regarding the parenting role experienced greater difficulty with postpartum adjustment. Violations of expectations regarding postbirth division of labor were found by Ruble, Fleming, Hackel, and Stangor (1988) and by Benson (1991) to contribute to diminished marital satisfaction. Benson (1991) also reported that disconfirmation of prebirth expectations regarding relational efficacy (the extent to which partners believed they could personally affect the relationship) contributed to postbirth relationship change. Although support expectations were not addressed specifically in these studies, the results suggest that expectancy violation is related to postpartum outcomes.

Expectancy Disconfirmation and Relationship Change: Testing the Model

In our preliminary attempts to assess the validity of the proposed social expectancy model, we have focused specifically on the extent to which disconfirmation of expectations regarding support from close relationship partners predicts changes in relationship quality and postpartum affect. The initial problem encountered in designing research to test the model was that of measurement. We found no existing measures of support expectations, and no measures of relationship quality outside those designed to assess marital satisfaction or love relationships. Consequently, we conducted pilot research to develop appropriate measures.

Measurement of Support Expectations

With regard to support expectations, we first asked 103 undergraduate and graduate students of childbearing age and 55 women attending prebirth education classes to indicate their expectations for postbirth support. (Students were asked to indicate expectations that prebirth women would be likely to have regarding postbirth support.) Individual items from respondents were sorted according to commonality by two research assistants working independently, and these sorts were reviewed by Levitt. Expectations listed by students did not differ substantially from those listed by women attending prebirth classes. Expectation items endorsed by at least two individuals were included in a checklist and pretested on a second sample of 40 women attending prebirth classes. Items that were appropriate across different relationships (spouse, parent, etc.) and that were checked by at least 10% of the sample were retained in the present 14-item version of the Support Expectations Index and further pretested on a sample of 30 women in prebirth education classes. Alpha reliability for the index was .94.

A mother-to-be is asked to indicate, on 7-point scales, the extent to which she expects a specific relation to provide each of several types of support after the baby is born. Scale responses are time-based, with a score of 7 indicating that more support is expected. For example, the mother is asked the extent to which she expects help with household chores in the first weeks after birth, and responses range from (1) "not at all during this time" to (7) "at least 3-4 hours every day." The Support Expectations Index items are listed in Table 9.1. The index is designed to be administered prior to the infant's birth. With modified instructions, the index can also be used to assess the extent to which each support item was actually provided by the relationship partner subsequent to the birth of the infant.

Because subjective perceptions of support are often found to have greater predictive power than more objective measures (Antonucci & Israel, 1986), we also developed an index to measure perceived confirmation-disconfirmation of expectations. On the basis of the Support Expectations Index, a mother is asked to indicate, on a 5-point scale for each item, the extent to which the support received from a specific relation was (1) "much less than expected" to (5) "much more than expected." The Expectancy Confirmation Scale was pretested on a group of 25 mothers of infants attending an infant-mother play group. Alpha reliability for the pilot sample was .79.

Relationship Quality Measures

In developing measures of relationship quality, we were encouraged by research demonstrating comparability in the factor structures of marital satisfaction and love scales across different relations (parents, spouses,

TABLE 9.1. Support Expectations Index Items

1. Babysit or stay with the baby while you are out.
2. Spend time talking with you after the baby is born.
3. Provide financial support or assistance.
4. Purchase items for the baby.
5. Help you care for the baby in the first weeks after birth.
6. Help you care for the baby after the first few weeks.
7. Help with household chores in the first weeks after birth.
8. Help with household chores after the first few weeks.
9. Spend time playing with the baby, when the opportunity to do so is there.
10. Spend time teaching the baby to do things.
11. Show love or affection for the baby.
12. Show love or affection for you.
13. Indicate approval of, or agree with, the way you care for the baby.
14. Be generally helpful and supportive to you after the baby is born.

Note. Respondents are asked to indicate the extent to which they expect each type of support from specific relations on 7-point scales, with higher numbers indicating expectations for more support.

friends, etc.) (Davis & Todd, 1982; Sternberg & Grajek, 1984). Items included in a verbal Relationship Satisfaction Scale were drawn from three sources: the Rubin (1973) Liking and Loving Scale; the Campbell, Converse, and Rodgers (1976) Marital Satisfaction Scale from the Quality of American Life Study; and the marital satisfaction scales used by Belsky et al. (1983) in their longitudinal study of marital relations across the childbirth transition. The scale consisted initially of 42 items that were administered along with the Support Expectations Index to our first pilot sample. Of these, 30 items were retained on the basis of clarity and contribution to internal consistency, and pretested with our postbirth playgroup pilot sample. Reliability (alpha) was .81.

In addition to the verbal Relationship Satisfaction Scale, we developed a visual–spatial measure of relationship quality, the Relationship Closeness Scale, based on the work of Pipp, Shaver, Jennings, Lamborn, and Fischer (1985). These authors obtained retrospective data regarding the relationships of college students and their parents by asking the students to represent schematically, with two circles, their relations with their mothers and fathers during infancy, childhood, adolescence, and at present. Students tended to draw overlapping circles to represent the infancy period; distant, sometimes broken circles to represent their relations with parents at adolescence; and closer circles to represent their present relationships. Circle distance correlated with verbal descriptors of parent–child relations during the same time periods. We viewed this spatial representation technique as a promising means of assessing changes in relationship closeness that are difficult to capture with verbal indicators.

The spatial Relationship Closeness Scale consists of nine diagrams, each showing two circles, with the circles at progressively varying distances (Figure 9.2). Each respondent is asked to select the diagram that best represents the relationship with a target person. An earlier seven-choice version of the scale was pilot-tested with the expectation and relationship satisfaction measures. In line with the Pipp et al. (1985) research, respondents were asked to select the two-circle diagrams that best represented their relations with their mothers in infancy, childhood, adolescence, and the present. Respondents in both pilot samples selected circles that were significantly closer in infancy and further apart at adolescence, with greater closeness at present than during the adolescent period, providing convergent validation with the original unstructured Pipp et al. measure. As further evidence of validity, the spatial scale was highly correlated with the verbal Relationship Satisfaction Scale ($r = .70$).

Support Expectations, Relationship Change, and Postpartum Affect

We conducted a preliminary test of our expectancy model by querying 53 middle- income mothers of 13-month-old infants about their closest

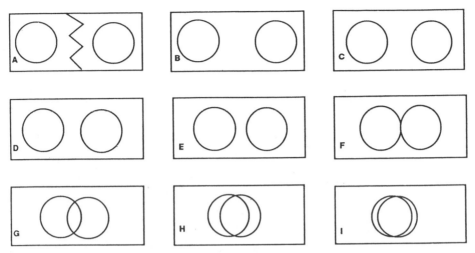

FIGURE 9.2. Relationship Closeness Scale. From Coffman, Levitt, and Guacci-Franco (1993). Copyright 1993 by Jannetti Publications. Reprinted by permission.

relationship. Of these, 43 had been interviewed 3 weeks after the birth of their infants (Coffman, Levitt, & Deets, 1991; Coffman, Levitt, Deets, & Quigley, 1991), and the remainder were selected from birth records to supplement the longitudinal sample. Prebirth support expectations were not obtained; consequently, the Expectancy Confirmation Scale was used to assess the degree to which mothers perceived that their support expectations had been confirmed or disconfirmed following their infants' birth.

The proposed link between expectancy disconfirmation and relationship change was assessed within the context of other variables that have been associated with postpartum outcomes in past research, including the general support provided to each mother by the close person; the degree of stress (daily hassles) reported by the mother (Kanner, Coyne, Schaefer, & Lazarus, 1981); and the difficulty of the infant's temperament (assessed with the Infant Characteristics Questionnaire of Bates, Freeland, & Lounsbury, 1979). These variables were included, along with the Expectancy Confirmation Scale scores, in the path model illustrated in Figure 9.3.

Our initial research with the 43 women who had been interviewed at 3 weeks postpartum indicated that relationship quality served to mediate the effect of support from a mother's closest relation on maternal well-being (Coffman, Levitt, Deets, & Quigley, 1991). That is, low support from the close relation was linked to relationship dissatisfaction, which was in turn related to depressed affect. Thus, relationship change was specified as a mediator of postpartum affect in the path model.

Affect was measured with the Bradburn (1969) Affect Balance Scale, which has been used frequently to assess affective well-being in nonclinical populations. To index relationship change, each mother was asked at 13

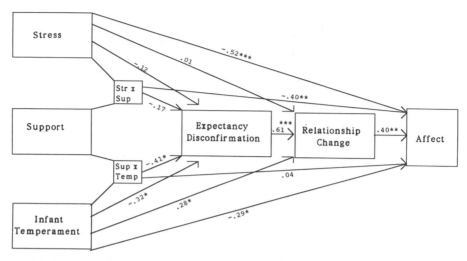

FIGURE 9.3. Path analysis of contributors to relationship change and affect balance following childbirth. *p < .05' **p < .01; ***p < .001.

months postpartum to indicate on the spatial Relationship Closeness Scale both the closeness of her current relationship with her closest person and the closeness of her relationship with that person prior to the infant's birth. A retrospective measure was created by subtracting current from prebirth Relationship Closeness. This measure was problematic, both because it was retrospective and because difference scores tend to be less reliable (Appelbaum & McCall, 1983). However, we validated the difference measure with a residual score analysis of actual change in scores on the verbal Relationship Satisfaction Scale, which had been administered at both 3 weeks and 13 months postpartum to 43 of the mothers. The 3-week Relationship Satisfaction scores were regressed on the 13-month scores, with the residuals representing the degree of change in the relationship across that time period. The correlation of the retrospective Relationship Closeness difference scores with the residual Relationship Satisfaction scores was .71. Thus, we were reasonably confident that the retrospective measure could be used to index relationship change.

As can be seen in Figure 9.3, expectancy disconfirmation was the strongest predictor of relationship change, accounting for a highly significant 32% of the variance over and above that accounted for by the remaining predictors. Only one other variable, difficult infant temperament, was related directly to relationship change, and the relation was a comparatively modest one. There was also a significant interaction, indicating a compound effect of expectancy disconfirmation and infant temperament on relationship change. Relationship change, in turn, was a significant predictor of postpartum affect. Note, however, that affect was multiply determined: Both high stress and difficult infant temperament predicted affect, and there was an interaction of stress and support, indicating the classic "buffering effect" of support (i.e., support promoted more positive affect under high-stress conditions). As an additional check on the results, we conducted a second path analysis, including the support, stress, support × stress interaction, and perceived expectancy confirmation variables as predictors with the residualized Relationship Satisfaction change scores as the criterion. The results were comparable: Perceived expectancy confirmation accounted for a significant 24% of the variance in relationship change, over and above the 9% accounted for by the remaining predictors.

The results affirm that postbirth relationship change is related to perceived expectancy disconfirmation, providing some support for the proposed model. However, sample limitations and the retrospective nature of the data preclude drawing firm conclusions. We have recently collected data for a more extensive study, in which both prebirth and postbirth questionnaires were completed by 105 women recruited through childbirth education classes (Coffman, Brown, & Levitt, 1992). The Support Expectations Index was completed 2 months prior to the infants' birth, along with the verbal and spatial relationship indices. Three months after their infants were born, participants again completed questionnaires including the relationship measures, the Expectancy Confirmation Scale, and the Received Support version of the Support Expectations Index. An index of support–expectation discrepancy was calculated by subtracting scores for each item on the Received Support Index from the corresponding item on the Support Expectations Index.

Preliminary analyses indicate that mean scores on the subjective Expectancy Confirmation Scale and on the more objective support–expectation discrepancy index were highly correlated ($r = .53$). Table 9.2 includes both the mean support–expectation discrepancy for each item and the partial correlation of each discrepancy with postbirth Relationship Closeness. Prebirth Relationship Closeness was partialed from the analyses, so that the tabled correlations represent the association of disconfirmed support expectations with change in relationship closeness across the childbirth transition.

The major discrepancies between prebirth expectations and postbirth support (column 1) were for items concerned with time spent caring for the child in the mother's absence (babysit), purchasing items for the baby, help with chores after the first few weeks, time spent playing with the baby, time spent teaching the baby, and showing the mother love and affection. (The marked discrepancy for the item regarding teaching the infant no doubt reflects the young age of the infant [3 months] at the time of the

TABLE 9.2. Discrepancy of Received Support from Expected Support, and Relationship Change

Item	1. Received–expected support discrepancy score[a]	2. Discrepancy and relationship change partial correlation[b]
Babysit	-.64	.32**
Time/talk	-.36	.54**
Financial	.00	.17
Buy items	-.63	.19
Care/first weeks	-.31	.24*
Care after	-.16	.34**
Chores/first weeks	-.34	.20*
Chores after	-.61	.35**
Play with baby	-.81	.26*
Teach baby	-1.42	.15
Show love for baby	-.53	.18
Show love for mother	-1.18	.40**
Approval	.27	-.08
General support	-.59	.38**
Mean of items	-.52	.48**

[a]Expected support subtracted from received support.
[b]Correlation of Relationship Closeness with received–expected support discrepancy after partialing prebirth Relationship Closeness.
$*p < .05; **p < .01.$

follow-up; this item would be more appropriate for older infants.) Expectations least likely to be discrepant from actual support were for providing financial support, helping with child care after the first few postbirth weeks, and approving the mother's child care methods.

As revealed in the partial correlations in Table 9.2 (column 2), significant predictors of relationship change included support-expectation discrepancies in the areas of baby care and playing with the baby, time spent talking with the mother, help with household tasks, demonstrating affection for the mother, and general support. The results are consistent with research indicating that violations of expectations regarding division of postbirth labor affect relationship satisfaction (Ruble et al., 1988), and suggest further that violations of emotional support expectations are important as well. These prospective findings regarding the association of expectancy disconfirmation with relationship change replicate the retrospective findings from our earlier study, and provide further support for the proposed model.

Thus, with regard to at least one major life transition—that precipitated by the birth of a child—the proposed expectancy model has received some confirmation. However, much work remains to be done with regard to unraveling the processes involved in the transformation of social relationships and the consequent evolution of convoy structure and function across the life span.

FUTURE DIRECTIONS

The proposed model of processes underlying relationship continuity and change across the life span is intended not as a formal theory, but as a point of departure for further study of life-span attachment processes within the context of the social network perspective. A number of avenues might be taken by researchers interested in pursuing this objective. First, additional studies of the childbirth transition might be undertaken with childless control groups, to ensure that the observed pattern of expectancy disconfirmation and relationship change is associated with the transition, and is not simply a function of the passage of time (Cowan & Cowan, 1988). Second, we need to learn how the direction of expectancy disconfirmation might affect relationship outcomes. The current analyses were focused only on the extent to which change occurred; the influence of negative versus positive instances of expectancy violation on relationship change has not been determined. Given research suggesting that conflict has a greater impact on relationship outcomes than positive interactions do (e.g., Gottman, 1979; Gottman & Krokoff, 1989), further exploration of this issue is essential.

Third, the childbirth transition represents only one significant transition in a lifetime of relatively ordered and predictable life events. Other events that occur with sufficient frequency to afford prospective study include school entry and departure, leaving home in early adulthood, marriage, job entry, and retirement. Non-normative events that might be analyzed prospectively include surgical procedures, geographic relocation, and divorce. It is important to extend the present analyses to other life transitions, in order to assess the generality of the association between disconfirmed support expectations and relationship/well-being outcomes. From the perspective of the proposed model, it would also be worthwhile to explore culturally based normative expectations regarding support from close relations at various stages of the life cycle. How such normative expectations interact with those derived through individual experience in the formulation of expectancies regarding support from specific social network members could then be explored.

Finally, even if the present results are replicated across various life transitions, only limited conclusions can be drawn from correlational research. It may be the case, for example, that individuals revise their estimates of received support as a result of changes in their relationships, so that relationship change leads to reports of expectancy disconfirmation rather than resulting from it. Intervention studies involving direct manipulation of support expectations are needed to supplement longitudinal efforts linking expectancy disconfirmation to relationship change.

In our recent study, in addition to collecting prospective correlational data, we attempted a minor intervention with participating couples during one of their prebirth education classes (Coffman et al., 1992). Couples in the intervention group completed the Support Expectations Index, shared their expectations with each other, and participated in a class discussion on the topic of support expectations. Couples in one control group completed the Support Expectations Index and an unrelated child-rearing attitudes questionnaire. Those in a second control group completed only the child-rearing attitudes questionnaire. Control group members shared their answers only on the child-rearing attitudes questionnaire and participated in a class discussion on child rearing. Preliminary results suggest that the intervention had a positive effect on couples, who indicated that they found the exercise to be worthwhile. The overall effects were not strong; however, considering the limited nature of the intervention, the results encourage further efforts.

Future interventions might include, in addition to clarification of support expectations held by relationship partners, the provision of information regarding the extent to which expectations are realistic, and attempts to modify unrealistic partner expectations prior to potentially disruptive life transitions. Should such interventions achieve their objective of forestalling the disruption of close supportive relationships, they not only would lend credence to the proposed expectancy model, but would provide a template for the implementation of community-based intervention programs designed to maintain the supportive social attachments that are so essential to well-being.

ACKNOWLEDGMENTS

This chapter is dedicated to the memory of our good friend and colleague, Steve Loveless, whose contributions to the conceptualization and analysis of the research reported herein were invaluable. We thank Toni Antonucci and Daniel Smothergill for their comments on an earlier version of this chapter.

REFERENCES

Ainsworth, M. D. S. (1989). Attachments beyond infancy. *American Psychologist, 44,* 709–716.

Ainsworth, M. D. S., Blehar, M., Waters, E., & Wall, S. (1978). *Patterns of attachment.* Hillsdale, NJ: Erlbaum.

Altman, I., & Taylor, D. A. (1973). *Social penetration: The development of interpersonal relationships.* New York: Holt, Rinehart & Winston.

Antonucci, T. C. (1976). Attachment: A life span concept. *Human Development, 19,* 135-142.

Antonucci, T. C. (1986). Social support networks: A hierarchical mapping technique. *Generations, 10*(4), 10-12.

Antonucci, T. C. (1990). Social supports and social relationships. In R. H. Binstock & L. K. George (Eds.), *Handbook of aging and the social sciences* (pp. 205-226). New York: Academic Press.

Antonucci, T. C., & Akiyama, H. (1987). Social networks in adult life and a preliminary examination of the convoy model. *Journal of Gerontology, 42*(5), 519-527.

Antonucci, T. C., & Israel, B. (1986). Veridicality of social support: A comparison of principal and network members' responses. *Journal of Consulting and Clinical Psychology, 54,* 432-437.

Appelbaum, M. I., & McCall, R. B. (1983). Design and analysis in developmental psychology. In W. Kessen (Ed.), *Handbook of child psychology* (4th ed.): *Vol. 1. History, theory, and methods* (pp. 415-476). New York: Wiley.

Bates, J. E., Freeland, C. A., & Lounsbury, M. L. (1979). Measurement of infant difficultness. *Child Development, 50,* 794-803.

Belsky, J. (1985). Exploring individual differences in marital change across the transition to parenthood: The role of violated expectations. *Journal of Marriage and the Family, 47,* 1037-1044.

Belsky, J., Spanier, G. B., & Rovine, M. (1983). Stability and change in marriage across the transition to parenthood. *Journal of Marriage and the Family, 45,* 567-577.

Benson, P. R. (1991, April). *Predicting relationship adaptation among new parents.* Paper presented at the biennial meeting of the Society for Research in Child Development, Seattle.

Berman, W. H. (1988a). The role of attachment in the post-divorce experience. *Journal of Personality and Social Psychology, 54,* 496-503.

Berman, W. H. (1988b). The relationship of ex-spouse attachment to adjustment following divorce. *Journal of Family Psychology, 1,* 312-328.

Berman, W. H., & Sperling, M. B. (1991). Parental attachment and emotional distress in the transition to college. *Journal of Youth and Adolescence, 20*(4), 427-440.

Boukydis, C., Lester, B., & Hoffman, J. (1987). Parenting and social support networks in families of term and preterm infants. In C. Boukydis (Ed.), *Research on support for parents and infants in the postnatal period* (pp. 61-83). Norwood, NJ: Ablex.

Boyce, W. T. (1985). Social support, family relations, and children. In S. Cohen & S. L. Syme (Eds.), *Social support and health* (pp. 151-173). New York: Academic Press.

Bradburn, N. (1969). *The structure of psychological well-being.* Chicago: Aldine.

Bretherton, I. (1990). Open communication and internal working models: Their role in the development of attachment relationships. In R. A. Thompson (Ed.), *Nebraska Symposium on Motivation: Vol. 36. Socioemotional development* (pp. 57-113). Lincoln: University of Nebraska Press.

Cairns, R. B. (1977). Beyond social attachment: The dynamics of interactional development. In T. Alloway, P. Pliner, & L. Krames (Eds.), *Attachment behavior* (pp. 1-24). New York: Plenum.

Campbell, A., Converse, P., & Rodgers, W. (1976). *The quality of American life*. New York: Russell Sage Foundation.

Clark, M. S. (1984). A distinction between two types of relationships and its implications for development. In J. C. Masters & K. Yarkin-Levin (Eds.), *Boundary areas in social and developmental psychology* (pp. 241-270). New York: Academic Press.

Coffman, S., Brown, L., & Levitt, M. J. (1992, February). *Clarifying support expectations in prenatal couples*. Paper presented at the meeting of the Southern Nursing Research Society, Nashville, TN.

Coffman, S., Levitt, M. J., & Deets, C. (1991). Personal and professional support for mothers of NICU and healthy newborns. *Journal of Obstetric, Gynecologic, and Neonatal Nursing, 20*, 406-413.

Coffman, S., Levitt, M. J., Deets, C., & Quigley, K. L. (1991). Close relationships in mothers of at-risk and normal newborns: Support, expectancy confirmation, and maternal well-being. *Journal of Family Psychology, 5*, 93-107.

Coffman, S., Levitt, M. J., & Guacci-Franco, N. (1993). Mothers' stress and close relationships: Correlates with infant health status. *Pediatric Nursing, 19*, 135-142.

Cohen, S., & Wills, T. A. (1985). Stress, social support, and the buffering hypothesis. *Psychological Bulletin, 98*, 310-357.

Cowan, P. A., & Cowan, C. P. (1988). Changes in marriage during the transition to parenthood: Must we blame the baby? In G. Y. Michaels & W. A. Goldberg (Eds.), *The transition to parenthood* (pp. 114-154). New York: Cambridge University Press.

Crnic, K., & Greenberg, M. (1987). Maternal stress, social support, and coping: Influences on the early mother-infant relationship. In C. Boukydis (Ed.), *Research on support for parents and infants in the postnatal period* (pp. 25-40). Norwood, NJ: Ablex.

Crnic, K. A., Greenberg, M. T., Ragozin, A. S., Robinson, N. M., & Basham, R. B. (1983). Effects of stress and social support on mothers and premature and full term infants. *Child Development, 54*, 209-217.

Cutrona, C. E. (1984). Social support and stress in the transition to parenthood. *Journal of Abnormal Psychology, 93*, 378-390.

Davis, K. E., & Todd, M. J. (1982). Friendship and love relationships. *Advances in Descriptive Psychology, 2*, 79-122.

Fiske, S. T., & Taylor, S. E. (1991). *Social cognition*. New York: McGraw-Hill.

Furman, W., & Buhrmester, D. (1985). Children's perceptions of the personal relationships in their social networks. *Developmental Psychology, 21*, 1016-1024.

Gotlib, I. H., Whiffen, V. E., & Wallace, P. M. (1991). Prospective investigation of postpartum depression: Factors involved in onset and recovery. *Journal of Abnormal Psychology, 100*, 122-132.

Gottman, J. M. (1979). *Marital interaction: Experimental investigations*. New York: Academic Press.

Gottman, J. M., & Krokoff, L. J. (1989). Marital interaction and satisfaction: A longitudinal view. *Journal of Consulting and Clinical Psychology, 57*, 47-53.

Hinde, R. A., & Stevenson-Hinde, J. (1987). Interpersonal relationships and child development. *Developmental Review, 7,* 1-21.

Holmes, J. G., & Boon, S. D. (1990). Developments in the field of close relationships: Creating foundations for intervention strategies. *Personality and Social Psychology Bulletin, 16,* 23-41.

Hopkins, J., Marcus, M., & Campbell, S. B. (1984). Postpartum depression: A critical review. *Psychological Bulletin, 95,* 498-515.

Kach, J., & McGhee, P. (1982). Adjustment of early parenthood: The role of accuracy of preparenthood experiences. *Journal of Family Issues, 3,* 375-388.

Kahn, R. L., & Antonucci, T. C. (1980). Convoys over the life course: Attachment, roles, and social support. In P. B. Baltes & O. G. Brim (Eds.), *Life span development and behavior* (Vol. 3, pp. 253-286). New York: Academic Press.

Kanner, A., Coyne, J., Schaefer, C., & Lazarus, R. (1981). Comparison of two modes of stress measurement: Daily hassles and uplifts versus major life events. *Journal of Behavioral Medicine, 4,* 1-37.

Kelley, H. H., Berscheid, E., Christensen, A., Harvey, A. H., Huston, T. L., Levinger, G., McClintock, E., Peplau, L. A., & Peterson, D. R. (1993). *Close relationships.* New York: W. H. Freeman.

Levitt, M. J. (1980). Contingent feedback, familiarization, and infant affect: How a stranger becomes a friend. *Developmental Psychology, 16,* 425-432.

Levitt, M. J. (1991). Attachment and close relationships: A life span perspective. In J. L. Gewirtz & W. F. Kurtines (Eds.), *Intersections with attachment* (pp. 183-206). Hillsdale, NJ: Erlbaum.

Levitt, M. J., & Clark, M. C. (1982, April). *Mother-infant reciprocity, causality, and response to contingent feedback.* Paper presented at the meeting of the International Conference on Infant Studies, Austin, TX.

Levitt, M. J., Guacci, N., & Coffman, S. (1993). Social networks in infancy: An observational study. *Merrill-Palmer Quarterly, 39,* 233-251.

Levitt, M. J., Guacci-Franco, N., & Levitt, J. L. (1993). Convoys of social support in childhood and early adolescence: Structure and function. *Developmental Psychology, 29,* 811-818.

Levitt, M. J., Weber, R. A., & Guacci, N. (1993). Convoys of social support: An intergenerational analysis. *Psychology and Aging, 8,* 323-326.

Levitt, M. J., Weber, R. A., & Clark, M. C. (1986). Social network characteristics as sources of maternal support and well-being. *Developmental Psychology, 22,* 310-316.

Lewis, M. (1987). Social development in infancy and early childhood. In J. D. Osofsky (Ed.), *Handbook of infant development* (2nd ed., pp. 419-493). New York: Wiley

Lewis, M., Alessandri, S. M., & Sullivan, M. (1990). Violation of expectancy, loss of control, and anger expressions in young infants. *Developmental Psychology, 26,* 745-751.

Masters, J. C., & Yarkin-Levin, K. (Eds.). (1984). *Boundary areas in social and developmental psychology.* New York: Academic Press.

McCall, R. B. (1990). Infancy research: Individual differences. *Merrill-Palmer Quarterly, 36*(1), 141-158.

Mead, M. (1962). A cultural anthropologist's approach to maternal deprivation. In World Health Organization, *Deprivation of maternal care: A reassessment of its effects* (Public Health Papers No. 14, pp. 45-62). Geneva, Switzerland: World Health Organization.

Mutran, E., & Reitzes, D. C. (1984). Intergenerational support activities and well-being among the elderly: A convergence of exchange and symbolic interaction perspectives. *American Sociological Review, 49,* 117-130.

Pipp, S., Shaver, P., Jennings, S., Lamborn, S., & Fischer, K. (1985). Adolescents' theories about the development of their relationships with parents. *Journal of Personality and Social Psychology, 48,* 991-1001.

Reedy, M. N., Birren, J. E., & Schaie, K. W. (1981). Age and sex differences in satisfying love relationships across the adult life span. *Human Development, 24,* 52-56.

Rossi, A. S., & Rossi, P. H. (1990). *Of human bonding.* New York: Aldine/de Gruyter.

Rubin, Z. (1973). *Liking and loving.* New York: Holt, Rinehart & Winston.

Ruble, D. N., Fleming, A. S., Hackel, L. S., & Stangor, C. (1988). Changes in the marital relationship during the transition to first time motherhood: Effects of violated expectations concerning division of household labor. *Journal of Personality and Social Psychology, 55,* 78-87.

Schellenberg, J. A. (1990). William James and symbolic interactionism. *Personality and Social Psychology Bulletin, 16*(4), 769-773.

Shaver, P. R., & Hazan, C. (1988). A biased overview of the study of love. *Journal of Social and Personal Relationships, 5,* 473-502.

Smith, E. R., & Zarate, M. A. (1992). Exemplar-based model of social judgment. *Psychological Review, 99*(1), 3-21.

Sternberg, R. J., & Grajek, S. (1984). The nature of love. *Journal of Personality and Social Psychology, 47,* 312-329.

Takahashi, K. (1990). Affective relationships and their lifelong development. In P. B. Baltes, D. L. Featherman, & L. R. Sherrod (Eds.), *Life span development and behavior* (Vol. 10, pp. 1-29). Hillsdale, NJ: Erlbaum.

Tietjen, A. & Bradley, C. (1985). Social support and maternal psychosocial adjustment during the transition to parenthood. *Canadian Journal of Behavioral Science, 17*(2), 109-121.

Tronick, E. Z. (1989). Emotions and emotional communication in infants. *American Psychologist, 44*(2), 112-119.

Tronick, E. Z., Morelli, G. A., & Ivey, P. K. (1992). The Efe forager infant and toddler's pattern of social relationships: Multiple and simultaneous. *Developmental Psychology, 28*(4), 568-577.

Van IJzendoorn, M. H. (1992). Intergenerational transmission of parenting: A review of studies in nonclinical populations. *Developmental Review, 12,* 76-99.

Van IJzendoorn, M. H., & Tavecchio, L. W. C. (1987). Attachment theory as a Lakatosian research program. In L. W. C. Tavecchio & M. H. van IJzendoorn (Eds.), *Attachment in social networks.* Amsterdam: Elsevier.

Watson, J. S. (1979). Perception of contingency as a determinant of social responsiveness. In E. B. Thoman (Ed.), *Origins of the infant's social responsiveness* (pp. 33-64). Hillsdale, NJ: Erlbaum.

Weisz, J. R. (1986). Understanding the developing understanding of control. In M. Perlmutter (Ed.), *Minnesota Symposia on Child Psychology: Vol. 18. Cognitive perspectives on children's social and behavioral development* (pp. 219-285). Hillsdale, NJ: Erlbaum.

Zajonc, R. B. (1968). Attitudinal effects of mere exposure. *Journal of Personality and Social Psychology, 9,* 1-27.

CHAPTER 10

Attachment in Adulthood and Aging

TONI C. ANTONUCCI

The consideration of attachment as a life-span concept is not new. Both Bowlby and Ainsworth considered attachment from this perspective (Ainsworth, 1989, 1991; Ainsworth & Bowlby, 1991; Bowlby, 1969; see also Bretherton, 1992). As early as 1976, a special edition of the journal *Human Development* entitled "Attachment: A Life-Span Concept" (Antonucci, 1976) was published with representative authors from infancy, adulthood, and aging—each advocating the usefulness of the concept. Lerner and Ryff (1978) used attachment as the model case for a life-span concept. More recently, infant researchers have increasingly turned to the study of attachment as a life-span concept; for example, contributors to the monograph by Bretherton and Waters (1985), especially Main, Kaplan, and Cassidy (1985), and Ricks (1985), have considered adult attachment. Still others whose work has focused on adulthood and old age, such as Weiss (1982), Hazan and Shaver (1987), Blazer (1982), and Cicirelli (1989, 1991), have found the concept useful. The concept of attachment has been shown to have clinical and psychopathological implications (see Belsky & Nezworski, 1988) and to be cross-cultural, although the latter area is not without some controversy (van IJzendoorn, 1990). Several books have explored this topic explicitly, including Parkes and Stevenson-Hinde (1982), Parkes, Stevenson-Hinde, and Marris (1991), and the present volume. The current chapter proposes a further extension of attachment theory using the convoy model, which offers an integration of life-span developmental psychology and research on social relations. This extension is especially useful with older adults, but may also serve to integrate the plethora of research that has been emerging on the longitudinal effects of mother-infant attachment.

LIFE-SPAN DEVELOPMENT

Life-span developmental psychology argues that the individual is constantly and continually progressing through developmental sequences that are cumulative, although not always progressive. Ainsworth's (1989, 1991) emphasis on the importance of her early longitudinal work, both in Uganda and in Baltimore, highlights the degree to which attachment theory is fundamentally consonant with the basic tenets of life-span developmental psychology. Ainsworth has always argued that it is possible to ascertain the developmental progression of attachment in the infant by observing the mother's behaviors toward her infant over the first year of life, and, to a lesser extent (at least in the early months), the infant's behaviors toward his or her mother.

Basic to this perspective is the view that the mother's and infant's behaviors influence each other and show an underlying continuity, which may not always be identified through continuity in behaviors. For example, the young infant whose mother responds quickly to his or her cries tends to cry less at the end of the first year (Ainsworth, Blehar, Waters, & Wall, 1978; Ainsworth, 1991). The behaviors of the infant may seem inconsistent or noncumulative, but Ainsworth has argued that the mother's underlying behavior—that is, her responsiveness to her infant—provides the continuity, consistency, and predictability that lead from the mother's behavior to the infant's. Hence, in the language of life-span developmental psychologists, Ainsworth and Bowlby proposed both life-span continuity and intergenerational transmission. Both concepts are central to life-span developmental psychology and social gerontology.

Intraindividual Development

Life-span developmental psychology emphasizes both the intra- and interindividual development of the person. By "intraindividual development" is meant the ontogenetic development that occurs within the individual over time. In attachment research, intraindividual development is critical in several dimensions. The first of these is the behavior of the child or mother over time. All attachment research emphasizes the importance of these longitudinal behaviors. The classic works in this field have empirically examined longitudinal attachment behaviors of both the infant and the mother. The case for the infant is perhaps obvious, since it is the much more common example of development studied by child psychologists. The baby is developing quite dramatically in many ways—physically, cognitively, emotionally, socially—and this intraindividual development is so significant as to be readily observable. Even though attachment research has been much less concerned with adult development in the manner of usual interest to gerontologists, the change and continuity in the mother's behaviors over time constitute a clear example of adult development. The evolution of these behaviors in both the adult and infant members of the dyad are clear examples of intraindividual development.

Attachment researchers have always recognized that the baby is a developing being. It is important to note that attachment researchers have similarly appreciated the fact that the mother is a developing individual. The study of the continuity and evolution of maternal attachment behavior is, in fact, the study of adult intraindividual development in addition to the interindividual development of the mother–child relationship. Although the emphasis in attachment research has mostly been on the child, it is clear that this examination of the mother's behaviors represents a realization of, and indeed a commitment to, life-span development. By simple extension, one can see that the mother is still a mother throughout the child's infancy, childhood, and adolescence, as well as throughout her own young adulthood, middle age, and old age. Through all these years and experiences, her own development continues. Of course, at any specific time the possibility exists of specific emphasis on different issues, different relationships, and the addition of other attachment figures.

Interindividual Development

As intraindividual development occurs, the individual continues to maintain relationships with other people. These interactions constitute the basis for interindividual development. For the purposes of this chapter, it is useful to focus on social and emotional interactions. Indeed, it might be clearest to consider interindividual social development as the result of the cumulative impact of the interacting parties' intraindividual development, as well as their interindividual interaction. It is probably simplest to think of these as bidirectional influences. Just as the early 1970s saw increased recognition of the infant's effect on his or her mother, which was later generalized to the bidirectionality of all child–attachment figure relationships, this bidirectionality can also be seen to operate among adults. With adults, however, it is very likely that the situation is considerably more complex.

Intra- and Interindividual Development

As we seek to understand attachment among older adults, it is critical to recognize that as individuals age, they accumulate a greater number of experiences. People become more different, not less different. The lifetime accumulations of both intra- and interindividual interactions are what evolve into the attachments of older adults. Therefore, these interpersonal experiences are critical to the understanding of attachment among adults.

A major issue to consider in the extension of the concept of attachment into old age is the integration of multiple attachment relationships.

Several points are relevant. On the one hand, the older a person is, the longer he or she is likely to have had specific attachment relationships. Similarly, the older an individual is, the more attachment relationships he or she is likely to acquire. Both issues have already been addressed to some limited degree in the literature on infant-child attachment (see Sroufe & Fleeson, 1986).

Early longitudinal attachment studies, including Ainsworth's original studies, examined how relationships evolved. In fact, the behaviors of both the adult and the child were closely followed. This research was able to demonstrate both consistency over time and the evolution of behavior over time. In addition to the example mentioned above concerning early maternal response to crying, there is the literature considering proximal and distal attachment behaviors among infants (see, e.g., Ainsworth et al., 1978). Thus, it was demonstrated that infants who were securely attached, as demonstrated through their proximal attachment behaviors, were able to substitute distal attachment behaviors as they got older. Young children who felt threatened sought physical contact with their mothers (i.e., proximal attachment behaviors), but older securely attached children could be reassured by a simple glance toward their mother (i.e., distal attachment behaviors). The concept is easily extended through the life cycle, but much less is known about the appropriate assessments of such behaviors.

The bidirectionality of influence should also be reiterated. Thus, the growing child affects the mother, just as the maturing mother affects the child. It may be that the child can now use new abilities to maintain the relationship with the mother, or that the mother has new confidence in her own abilities, which in turn influences her interaction with her infant. As each member of the dyad ages, the relationship continues, but the specific behaviors that exemplify the relationship change.

EXTENDING ATTACHMENTS OVER TIME AND ACROSS DIMENSIONS

Bowlby, Ainsworth, and their colleagues have argued that secure attachment has a pervasive influence on the child's development. Attachment is said to provide a "secure base" from which the child explores the world. This concept may be seen as one inherent in child or early development, but it is equally relevant for the challenges that the individual faces over the life course. If both the child and the mother are attached, does attachment also provide the adult with a secure base from which to explore the world? I would propose that it does, though certainly not exclusively, through a secure attachment relationship with an infant. Nevertheless, it is useful to think of a number of secure attachment relationships providing the adult with a "convoy" through life, though in a manner somewhat more complicated than is true for the simpler attachment relationships of the child.

The first question to consider is the role of childhood attachments in lifelong attachments (e.g., to one's parents) in adult peer attachments (e.g., to one's spouse), and still later in adult–young child and elder–adult child attachments (e.g., to one's own infant, child, and adult child). All of these can clearly be seen as attachment relationships. The fundamental nature of these relationships to other aspects of life, as well as their interrelationship with one another, is critical. Their cumulative effect is also recognized by Levitt and colleagues (e.g., see Levitt, Coffman, Guacci-Franco, & Loveless, Chapter 9, this volume) who emphasize the importance of expectancies that develop over time and the devastating effect of expectancies of others that are not met.

The "graying" of attachment is a complicated affair that builds on the development of a lifetime of accumulated relationships and expectancies. The convoy model of social relations provides a framework for integrating these relationships, as well as for understanding and conceptualizing the nature of attachment relationships and distinguishing them from other social relationships commonly experienced among adults.

CONVOYS OF SOCIAL RELATIONS

In order to describe the multifaceted nature of social relations and their function in the individual's life, Robert Kahn and I (Kahn & Antonucci, 1980; Antonucci, 1985, 1990) have borrowed the anthropologist David Plath's (1980) term "convoy" to describe the conglomerate of social interactions and relationships within which most people exist. The term is especially useful because in the colloquial sense it conjures up the image of safe passage through difficult times, much as attachment theory argues that the attachment figure provides a secure base from which to explore the world. The "convoy of social relations" describes the close and significant relationships within which an individual is enmeshed. These convoy members provide aid and protection–indeed, safe passage through difficult times, be they developmental milestones, personal crises, or significant life events. However, even from the earliest conceptualizations of the convoy model, we recognized that the ideal may not always be realized. Thus, a convoy can shelter and protect *or* endanger and make vulnerable the individual, depending on the nature of the relationship. And with age, at least to a certain extent, the number of relationships with which the individual is engaged is certainly likely to increase.

The convoy model has been conceptually and diagrammatically presented as a hierarchical model of three concentric circles with the individual in the center (Antonucci, 1986). Each circle represents a different level of closeness. The inner circle is described as representing the most close and important relationships; usually (but not always), these are relationships with parents, spouse, and children. The middle circle represents relationships that are less close but still very close. These are likely to be other relatives and friends with whom one has multilevel relationships. The third circle is conceptualized as including people with whom one has special social relationships, but relationships that are role-specific and singular; examples of such people might include coworkers or the friends of close relatives. Thus, such a relationship is important and potentially influential, but is dependent upon a specific role relationship or connection and is likely to be terminated if that connection is not sustained. In attachment terminology, it might be said that one's relationships with inner-circle members are primary attachments; with middle-circle members, secondary attachments; and with outer-circle members, more generalized social relations. The convoy model is especially designed to give precedence to the importance of attachment relationships (such as the mother-infant attachment relationship), but to recognize that for normal adult development, other social relationships also play a critical role in the life of the individual in a manner that is much more likely to be both reciprocal and bidirectional.

The basic idea of the convoy model is to integrate the accumulation of intra- and interindividual interpersonal interactions that the individual experiences over time. As the convoy encircles individuals over their lifetime, it influences them in fundamental ways. Here, too, we can draw from the attachment literature. The same secure base provided by the attachment figure to the infant can be generalized to provide a secure base for the adult. But in defining what the secure base provides, instead of the opportunity for the child to explore his or her environment, we may turn to the more fundamental notion that is implied—namely, the interest, ability, and security to seek and meet the challenges that a person faces during the course of his or her lifetime.

Through adulthood, these challenges evolve and multiply. A young adult must develop the ability to initiate and sustain adult relationships; this includes choosing a partner with whom he or she can sustain a close and significant relationship. We might think of this in attachment terms as well (Feeney & Noller, 1990; Hazan & Shaver, 1987; Sperling & Berman, 1991). Thus, the young adult faced with the challenge of choosing a partner who will provide support as he or she faces the other challenges of life—in other words, a secure base from which to explore the world. In adult terms, we might speak of the support provided by a significant other that enables the individual to develop his or her potential optimally. This could be the challenge of school, a career, or parenthood. An attachment relationship with a peer is likely to be just as beneficial and cumulatively advantageous as the continued support of a secure life-long parent–child attachment. However, it seems likely that these peer–peer relationships serve particular functions that cannot be met by the parent–child attachment. The examination of attachment within a life-span perspective allows us to extend our clinical awareness of the importance of these relationships to normal development by understanding that they must continue to evolve not only within the context of the original (i.e., parent–child) relationship, but also outside that context, and must enable the individual to continue to expand the base of his or her primary attachment relationships to meet the tasks, needs, and goals of normal development.

These attachment relationships, of course, continue to evolve, develop, and be enumerated through the life span. The young adult, having successfully acquired a peer adult attachment, often next turns to the challenge of parenting and establishing a significant relationship for the first time with a person many years his or her junior. The bulk of the attachment literature has focused on the mother as the guiding force of the relationship, but placing this new relationship in the life-course sequence of attachments makes it eminently clearer how developmental and cumulative the relationship is, both for the mother and her infant.

ETIOLOGICAL ISSUES IN ATTACHMENT

A basic question in the study of attachment is the etiological one: What causes secure attachment? Or, to put it another way, how is secure attachment most successfully developed? At the clinical level, Ainsworth has basically responded that although attachment is clearly a bidirectional phenomenon, the most critical aspect of its development is the responsiveness of the mother to the child.

Ainsworth's careful longitudinal studies, as well as our own and those of others (e.g., Antonucci & Levitt, 1984; Sroufe, 1985), indicate that the mother's responsiveness is the most consistent and predictive characteristic of later infant attachment security. This being the case, is it possible to dissect the concept of maternal responsiveness or to speculate about how and why maternal responsivity translates into infant attachment security, and, furthermore, to extrapolate from this relationship to adult attachments?

This is not a simple question. Indeed, the very example of the mother's responding quickly to the cries of her young infant has been a controversial one. At various times it has been argued that responding so quickly to infants' cries will create spoiled children—ones who will require constant attention and be unable or unwilling to meet their own needs as they mature. The evidence has been to the contrary. What psychological constructs might explain the fact that infants who are responded to quickly are less likely to continue to make the same types of requests as they get older? Attachment theorists have argued that a responsive mother teaches the child that he or she can have confidence that reasonable requests will be responded to appropriately, and that this responsiveness of the attachment figure develops in the child a sense of trust and empowerment. The child learns to trust that the world is a kind and benevolent place, made so by responsive others who help the child achieve his or her goals. But the child also develops through attachment relationships a sense of empowerment—a sense that he or she can influence, affect, even control the world. It is the combination of trust and empowerment that is interpreted as secure attachment and that eventually allows the infant to develop optimally. This combination is also a powerful base for adults.

We (Antonucci & Jackson, 1987), building upon a variety of research—including the literatures on attachment, control (see Baltes & Baltes, 1990; Langer & Rodin, 1976; Skinner, 1985), efficacy (see Bandura, 1986; Ewart, 1992), and psychommunological functioning (Kiecolt-Glaser et al., 1987; Jemmott & Locke, 1980)—have speculated on the etiological basis for the power of significant social relationships over time. To summarize briefly, we know from these literatures that the perception of control can fundamentally influence individuals' feelings about themselves and, indeed, their health. Langer and Rodin (1976) gave house plants to institutionalized elderly individuals. Some were asked to take care of the plant—in other words, to take control of and responsibility for them. Others were told simply to enjoy the plants in their rooms; others would care for the plants. The people who were told they had responsibility for the care of their plants showed improvements in general affect and were less likely to have died at the time of follow-up several months later. Margaret Baltes (Baltes & Baltes, 1990) has shown that institutionalized elderly people have clever and diverse ways of controlling their environment, often with "dependent" behaviors. Bandura's (1986) work adds still another dimension. In a series of studies of men recovering from mild myocardial infarctions, Bandura was able to show that among those with objectively similar health status, men with wives who thought their husbands would recover were much more likely to recover than men whose wives did not think they would recover.

Each of these examples might easily be explained in terms of adult attachments. One might argue that secure adult attachments provide individuals with feelings of competence, a perception of control, and a belief in their own ability to meet the challenges of the world successfully— in short, a secure base from which to explore or to take control of some aspects of their lives. In the example of caring for house plants, this activity provided institutionalized elderly individuals with total control over some small portion of their otherwise externally controlled lives. In the case of Bandura's cardiac rehabilitation patients, we might argue that some wives were able to provide their husbands with a secure base, which translated into a sense of being able to control and successfully direct their own recovery. It seems likely that the relationships between Bandura's wives and their husbands, and the effects of these relationships, were more cumulative than this particular explanation might suggest. Indeed, adult attachments in general seem likely to be more cumulative and more multi-faceted than early attachments.

We (Antonucci & Jackson, 1987) have explicitly tried to specify the nature of these interactions more precisely. We have argued that continual cumulative interactions first with primary and then with secondary attach-ment figures, and later in other social relationships, provide and then contribute to this base. In effect, the infant, child, or adult is not only re-sponded to, as is the case with maternal responsiveness; in a more gen-eralized sense, he or she is provided with accurate, supportive, contingent feedback. This feedback assures the individual that he or she is a worthy and competent individual, in addition to being specific to the event. As in the role of the responsive mother, the individual experiences inter-actions that are responsive to his or her behaviors. In optimal settings, the individual accumulates helpful, supportive interactions over time, which lead first to secure attachment with the primary attachment figure(s) but then generalize to other relationships.

Of course, the situation is neither this simple nor this linear. It begins with the mother–child relationship, which is likely to become increasingly complex as the child and mother mature. The optimal situation is one in which a mother is responsive to her young infant and maintains that responsiveness to her child as the child matures and develops different requirements. Thinking of the changing infant and recognizing that this relationship is usually sustained over 50 years, we cannot help being impressed by the complexity of this relationship. In keeping with the dyadic research on attachment, it is important to recognize that both the child and parent are developing, evolving, and changing over time.

In some ways the attachment literature thus far has focused on rela-tively simple cases, although it did not seem so at the time. In defining infant attachment security, we can rely primarily on the mother's respon-sivity to her child and her child's response to separation and to threats in security. As the infant matures through childhood, adolescence, and adulthood, the types of responsiveness required by the child become increasingly complex but are likely to have similarly far-reaching effects on the individual. We (Antonucci & Jackson, 1987) have argued, however, that secure relationships will provide the individual with a feeling of personal efficacy that permits him or her to meet the challenges of life successfully.

Meeting the challenges of life successfully, it should be pointed out, does not always mean being successful. In fact, the securely attached adult may be the one who is able to garner the appropriate feedback permitting him or her to make a decision that "success" is impossible, unsuitable, or too interpersonally costly. The complication of later attachments is that the appropriate feedback may not be so universal. Thus, with an infant, good adult attachment figures maximize the probability that the infant will be securely attached. "Securely attached" can be assessed in a relatively universal manner as the ability to withstand separation from the attachment figure and to seek and explore (usually physically) new aspects of the environment. As the individual gets older, the appropriate way to explore the challenges of the environment becomes increasingly person-specific. Thus, a base of secure attachment relationships may mean that the individual strives for the goal of being a rocket scientist, or it may mean recognizing that he or she does not have the ability to be one. The broader challenges adults face require a closer matching of individual ability and goal setting.

In social relationships, it is likely that there is greater specific continuity. Individuals who did not enjoy secure attachments as children will have much greater difficulty achieving secure adult attachments. However, as the work of Main et al. (1985) suggests, some individuals are able as adults to recognize limitations in their early attachment relationships and to recover from them. These findings caution us to avoid assuming a fatality of life-span continuity in attachment relationships, although one must not underestimate their potential negative impact. As the convoy model of social relations makes clear, individuals can move through their lives surrounded by a number of other individuals, each of whom can affect them in significant negative or positive ways over time.

Although many of the causal factors of attachment and other social relationships remain purely speculative, an accumulating body of evidence is becoming available that highlights intra- and interindividual aspects of attachment and other support relationships, and documents their significant impact on health and well-being. I now turn to a brief review of available evidence from our own program of research on adult social relationships.

EMPIRICAL EVIDENCE

During the past 15 years, my colleagues and I have undertaken a series of studies focusing on the social relationships of older people. These studies in many ways constitute an empirical examination of the convoy model. Among the more novel aspects of this research program is the attempt to use survey methodology to assess qualitative as well as quantitative aspects of older adults' social relationships.

Our preliminary efforts began with a study entitled "Supports of the Elderly: Family, Friends and Professionals" (Kahn & Antonucci, 1984). The initial study consisted of a national probability sample of 718 men and women over 50 years of age interviewed in 1980. A second wave of the study was conducted in 1984 (Antonucci, Kahn, Harrison, & Payne, 1986). These data were useful for confirming who were nominated as partners in close social relationships (i.e., the subjects' attachments and other social relations), as well as the stability of these relationships over time. Evidence was also made available about the association between these relationships and the general well-being of the individuals.

Stability of Close Social Relationships

Although some important aspects of the methodology were different in the two studies—for example, the 1980 data were collected in face-to-face interviews, whereas the 1984 data were collected by telephone (see Antonucci & Akiyama, 1987b, for details)—the evidence indicated significant stability over time concerning the people mentioned, as well as the number, frequency of contact, and perceived adequacy of these relationships. There was also significant stability in the report at both time periods of most support behaviors—for example, "reassure you," "care for you when sick," "talk with you about your health," and "talk with you when you are upset" (and, to a slightly lesser degree, "confide in you" and "respect you"). This pattern of stability in adult relationships seems to parallel the type of continuity that has been documented in mother–child relationships. I turn now to a more detailed consideration of whom the elderly nominated as their primary attachment figures.

Nature of Close Social Relationships

Using a hierarchical mapping technique (detailed in Antonucci, 1986), we asked individuals to generate the group of people so close and important to them that it would be hard to imagine life without them—people who might easily be considered adult primary attachment figures. The data are detailed in Antonucci and Akiyama (1987a) but are summarized here. The data indicated that almost the entire sample could nominate members of this inner circle, but that the average number of people nominated for this category was in fact only 3.5. In general, there were no age differences; that is, people over 75 nominated about the same number of people as those in their 50s. Additional characteristics of this inner circle that were suggestive of their primary attachment quality were the average duration of these relationships (more than 30 years) and the predominance of family relationships (primarily spouses and children).

Apropos of the nature of these relationships, we examined the proportion of types of support exchanged with inner-circle ("primary") attachment figures as compared to those in middle- and outer-circle ("other") social relationships. These supports included confiding, respect, reassurance, sick care, talking about their health, and talking about things that worried or upset them. The data were clear: People both received and provided these things in their primary attachments/inner-circle relationships much more than in any other of their social relationships. To reinterpret this in the language of attachment theory, we might argue that such exchanges continue to provide adults with the type of secure base that mothers provide their infants in the secure attachment relationship. Mothers hold, look at, talk to, smile at, soothe, and attend to the physical needs of their infants; in other words, they care for and comfort them. We could similarly argue that adults turn to their primary attachment figures for the same care and comfort (in the form of sharing of confidence, problems, and worries; care when sick; and reassurance and respect). But just as early proximal attachment behaviors are replaced by distal attachment behaviors in the first years of life, remaining specific to the primary attachment figure while at the same time expanding to other attachment figures, adults appear to maintain certain behavioral links with their primary adult attachment figures but also to include others for specific support exchanges.

Close examination of the pattern of these exchanges, especially their evolution through old age, will be revealing. Certain patterns are already evident. For example, we (Antonucci, Kahn, & Akiyama, 1989) were able to show that elderly people who spoke to close supportive others about symptoms they were experiencing were more likely to make appropriate inquiries to health care professionals about those symptoms than elderly people who did not. Thus, in behavior patterns that are increasingly important among the elderly, primary attachment relationships seem to provide individuals with the secure base to take the appropriate next step, and thereby to meet the challenges of age successfully.

Intergenerational Patterns of Social Relations

One additional aspect of the original "Supports of the Elderly" study was interviewing the partners in the closest social relationships mentioned by people over 70 years of age, including, if possible, the intergenerational intrafamily members nominated as close social relations. These data are reported in detail in Antonucci and Akiyama (1991). We were able to document intergenerational, intrafamilial continuity in these adult attachment relationships. These data showed strong similarity in the inner circles of grandparents and their adult children, but much less similarity among their grandchildren. In fact, a large number of characteristics of the close social relationships of grandparents and adult children were quite similar. The nature of the relationships and the degree to which specific characteristics of the relationships existed were also quite similar among adult children and their parents (i.e., among the parents and grandparents). This was true for both giving and receiving of reassurance, respect, and either giving or receiving of all the other social exchanges. It should be noted that these data simply provide information about the descriptive aspects of close social relationships. In many ways the data can still only be considered preliminary, since they do not yet provide information about the quality of the relationships. Thus, in terms of the attachment literature, it may be the case that families exhibit similar attachment behavior patterns; however, this does not necessarily translate into information about the quality or security of these relationships. Data on negative aspects of social relationships in adulthood from these studies are suggestive.

Significant Negative Close Social Relationships

Some data are available on negative close social relationships which might be interpreted as attachment relationships of poor or ambivalent quality. Two recent analyses are relevant. We (Schuster, Antonucci, & Akiyama, 1993) used three questions to assess the negative aspects of social relationships: (1) "Do people in your network get on your nerves?" (2) "Are there people in your network who don't understand you?" and (3) "Are there people in your network who make too many demands on you?" Although the analyses are extensive, a brief summary is presented here. Examination of an index of these measures among the young-old, middle-old, and old-old indicated that negative support relationships had a more significant negative effect on well-being than did reports of positive feelings of support. Much as we have seen the powerful effect of insecure attachment relationships among infants influencing social competence, ego resilience, and even pathology, it may be the case that negative support relationships among older adults have a similarly strong effect on their overall well-being.

Another set of analyses examined the connection between primary attachments/inner-circle membership and well-being. We (Antonucci & Akiyama, 1993) found that among women, but not men, number of people in the inner circle was negatively related to happiness. We have speculated that for women, more close relations may translate into more burdensome relationships because of the more active exchange of supports among women. Thus, for women but not for men, having more close relationships may mean having too many demands made upon them by others. This finding serves as a reminder that, just as is the case with infant attachment relationships, it should not be assumed that the presence of a primary attachment relationship necessarily implies that this is a secure attachment relationship or that it always leads to positive outcomes.

SUMMARY

In this chapter, I have tried to make the case for attachment across the life span and to examine the special case of close social relations (i.e., primary attachment relationships) among the elderly. Theoretically, it is suggested that the convoy model of social relations offers a useful integration of primary and secondary attachment relationships with other social ties. Some evidence is already available and generally supportive of these theoretical notions; however, much work needs to be done. It still remains to be seen, for instance, how primary attachment relationships can help or hinder the individual in successfully meeting the challenges of aging. Some of our data (Antonucci et al., 1989) provide suggestive and potentially critically important clues. It may be that the presence of secure primary attachments provides a secure base that leads to feelings of personal control and self-efficacy over a lifetime, and that such feelings allow the older adult to make appropriate and successful choices when confronted with the challenges of aging.

ACKNOWLEDGMENTS

This chapter was written with the support of a Senior International Fogarty Fellowship while I was a visiting scholar at the Institut National de la Santé et de la Recherche Médicale in Paris, France. I thank Dr. Mary Levitt for her comments on an earlier draft of this chapter, and Ms. Kelly Everding for her assistance in the preparation of the manuscript.

REFERENCES

Ainsworth, M. D. S. (1989). Attachments beyond infancy. *American Psychologist, 44,* 709-716.

Ainsworth, M. D. S. (1991). Attachments and other affectional bonds across the life cycle. In C. Parkes, J. Stevenson-Hinde, & P. Marris (Eds.), *Attachment across the life cycle* (pp. 33-51). London: Routledge & Kegan Paul.

Ainsworth, M. D. S., Blehar, M. C., Waters, E., & Wall, S. (1978). *Patterns of attachment: A psychological study of the Strange Situation.* Hillsdale, NJ: Erlbaum.

Ainsworth, M. D. S., & Bowlby, J. (1991). An etiological approach to personality development. *American Psychologist, 46*(4), 333-341.

Antonucci, T. C. (Ed.). (1976). Attachment: A life-span concept [Special issue]. *Human Development, 19*(3).

Antonucci, T. C. (1985). Personal characteristics, social support, and social behavior. In R. H. Binstock & E. Shanas (Eds.), *Handbook of aging and the social sciences* (2nd ed., pp. 94-128). New York: Van Nostrand Reinhold.

Antonucci, T. C. (1986). Social support networks: A hierarchical mapping technique. *Generations, 10*(4), 10-12.

Antonucci, T. C. (1990). Social supports and social relationships. In R. H. Binstock & L. K. George (Eds.), *Handbook of aging and the social sciences* (3rd ed., pp. 205-227). New York: Academic Press.

Antonucci, T. C., & Akiyama, H. (1987a). Social networks in adult life and a preliminary examination of the convoy model. *Journal of Gerontology, 42*(5), 519-527.

Antonucci, T. C., & Akiyama, H. (1987b). An examination of sex differences in social support among older men and women. *Sex Roles, 17*(11-12), 737-749.

Antonucci, T. C., & Akiyama, H. (1991). Convoys of social support: Generational issues. *Marriage and Family Review, 16*(1-2), 103-112.

Antonucci, T. C., & Akiyama, H. (1993). *The negative effects of intimate social networks among older women as compared with men.* Unpublished manuscript.

Antonucci, T. C., & Jackson, J. S. (1987). Social support, interpersonal efficacy, and health. In L. L. Carstensen & B. A. Edelstein (Eds.), *Handbook of clinical gerontology* (pp. 291-311). Elmsford, NY: Pergamon Press.

Antonucci, T. C., Kahn, R. L., & Akiyama, H. (1989). Psychosocial factors and the response to cancer symptoms. In R. Yancik & J. W. Yates (Eds.), *Cancer in the elderly: Approaches to early detection and treatment* (pp. 40-52). New York: Springer.

Antonucci, T. C., Kahn, R. L., Harrison, R. V., & Payne, B. C. (1986). *Cancer symptoms in the elderly.* Washington, DC: National Cancer Institute.

Antonucci, T. C., & Levitt, M. J. (1984). Early prediction of attachment security: A multivariate approach. *Infant Behavior and Development, 7,* 1-18.

Baltes, P. B., & Baltes, M. M. (Eds.). (1990). *Successful aging: Perspectives from the behavioral sciences.* Cambridge, England: Cambridge University Press.

Bandura, A. (1986). *Social foundations of thought and action.* Englewood Cliffs, NJ: Prentice-Hall.

Belsky, J., & Nezworski, T. (1988). *Clinical implications of attachment.* Hillsdale, NJ: Erlbaum.

Blazer, D. G. (1982). Social support and mortality in an elderly population. *American Journal of Epidemiology, 115,* 684-694.

Bowlby, J. (1969). *Attachment and loss: Vol. 1. Attachment.* New York: Basic Books.

Bretherton, I. (1992). The origins of attachment theory: John Bowlby and Mary Ainsworth. *Developmental Psychology, 28*(5), 759-775.

Bretherton, I., & Waters, E. (Eds.). (1985). Growing points of attachment theory and research. *Monographs of the Society for Research in Child Development, 50*(1-2, Serial No. 209).

Cicirelli, V. G. (1989). Feelings of attachment to siblings and well-being in later life. *Psychology and Aging, 4,* 211-216.

Cicirelli, V. G. (1991). Adult children's help to aging parent: Attachment and altruism. In L. Montada & H. W. Bierhoff (Eds.), *Altruism in social systems* (pp. 41-57). Lewiston, NY: Hogefe & Huber.

Ewart, C. K. (1992). Role of physical self-efficacy in recovery from heart attack. In R. Schwarzer (Ed.) *Self-efficacy: Thought control of action* (pp. 298-304). New York: Hemisphere.

Feeney, J. A., & Noller, P. (1990). Attachment style as a predictor of adult romantic relationships. *Journal of Personality and Social Psychology, 58*(2), 281-291.

Hazan, C., & Shaver, P. (1987). Romantic love conceptualized as an attachment process. *Journal of Personality and Social Psychology, 52,* 511-524.

Jemmott, J., & Locke, S. E. (1980). Psychological factors, immunologic mediation, and human susceptibility to infectious disease: How much do we know? *Psychological Bulletin, 95,* 78-108.

Kahn, R. L., & Antonucci, T. C. (1980). Convoys over the life course: Attachment, roles, and social support. In P. B. Baltes & O. Brim (Eds.), *Life-span development and behavior* (Vol. 3, pp. 253-286). New York: Academic Press.

Kahn, R. L., & Antonucci, T. C. (1984). *Supports of the elderly: Family/friends/professionals.* Washington, DC: National Institute on Aging.

Kiecolt-Glaser, J. K., Glaser, R., Shuttleworth, E. C., Dyer, C. S., Ogrocki, P., & Speicher, C. E. (1987). Chronic stress and immunity in family caregivers of Alzheimer's disease victims. *Psychosomatic Medicine, 49,* 523-535.

Langer, E. T., & Rodin, T. (1976). The effects of choice and enhanced personal responsibility for the aged: A field experiment in an institutional setting. *Journal of Personality and Social Psychology, 34,* 191-198.

Lerner, R. M., & Ryff, C. (1978). Implementation of the life-span view of human development: The sample ease of attachment. In P. B. Baltes, D. L. Featherman, & R. M. Lerner (Eds.), *Life-span development and behavior* (Vol. 1, pp. 1-44). New York: Academic Press.

Main, M., Kaplan, N., & Cassidy, J. (1985). Security in infancy, childhood and adulthood: move to the level of representation. In I. Bretherton & E. Waters (Eds.), Growing points of attachment theory and research. *Monographs of the Society for Research in Child Development, 50*(1-2, Serial No. 209), 66-104.

Parkes, C., & Stevenson-Hinde, J. (Eds.). (1982). *The place of attachment in human behavior.* New York: Basic Books.

Parkes, C., Stevenson-Hinde, J., & Marris, P. (Eds.). (1991). *Attachment across the life cycle.* London: Routledge & Kegan Paul.

Plath, D. W. (1980). *Long engagements: Maturity in modern Japan.* Stanford, CA: Stanford University Press.

Ricks, M. H. (1985). The social transmission of parental behavior: Attachment across generations. In I. Bretherton & E. Waters (Eds.), Growing points of attachment theory and research. *Monographs of the Society for Research in Child Development, 50*(1-2), 211-227.

Schuster, T. L., Antonucci, T. C., & Akiyama, H. (1993). *Support and negativity in social networks and well-being in later life stages.* Unpublished manuscript.

Skinner, E. A. (1985). Action, control judgements, and the structure of control experience. *Psychological Review, 92*(1), 39-58.

Sperling, M. B., & Berman, W. H. (1991). An attachment classification of desperate love. *Journal of Personality Assessment, 55,* 45-56.

Sroufe, L. A. (1985). Attachment classification from the perspective of infant-caregiver relationships and infant temperament. *Child Development, 56*(1), 1-14.

Sroufe, A., & Fleeson, J. (1986). Attachment and the construction of relationships. In W. Hartup & Z. Rubin (Eds.), *Relationships and development* (pp. 51-71). Hillsdale, NJ: Erlbaum.

van IJzendoorn, M. H. (1990). Special topic: Cross-cultural validity of attachment theory. *Human Development, 33*(1), 2.

Weiss, R. S. (1982). Attachment in adult life. In C. Parkes & J. Stevenson-Hinde (Eds.) *The place of attachment in human behavior* (pp. 171-184). New York: Basic Books.

PART IV

Clinical Perspectives

CHAPTER 11

Suicidal Behavior and Attachment
A Developmental Model

KENNETH S. ADAM

> Whereas during later life it is often difficult to trace how a person's
> disturbed emotional state is related to his experiences, whether
> they be because of his current life or those of his past, during the
> early years of childhood the relationship between emotional state
> and current or recent experiences is often crystal clear. In these
> troubled states of early childhood, it is held, can be discerned the
> prototype of many pathological conditions of later years.
>
> —JOHN BOWLBY (1973)

The idea that the attachment paradigm might have a direct bearing on our understanding of psychopathology was at the center of John Bowlby's thought from the beginning. Although the essential connection between early childhood experience and personality formation had long been held by psychoanalysts, the notion that commonplace experiences such as separation from the mother might have long-term detrimental effects aroused much skepticism (Hill, 1972; Munro, 1969; Munro & Griffiths, 1969; Newcombe & Lerner, 1982). Much progress has been made over the past 30 years, however. Bowlby's brilliant insights about separation responses as the key to understanding attachment led to the development of the Strange Situation by Mary Ainsworth, which operationalized the study of separation in an experimental situation (Ainsworth, Blehar, Waters, & Wall, 1978; Bretherton, 1985; Goldberg, 1991). Subsequent longitudinal studies have shown insecure attachment to be related to a number of difficulties in later social and interpersonal functioning (Bretherton, 1985; Sroufe, 1983, 1988; Sroufe & Rutter, 1984). Further research on high-risk children has suggested that disturbed attachment may be a major contributor to risk in these children (Bowlby, 1988a; Carlson, Cicchetti, Barnett, & Braunwald, 1989; Crittenden, 1988; Schneider-Rosen, Braunwald, Carlson, & Cicchetti, 1985; Sroufe & Fleeson, 1986).

Despite these advances, convincing research support for the causal role of disturbed attachment in personality and psychiatric disorders has been slow in developing. One reason for this has been an overemphasis on the search for linear effects in research designs; this has oversimplified cause-and-effect relationships and produced inconsistent results. In addition, there has been little systematic study on the attachment effects of such experiences as parental rejection, divorce, and physical or sexual abuse. Furthermore, there has been a widespread tendency to treat the various types of events (loss, abuse, neglect, etc.) as if they are unique, rather than to examine the possibility that a variety of events in parent–child relationships might exert their effects through common developmental pathways such as the attachment system. Finally, few studies account for the role of moderating, protective, or confounding variables that might affect outcome following these events (Crook & Eliot, 1980; Lloyd, 1980; Tennant, Bebbington, & Hurry, 1980, 1981).

The goal of this chapter is to point out how disturbances in the early parent–child relationship may contribute to the development of a vulnerability to suicidal behavior, and how the attachment paradigm specifically may serve as a better framework for understanding suicidal behavior than existing theoretical models. I review some of my long-standing ideas about this problem, summarize some findings from my colleagues' and my previous research, and draw together other evidence from several sources, which suggests that suicidal behavior may well be a specific manifestation of pathological attachment behavior in later life. I then outline a general causal model for the development of suicidal behavior from an attachment point of view, and briefly outline an ongoing research project that is testing further aspects of this model, using newer measures of adult attachment. I hope to show not only that the attachment paradigm has value for understanding the common clinical problem of suicidal behavior, but also that suicidal behavior may be an ideal marker for tracing the developmental trajectory of at least some forms of insecure attachment over the life cycle.

ATTACHMENT AND SUICIDE:
HISTORICAL BACKGROUND

The idea that attachment difficulties might have a direct bearing on understanding suicidal behavior stems from psychoanalytic studies, which have long pointed to the role of loss in the etiology of depression and suicide. Freud (1917/1957), in his seminal paper "Mourning and Melancholia," differentiated between the normal process of mourning (in which a loved object is relinquished without loss of self-esteem or ego depletion) and the pathological process of melancholia (where object loss is followed by pathological mourning, self-blame, and aggression; when directed toward an internal representation of the lost object, this aggression leads to depression and ultimately suicide). Later writers of the traditional Freudian school (Abraham, 1924/1965; Menninger, 1933; Zilboorg, 1936) related the inability to tolerate current loss to earlier losses and frustrations in the oral period of development. Object relations theorists, following the lead of Melanie Klein, detailed other important aspects of the inner object relations of suicidal patients, such as the need to split off and destroy bad internal objects in order to preserve good objects (Asch, 1980; Guntrip, 1968; Klein, 1935; Masterson, 1976, 1983).

All of these theoretical perspectives view suicide as a problem of internal object relations and aggression, and all point to developmental difficulties in the early period of childhood. However, there is much disagreement about the nature of the deficit or traumatic events experienced, as well as whether the destructive aggression that arises originates within the infant himself or herself, or as a response to some critical failure of parenting on the part of the mother. Traditional psychoanalytic theory and Kleinian theory both emphasize the role of a natural aggressive instinct and "oral sadism," whereas the object relations theorists and self psychologists understand aggression as an inevitable and purposeful response to frustrations or failures within the relationship. All psychoanalytic theories assume that important aspects of the interactions between the child and his or her object world are internalized and structured, and that the interactions between these internalized representations and the external environment are major factors in shaping later behavior (Eagle, 1987; Greenberg & Mitchell, 1983; Mitchell, 1988).

Little attention, however, has been given in this literature to the important role of interactional or transactional processes between the suicidal person and his or her "external" or "real" object world. Menninger (1933) pointed out that attacking oneself may be an effective means of hurting another person, and both Zilboorg (1936) and Friedlander (1940) emphasized the importance of spite as a motive in suicide. Other psychoanalytic writers, observing that some suicidal patients had fantasies of joining an idealized lost object in death, have pointed to "libidinal aspects" in oral regressions (Friedlander, 1940; Hendin, 1963; Hendricks, 1940; Menninger, 1938). More recently, both Asch (1980) and Hale (1985) have noted the essentially dyadic nature of many suicidal acts, referring to these relationships as "sadomasochistic"; and Maltsberger (1986), using a self-psychological framework, has described suicidal patients as overly reliant on self-objects for comfort. However, like most psychoanalytic writers, they all frame their theoretical hypotheses within an exclusively intrapsychic framework.

EARLY PARENTAL LOSS/UNAVAILABILITY
AND SUICIDAL BEHAVIOR

Clinical and Empirical Studies

The importance of the role of current loss and rejection in social relationships as precipitants of suicidal behavior is well known, as it is commonplace clinically and well documented in empirical research. Clinical studies of attempted suicide have repeatedly pointed to the importance of interpersonal conflict, rejection, and loss as antecedent events in suicide attempts; although the events preceding actual suicide are inevitably more obscure, such evidence as exists points in the same direction. In adults, these events most often involve lovers, spouses, or other family members, but may also involve other significant persons, such as members of the nursing staff or psychotherapists. In children and adolescents, conflicts with parents, siblings, or boyfriends/girlfriends have been widely found as key events preceding suicidal actions (see Adam, 1990, for a review). A considerable body of evidence indicates that the interpersonal difficulties preceding suicidal behavior are not merely the result of transient conflicts, but are part of more pervasive and long-standing difficulties with relationships, indicating deep-seated personality problems (Crook, Raskin, & Davis, 1975; Farmer & Creed, 1986; Weissman, Fox, & Klerman, 1973).

Although the relationship of current loss and separation to suicidal behavior is generally accepted, the idea that earlier experiences create the vulnerability for this is much more controversial. Retrospective data on early events are always problematic, and the temporal relationship between these events and later behavior is greatly extended—often over many decades, or in the case of completed suicide, literally over a lifetime.

As with the study of depression, most attention has been given to the role of loss, and indeed a significant relationship between early parental loss and suicidal behavior has been established. Since 1941 more than 30 studies have been published, 22 of which have used a case–control design. Most of these studies have methodological problems; however, all 17 of the studies of attempted suicide found a higher incidence of parental loss in cases than controls, although in two of these (both with problematic control groups), the difference did not reach statistical significance (Adam, 1990). Studies of early parental loss in completed suicide are fewer than those of attempted suicide, presumably because of the greater difficulty in accessing information about childhood events for these persons, and all have serious methodological problems. Of five such studies reviewed, three found excesses of parental death or permanent separation in samples of suicides, and two found no such excess (Adam, 1990).

Although there appears little doubt that early parental loss is a significant risk factor in the etiology of suicidal behavior, a number of other serious difficulties in family and parent–child relationships have increasingly been reported in recent years, particularly in studies of children and adolescents. Parental strife, neglect, chronic physical and psychiatric illness, and child abuse have all been reported in this literature, and these problems are often multiple and long-standing (Friedman, Corn, & Hurt, 1984; Garfinkel, Froese, & Hood, 1982; Pfeffer, 1981; Stanley, & Barter, 1970; de Wilde, Kienhorst, Diekstra, & Wolters, 1992). Similar events have also been reported in adult studies, but have only recently begun to get systematic attention (Goldney, 1985; Ross, Clayer, & Campbell, 1983; Silove, George, & Bhavani-Sankaram, 1987; van der Kolk, Perry, & Herman, 1991).

Our Group's Previous Research

My colleagues and I have conducted several studies that have attempted to address the issues of early parental loss and the quality of the early family environment in suicidal individuals. In the first of these studies (Adam, Lohrenz, Harper, & Streiner, 1982), we compared 76 university students with a history of parental loss before age 17 (parental death or permanent separation) to 61 students from intact homes. We conducted a detailed inquiry into thoughts of suicide, taking care to differentiate serious and persistent preoccupations from the more transient and trivial thoughts common in this age group and to document any history of suicide attempts. Then, in a searching semistructured interview, we inquired about all aspects of early family loss events, including the stability of relationships prior to the breakup of a home, the availability of caretaking during the period of a year or so surrounding the event, and the family circumstances over the long term subsequent to this. Although we were particularly interested in the availability of caretakers to a child, we also paid close attention to the quality of caretaking, including responsiveness to both physical and emotional needs.

Forty-seven percent of the parental loss subjects were found to have experienced significant suicidal ideation, compared to only 15% from intact homes, and 14 of 17 subjects who had made suicide attempts fell into the parental loss group. Both findings were highly statistically significant. To our surprise, we found little difference in reported suicidal behaviors between subjects who had experienced the death of a parent and those whose parents had divorced or separated. Reviewing the transcripts of all parental loss subjects to see whether we could determine what might differentiate the suicidal from the nonsuicidal subjects, we found that though all the families had become disorganized during the immediate period of the breakup of the home, in the suicidal group the disorganization was considerably greater and persisted over the long term. The failure of recovery in the suicidal group was seen in a number of ways. Subjects who had experienced parental death reported more intense initial grief and more signs of unresolved mourning, such as a severe and prolonged bereavement reaction or the development of a major psychiatric illness (e.g., depression or alcoholism). Similarly, in cases where parental divorce had broken the home, there was more severe family disorganization surrounding the event and a failure to respond constructively to the crisis over the long term.

In the nonsuicidal group, on the other hand, bereavement reactions were less likely to have taken a pathological course; there was less evidence of continuing postdivorce strife between the parents; and responsive alternative caretakers were more readily available. Regardless of the cause of a family's breakup, the remaining parent was more likely to remarry successfully and to reconstitute a stable home. Nonsuicidal subjects generally spoke with greater warmth and understanding about their parents and stepparents, and perceived the effects of the breakup as having been less detrimental to their lives. This study concluded that, whereas parental loss in childhood appeared to be a significant risk factor in the development of suicidal ideation and behavior in these young subjects, this only appeared to be the case under certain conditions where the ongoing care of the children had been jeopardized.

As we were now interested more generally in the quality of care in the family life of suicidal individuals, we undertook a second study (Adam, Bouckoms, & Streiner, 1982) in which we compared the family backgrounds of 98 patients who had been hospitalized following a suicide attempt to 102 control patients recruited from a community general practice who had never made a suicide attempt. Using the same procedures as previously, we inquired in detail about the quality of each subject's early family life, including the availability, consistency, and adequacy of care given to the child (whether by parents, other family members, or alternative caregivers). In cases where parents had died or permanently separated, we inquired about conditions of family life before, during, and after these events. We also used specific criteria to assign a global rating (stable, unstable, or chaotic) of family life for all subjects, including those with "intact" homes. We found that whereas over 50% of the attempted-suicide sample had experienced parental loss (compared to 22% of general-practice controls), 92% overall were rated as having had an unstable or chaotic early family life (compared to 40% of controls). To look at the findings another way, the odds ratio (an approximation to relative risk) for suicide attempt in subjects with a history of parental loss was found to be 2.3; the same odds ratio in subjects with unstable homes was 2.2; and the same odds ratio in suicide attempt in subjects with chaotic homes (who constituted 55% of the total attempted-suicide sample) was 9.7. As in the previous study, we found that parental loss was only a risk factor when it had been preceded by instability and turmoil in the families and where the families had been unable to respond constructively to the crisis of loss and the tasks of family reorganization.

Taken together, these studies do not support the notion that any particular class of event, such as the death of a parent, is specific to the development of suicidal behavior; rather, they indicate that a wide variety of events and circumstances resulting in the unavailability of adequate parental care play a major role. These events range from the less obvious emotional unavailability of a depressed or otherwise ill parent to the more strikingly traumatic experiences associated with the unresolved death or separation of parents, physical or sexual abuse, or multiple changes of caretakers. Nor does the evidence support the idea that a specific, discrete period of childhood is involved. Quite the contrary: The family disturbances in suicidal subjects are usually present early on, and they tend to be enduring and often continuous throughout much of childhood and adolescence.

The idea that such profound and long-standing insecurities in the parent–child relationship could lead to serious attachment difficulties seems obvious to those informed of the findings of attachment research, but what evidence is there that links attachment mechanisms directly to suicidal behavior? For this, we must turn to studies of separation and attachment in children and to clinical observations in psychiatric settings.

ATTACHMENT MECHANISMS AND VULNERABILITY TO SUICIDAL BEHAVIOR

Attachment, Separation, and Aggression

Evidence that anger and aggression are predictable responses to separation from parents was thoroughly documented by John Bowlby (1969, 1973). A series of studies of normal children during brief separations from their parents showed that children between the ages of 18 and 30 months tended to respond to separation in a typical way, which Bowlby broke down into three phases. In the first, which Bowlby termed a phase of "protest," a child showed agitation and tearfulness, and threw himself or herself about with strong expressions of anger. If the mother did not reappear within a reasonable period of time, this protest phase was followed by a phase of "despair," in which the child might cry monotonously or intermittently, become withdrawn and inactive, and make no demands on people in the environment. After a more prolonged period of separation, the child entered a phase of "detachment," during which he or she showed increased interest in the surroundings and might even smile and become sociable, suggesting recovery. On being reunited with their mothers, children separated for several weeks appeared unresponsive and undemanding, and eventual recognition of their mothers was usually accompanied by feelings of intense ambivalence and anger. Bowlby noted that there was often oscillation between these phases, and that throughout the children were is prone to tantrums and episodes of destructive behavior, which he described as being "often of a disquietingly violent kind" (Bowlby, 1961, p. 483).

Maternal Rejection and Aggression

Although these early observations focused attention on children's responses to separation from attachment figures, other evidence has accumulated showing that rejection or the threat of rejection by parents is an equally potent cause of anxiety and anger. More recently, mothers' rejection of physical contact with their children has also been shown to be a powerful stimulus to anger and aggressive behavior. Bowlby suggested that children and adolescents who are subjected not only to repeated separations but to constant threats of abandonment may show the "most violently angry and dysfunctional responses of all" (Bowlby, 1973, p. 249).

In one report (Main & Stadtman, 1981) in which mother–infant interaction was observed in a mildly stressful laboratory situation, hitting, slapping, and threatening the mother were clearly associated with the mother's aversion to contact following approaches by the child. In another study, Main and Goldwyn (1984) noted that children who were avoidant of their mothers and showed unusually little anger in the Strange Situation showed "sudden out of context, inexplicable, bouts of angry behavior and attacks and threats of attack" on their mothers in the home and other settings (p. 209). In yet another study (George & Main, 1979), when physically abused toddlers 1–3 years of age were compared to matched nonabused controls from families experiencing stress, it was found that the abused children more frequently assaulted their peers, and "harassed" and assaulted their caregivers; they were also much less likely than controls to approach caregivers or peers in response to friendly overtures.

Main and Goldwyn (1984) have suggested that the difficulties these children have with control of aggression, their lack of empathy for the distress of others, and their tendency to avoid social contacts represent a "continuum of psychological process" from the experience of "normal rejection" seen in relatively maternally rejected infants in normal samples to the more profoundly rejected children who are subject to actual physical abuse. They have hypothesized that repeated experiences of rejection may lead to a deactivation of the attachment behavioral system, which leads an infant to shift his or her attention away from attachment figures in order to avoid the pain of rejection. Stressful or frightening events, which activate the attachment behavioral system, throw the infant into an approach-avoidance conflict and lead to outbursts of anger and aggression. A recent study by Lyons-Ruth, Repacholi, McLeod, and Silva (1991) would appear to confirm these observations. Infants classified as disorganized/disoriented in the Strange Situation were found to be significantly more likely than those with organized strategies to be rated as highly aggressive in the classroom at age 5.

Insecure Attachment, Aggression, and Suicidal Behavior

Although the self-directed aggression we see in suicidal behavior may seem remote from the anger and outward-directed aggression described previously in infants and toddlers who are insecurely attached, there is good reason to believe that there may be a close developmental link. No studies specifically focusing on the developmental aspects of self-destructive behavior in children from the attachment point of view have been carried out, but some findings by Main, Kaplan, and Cassidy (1985) in a longitudinal study of normal children are of interest. Forty children, previously classified in the Strange Situation at 12–18 months, were reassessed at 6 years of age. The Klagsbrun–Bowlby adaptation of Hansburg's Separation Anxiety Test was administered, in which the subjects were asked to respond to a series of photographs of children undergoing various types of separation from parents. The strongest of the separation experiences portrayed, in which parents were seen to be leaving for a 2-week period, was followed by a question: "What's the little girl/boy gonna do?" Children who had been rated as securely attached in the Strange Situation 5 years earlier usually reported constructive responses, such as those that called on others for help, or that might lead to a termination of the separation situation. Those rated as insecure in infancy (the avoidant, anxious/ambivalent, or disorganized/disoriented children) often responded with silence or stated that they didn't know what to do. Of great interest here is the fact that a number of these (who were given the lowest scores) said that they would kill either themselves or their parents in order to deal with the situation.

Clinical Studies

The idea that such responses might form the nucleus of a vulnerability to actual suicidal behavior seems incredible in children so young, but direct support for the notion is found in a recent study by Rosenthal and Rosenthal (1984). Sixteen preschool children ranging in age from 2½ to 5 years, who were referred after seriously injuring themselves or attempting to do so, were compared with a matched group of 16 nonsuicidal preschoolers who had serious behavior problems. Whereas equal numbers of the suicidal and nonsuicidal children had experienced parental divorce or parental death, there was a significantly higher incidence of physical abuse and neglect among the suicidal children. Moreover, most of them were clearly unwanted by their parents, who considered them to be burdensome. Compared to the behavior problem children, the suicidal children were found to be more likely to have run away from home and to have demonstrated nonsuicidal aggression to themselves, were more likely to have shown depressive symptoms, and were less likely to show pain and crying after injury. Regardless of whether or not they had experienced physical abuse, the loss of a parent (through divorce, alternative placement, or death), or parental unavailability because of depression, the suicidal children expressed profound feelings of abandonment, yearning for reunion, despair, and lack of hope of remedying their lot—all feelings that were absent in the behavior problem group. Although the authors did not give their classification criteria, all the suicidal children were reported to have "disturbed attachment behavior," and all suffered from overwhelming disturbances in their relations with key figures; these difficulties were found to have been present before they became suicidal.

Although not framed within the attachment paradigm, many case reports on suicidal adolescents contain examples that are consistent with the observations reported above. Schrut (1964), in a clinical study, interviewed 19 suicidal children and adolescents whose parents appeared to feel intense ambivalence and strong resentment toward their children. In over half the cases the children were felt to be a burden—an attitude that was often conveyed by coldness and hypercritical discipline or by an "absence of mothering." The author used the diagnostic terms of the time to describe the children as "hyperactive" or "schizoid," but he provided several detailed case descriptions to illustrate how misbehavior and self-destructive behavior in the children, arising out of anxiety and anger about being unable to "reach mother," were able to arouse the concerned responses that had otherwise been unavailable. In some cases this appeared to lead to retaliatory resentment on the mothers' part, with further emotional distancing, repeated cycles of the children's suicidal threats and attempts, and provocations and counterprovocations passing back and forth between parents and children. The cycles described are strongly reminiscent of the "specific syndrome" of approach-avoidance described by Main and Stadtman (1981), in which infants, frustrated in their attempts to achieve contact with rejecting mothers, reacted with anger and renewed determination as their attachment needs were activated. It is interesting to note in this regard that 15 of Schrut's 19 patients were described by their mothers as having been "anxious, difficult to handle, and never satisfied" in their earlier years and "generally hostile and aggressive" in their later years. In another clinical study, Crumley (1979) noted that the suicidal adolescents he studied tended to become involved in clinging, overpossessive relationships with boyfriends/girlfriends, and characteristically displayed excessive rage and anger when these persons were unavailable for whatever reason. Although neither Schrut nor Crumley used the term, their descriptions are strongly suggestive of insecure attachment behavior.

We (Adam & Adam, 1978) reported a number of clinical cases of attempted suicide in adults, in which striking similarities were observed between the behavior of attempted suicide patients during the acute suicidal crisis and the behavior of children following brief separations from attachment figures as described by John Bowlby. What is unique about these observations is that they were made within the context of a crisis intervention service that routinely assessed patients with their spouses and/or families within hours of their admission when the family members and/or significant others were intensely involved in the suicidal crisis. As the case examples speak for themselves, two are recounted here.

Case 1
    Following an argument with his wife, who had threatened him with separation, an otherwise responsible 40-year-old man became violent—breaking up furniture in his home, taking an overdose of tranquilizers, and then smashing his car against his garage. On admission to the hospital, he was depressed, angry, and uncommunicative except for persistent threats of suicide. When a member of the crisis team staff who was called to assess him summoned his family, he refused to talk to them, curled up in a ball in his bed, and remained petulant and silent throughout most of the initial family interview. He eventually broke into the conversation with angry accusations about their lack of concern, made further suicidal threats, and refused to go home. A tearful scene followed, and the next day the family members came to the hospital and begged him to come home with them.

Case 2
    Mr. M, a 38-year-old man, was admitted to the hospital with a drug overdose after finding his wife, who had been talking of separa-

tion for several months, in bed with another man. On making the discovery he abused her verbally, pleaded with her to return to him, and then swallowed the pills in her presence. When seen initially in the hospital he was cold and detached, expressed his belief that no one cared for him, and rejected the approaches of the crisis team staff. He repeatedly threatened suicide and asked whether his wife was inquiring after him. When it became clear that she refused to see him and was taking taken further steps toward formalizing a legal separation, his aloofness and control gradually gave way to hostile and belligerent behavior. He talked of leaving the hospital, and threatened to assault anyone who spoke to him. The use of these means to avoid his sadness was pointed out to him by the staff members, who persisted in their efforts to approach him; after a few visits, he began grieving openly amidst loud proclamations of his sense of loss, which were accompanied by intense physical distress. Following this he became markedly dependent on and clung to the crisis team staff, anxiously awaiting their daily visits and attempting to prolong the interviews. He openly sought physical contact with his staff therapist, and at one point asked to hold her hand during an interview.

In each of these cases, background information revealed a story of traumatic loss of a parent in early life, followed by the failure of alternative care and by later marital and family relationships that were troubled by persistent conflicts over dependency, jealousy, and concerns about being loved. These observations, which are typical of those seen in countless hospital emergency rooms around the world, are strongly suggestive of an attachment process linking early insecurity with attachment figures to later crises with current attachment figures.

Animal Studies

Corroborating evidence supporting these ideas can be found in some recent animal research. Observations of primates in the laboratory have provided convincing evidence that deficits in the early social environment can have a profound and enduring influence on social behavior (Suomi, 1977). Rhesus monkeys raised under various conditions of isolation show important social deficits and abnormal behaviors, which do not disappear spontaneously, but continue to plague them throughout their lives. Important among these are behavior and physiological symptoms similar to those observed in depression in humans. Moreover, disturbances in the control of aggression are a regular feature of monkeys raised in isolation, often taking the form of self-aggression and, when the monkeys are reunited with their peers, inappropriate aggression toward them

(Suomi 1985). Jones and Barraclough (1978) have noted extensive evidence linking self-injurious behavior in nonhuman mammals to a number of biological and social variables, including stressful events, interference with sexual bonding, and isolation or confinement. In an interesting study, Jones, Congiu, and Stevenson (1979) have pointed to similarities between the affective state and social situation preceding suicidal acts in humans and those in animal self-injury, suggesting that they may be homologous behaviors. These authors have argued that the feelings of depression and tension preceding suicidal acts in humans are similar to the agitation and depression-like behavior observed in animals prior to self-injurious acts, and note that conditions of bond disruption, isolation, and confinement are similar in both cases. Although the similarities appear to be particularly strong for self-mutilators, they hold for self-poisoners as well. Equally significant in terms of our own observations is the fact that these effects in animals can be mediated and modified by varying the interactional conditions of rearing. Factors before, during, and following reunion alter the response of infant monkeys, and among high-risk primate infants, individual responsiveness shows considerable variability (Cairns, 1977).

A DEVELOPMENTAL MODEL

Causal models are attempts to understand how a variety of influences act together to produce illness or disorder. Linear effects models, which attribute a disorder uniformly and directly to an antecedent cause, are adequate for an understanding of simple causal relationships (e.g., the effect of a severe blow to the head on consciousness); however, they are totally inadequate for explaining the complexities of causality involved in most human disease processes. The epidemiological triad of the agent, host, and environment, widely applied to the understanding of infectious disease earlier in this century, has led to the useful notions of "necessary" and "sufficient" causes. However, contemporary epidemiological studies of causality, dealing with more complex disease processes, have paid increasing attention to the effects of intervening variables that may augment or mitigate against the effects of specific causal variables, confounding relationships and obscuring our understanding of them (Schlesselman, 1987). No contemporary causal model can be considered adequate unless it considers both risk and protective factors, or, in Rutter's terms, both "vulnerability" and "resilience" (Pellegrini, 1980; Rutter, 1985, 1987). Nowhere are these considerations more important than in the study of psychiatric and behavioral disorders, where constitutional factors invariably unfold within a social context and the environment is often critical in determining whether the constitutional potential is realized. As Lewontin (1992), speaking about the interaction of internal and external forces on the development of living organisms generally, points out,

> The external forces [that] we usually think of as "environment" are themselves partly a consequence of the activities of the organism itself as it produces and consumes the conditions of its own existence. Organisms do not simply find the world in which they develop. They make it. Reciprocally, the internal forces are not autonomous, but act in response to the external. (p. 34)

It is important to point out, when one looks at the effects of early experience on development, the obvious but often overlooked fact that *events* are not the same as *experiences*. To become experiences, events must be perceived (both affectively and cognitively), interpreted, and remembered. All this depends on a multitude of factors, not the least of which are the individuals' prior experiences and the modifying effects of others in the environment who share, confirm, or disconfirm what has been experienced and its meaning (Bowlby, 1988b; Miller, 1979/1981; Stern, 1985). Furthermore, to have long-term effects, early experiences must be internalized and structured in some way if they are to affect the experience of later events, as Freud pointed out long ago (Freud, 1916–1917/1963).

Figure 11.1 illustrates a complex vulnerability model outlining the role of insecure attachment as a risk factor for suicidal behavior, which I have been elaborating for some time (Adam, 1982). In developing this model I have attempted to differentiate between "predisposing factors," which I understand to produce a more or less specific vulnerability to suicidal behavior through their effects on the attachment system, and "precipitating factors" in the current life of the individual, which act to unmask this vulnerability, leading to the expression of overt suicidal ideation or behavior. The central line of the model in Figure 11.1 contains the hypothesis that early attachment experiences produce vulnerability to suicidal behavior through their effects on the attachment system, mediated through the internal working models of self and attachment figures. The effects of these internal structures are seen as being manifested in various personality difficulties involving the sense of self-worth, affect regulation, and the capacity to form and maintain relationships, which are seen as the keys to understanding vulnerability or resilience to later attachment stress. The outer lines of the model trace the pathways from secure attachment to resilience and the capacity to contain anxiety, mourn loss, and cope with crisis, and from insecure attachment to vulnerability and a propensity to react to loss or threatened loss with immobilizing anxiety, destructive anger, hopelessness, and ego decompensation.

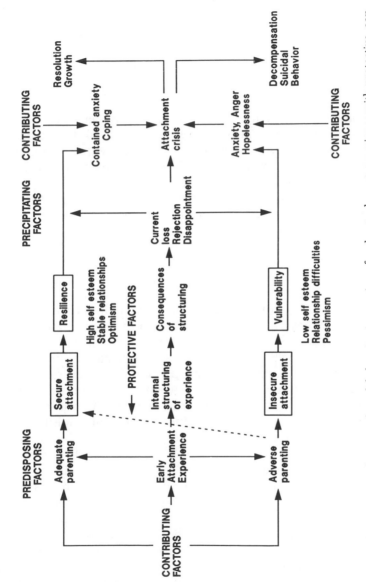

FIGURE 11.1 Developmental model showing interaction of early attachment experience with protective, contributing, and predisposing factors in producing vulnerability to suicidal behavior.

289

"Contributing factors" within this model are moderating variables, which act in a more general way on both predisposing or precipitating factors to augment, facilitate, or suppress their expression (Bebbington, 1980). These may act indirectly, as has been suggested by Brown and Harris (1978), to increase the likelihood of exposure to specific precipitating or predisposing variables, or more directly, affecting the individual's internal controls and decreasing his or her ability to cope with crisis. Living in an area of high social disorganization, which increases the likelihood of the individual's being exposed to a chaotic or broken home, is an example of the first kind of effect; the intake of intoxicating drugs or alcohol, which may have disinhibiting or depressant effects on the central nervous system of the individual, is an example of the second kind of effect. The coexistence of major mental disorder, which interferes with judgment, disrupts the control of impulses, and often affects social relationships, may contribute in several ways.

At any point in this model, "protective factors," which mitigate against the effects of adverse experience or an accretion of further adverse attachment experiences compounding an earlier adverse experience, may modify the pathway taken. They may sometimes move the individual toward a more resilient pathway, and at other times toward a more vulnerable pathway. All of this is in keeping with the general considerations of contemporary developmental psychopathology (Sroufe & Rutter, 1984; Cicchetti, 1984; Bowlby, 1988a). Studies of attachment in children have shown that while the attachment patterns in early life tend to remain stable, they are not unalterable, and changes for good or ill can occur if circumstances change (Bretherton, 1985). This possibility is reflected in the model by the broken lines indicating an alternate pathway from adverse parenting to secure attachment, such as can occur when a displaced child has been successfully adopted. Similarly, an alternative pathway (not indicated in the figure) from adequate parenting to insecure attachment is possible in the face of subsequent adverse experience, such as that which can result from a major traumatic loss. The balance of accretion between favorable and unfavorable experiences undoubtedly influences the final outcome.

Looked at in this way, the acute suicidal crisis can be better conceptualized as an acute attachment crisis, and suicidal behavior as extreme attachment behavior that takes both its form and function from the childhood separation response. Although the evidence linking attachment mechanisms to suicidal behavior as outlined above is incomplete, it fulfils many of the scientific criteria for proof of cause and effect (Hill, 1965; Schlesselman, 1987). A strong association has been shown to exist between inadequate parental care in childhood and suicidal behavior, and this evidence is consistent across a variety of studies, with no convincing methodologically sound negative studies. The temporal relationships between the causal factor (inadequate care) and the outcome (suicidal behavior) are appropriate in term of both past experience and current experiences. Moreover, the severity of exposure to adverse childhood experiences has been correlated with the severity of suicidal behavior for both frequency and intent in two separate studies (Adam, Lohrenz, et al., 1982; Hawton, Osborn, O'Grady, & Cole, 1982). A solid body of evidence has demonstrated that the attachment organization of infancy tends to remain stable over time and that it has important long-term consequences on development (Cicchetti, Cummings, Greenberg, & Marvin, 1990). Insecurely attached children appear to be compromised in many areas of social and interpersonal functioning, and a growing body of data suggests that they may be at greater risk for depression and behavioral disturbance (Sroufe, 1988). Kobak and Sceery (1988) showed that college students classified as "autonomous" (secure) on the Adult Attachment Interview (AAI; George, Kaplan, & Main, 1985) were more ego-resilient, were less hostile and anxious, and had higher self-regard and expectations of support from others than those classified as "preoccupied" or "dismissing" (insecure). In a more recent study, Kobak, Sandler, and Gamble (1991) found that teenagers classified as preoccupied on the AAI reported more depressive symptoms and had higher levels of dysfunctional anger than those rated as autonomous.

It would appear that those who have experienced their caretakers as sensitive and available are likely to develop a high regard for themselves and to have optimistic expectations of others—conditions that favor the formation and maintenance of relationships. Those who have experienced their caretakers as insensitive and unavailable, or whose childhood experience has been intruded upon by parental needs, are more likely to have poor regard for themselves and pessimistic and hostile expectations of others, both of which are likely to contribute to difficulties in forming and maintaining relationships. Extensive evidence shows just these characteristics to be present in patients making suicide attempts. Personality studies have repeatedly found suicidal individuals to show a high degree of social withdrawal and interpersonal difficulty; they exhibit greater aggression and hostility toward others, and higher dependency and lower self-esteem, than a variety of control groups (Frances, Fyer, & Clarkin, 1986; Blumenthal & Kupfer, 1988; Goldsmith, Fyer, & Frances, 1990).

The similarities I have described between the behavior of children following brief separations and the behavior of adults in an acute suicidal crisis are strongly suggestive of a process link between the two, mediated by internal working models of attachment. The interpersonal crisis that so frequently precipitates suicidal behavior is characterized by dramatic outbursts of anger, accompanied by destructive physical or verbal attacks on the significant person concerned; these are often intermingled with pleading, clinging, and explicit demands for love and attention. In the face of irretrievable loss or continuing uncertainty about the relationship, there may be withdrawal into hopelessness and depression, with renewed suicidal threats or actions.

The severity of the suicidal behavior that ensues in such crises and the likelihood of its being repeated may well be functions of both the responsiveness of the significant others in the interpersonal world of the person concerned, and specific organizational characteristics of the internal working model as reflected in the personality configuration. Individuals with borderline personality disorder, for example, who are known to be at high risk for suicidal behavior, probably have a characteristic attachment organization (Frances et al., 1986; West, Keller, Links, & Patrick, 1993). The continuum of suicidal behavior from suicidal ideation to suicide attempt to completed suicide may well represent both a developmental continuum of attachment (from relatively insecure to grossly insecure), and a psychological continuum of internalization (from external to internal worlds of experience). At one end of this continuum are predominantly interpersonal and "manipulative" suicidal actions, which appear primarily motivated by an urgent and more hopeful appeal to a threatened attachment relationship; at the other are more despairing and potentially lethal communications, with deeply disappointing and strongly negative internal models of self and attachment figures.

RESEARCH IN PROGRESS TO ASSESS THE MODEL

My colleagues and I are currently completing a study of attachment patterns in suicidal adolescents, using three standardized measures of adult attachment. The Parental Bonding Instrument (PBI; Parker, Tupling, & Brown, 1979) is a self-report scale measuring the subject's perceptions of parents on two dimensions—care and protection—derived from attachment theory and related research. The Attachment Questionnaire (AQ; West & Sheldon, 1988) is a self-report questionnaire that classifies current attachment relationships into four patterns and seven dimensions consistent with Bowlby's descriptions. The AAI (George et al., 1985) is a semistructured interview focused on early attachment experiences, which allows the current mental organization of adults with regard to their primary parental attachment figures to be classified into categories that closely correlate with the Ainsworth Strange Situation classifications of attachment in children.

Both the AAI and AQ are constructed to differentiate representational models of attachment by assessing an adult's attachment strategies. The AAI not only explores the adult's experience with attachment figures in a systematic way, but it allows for the assessment of the outcome of this experience (a function of the interaction of vulnerability and protective factors) in terms of internal attachment organization. The AQ elicits information about current attachment-relevant experiences, cognitions, and affects, yielding ratings for both the degree of insecurity associated with each component of attachment and the overall attachment pattern of the respondent. Concurrent use of several instruments should provide a more complete description of attachment-relevant information than the use of one instrument alone.

Our present study is comparing a sample of adolescents with lifetime histories of suicidal ideation or suicide attempt to a control group of adolescents who have never seriously thought of suicide or made a suicide attempt. Because both cases and controls are from a clinical population, where one would expect a high incidence of attachment insecurity, the design poses a stringent test of the specificity of attachment as a risk factor for suicidal behavior. Thus far, our data suggest that attachment variables do indeed clearly distinguish cases from controls; there are also important gender differences in both suicidal activity and attachment patterns. Analysis of the data is as yet incomplete, but we will be interested to see whether any particular attachment category or combination of categories differentiates suicidal from nonsuicidal subjects, and whether the pattern of internal organization revealed in the AAI correlates in a meaningful way with the patterns derived from the AQ and PBI. If we do confirm that attachment measures strongly differentiate the suicidal from the nonsuicidal subjects, then further studies examining attachment patterns in other suicidal populations over the life cycle will be indicated, to determine the generalizability of the findings. Gender differences in attachment patterns will require close scrutiny in any such studies, in view of the well-known differences in both sex and age distribution between fatal and nonfatal suicidal behavior. Studies of attachment patterns in suicidal and nonsuicidal members of specific psychiatric patient groups would help to sort out the important question of whether the suicidal behavior in these populations is a function of the clinical condition or a common underlying attachment disturbance.

REFERENCES

Abraham, K. (1965). A short study on the development of the libido in the light of mental disorders. In K. Abraham, *Selected papers on psychoanalysis* (pp. 418-501). London: Hogarth Press. (Original work published 1924)

Adam, K. S. (1982). Loss, suicide and attachment. In C. M. Parkes & J. Stevenson-Hinde (Eds.), *The place of attachment in human behavior* (pp. 269-294). New York: Basic Books..

Adam, K. S. (1990). Environmental, psychosocial and psychoanalytic aspects of suicidal behavior. In S. J. Blumenthal & D. J. Kupfer (Eds.), *Suicide over the life cycle: Risk factors, assessment and treatment of suicidal patients* (pp. 39-96). Washington, DC: American Psychiatric Press.

Adam, K. S., & Adam, G. (1978). *Attachment theory and attempted suicide.* Paper presented at the 15th Annual Congress of the Royal Australian and New Zealand College of Psychiatrists, Singapore.

Adam, K. S., Bouckoms, A., & Streiner, D. (1982). Parental loss and family stability in attempted suicide. *Archives of General Psychiatry, 39*(9), 1081-1085.

Adam, K. S., Lohrenz, J. G., Harper, D., & Streiner, D. (1982). Early parental loss and suicidal ideation in university students. *Canadian Journal of Psychiatry, 27,* 275-281.

Ainsworth, M., Blehar, M. C., Waters, E., & Wall, S. (1978). *Patterns of attachment: A psychological study of the Strange Situation.* Hillsdale, NJ: Erlbaum.

Asch, S. (1980). Suicide and the hidden executioner. *International Review of Psycho-Analysis, 7,* 51-59.

Bebbington, P. E. (1980). Causal models and logical inference in epidemiological psychiatry. *British Journal of Psychiatry, 136,* 317-325.

Blumenthal, S. J., & Kupfer, D. J. (1988). Overview of early detection and treatment strategies for suicidal behavior in young people. *Journal of Youth and Adolescence, 17,* 1-23.

Bowlby, J. (1961). Childhood mourning and its implications for Psychiatry. *American Journal of Psychiatry, 118,* 481-497.

Bowlby, J. (1969). *Attachment and loss: Vol. 1. Attachment.* New York: Basic Books.

Bowlby, J. (1973). *Attachment and loss: Vol. 2. Separation: Anxiety and anger.* New York: Basic Books.

Bowlby, J. (1988a). Developmental psychiatry comes of age. *American Journal of Psychiatry, 145,* 1-10.

Bowlby, J. (1988b). On knowing what you are not supposed to know and feeling what you are not supposed to feel. In J. Bowlby, *A secure base* (pp. 99-118). New York: Basic Books.

Bretherton, I. (1985). Attachment theory: Retrospect and prospect. In I. Bretherton & E. Waters (Eds.), Growing points of attachment theory and research. *Monographs of the Society for Research in Child Development, 50,* (1-2, Serial No. 209), 3-35.

Brown, G. W., & Harris T. (1978). *Social origins of depression: A study of psychiatric disorders in women.* London: Tavistock.

Cairns, R. B. (1977). Beyond social attachment: The dynamics of interactional development. In T. Alloway, P. Plinen, & L. Krames (Eds.), *Attachment behavior: Advances in the study of communication and affect* (pp. 1-21). New York: Plenum.

Carlson, V., Cicchetti, D., Barnett, D., & Braunwald, K. (1989). Disorganized/dissociated attachment relationships in maltreated infants. *Developmental Psychiatry, 25*(4), 525-531.

Cicchetti, D. (1984). The emergence of developmental psychopathology. *Child Development, 55,* 1-7.

Cicchetti, D., Cummings, E. M., Greenberg, M., & Marvin, R. (1990). An organizational perspective on attchment beyond infancy. In M. Greenberg, D. Cicchetti,

& E. M. Cummings (Eds.), *Attachment in the preschool years: Theory, research, and intervention* (pp. 3-49). Chicago: University of Chicago Press.

Crittenden, P. M. (1988). Relationships at risk. In J. Belsky & T. Nezworski (Eds.), *Clinical implications of attachment theory* (pp. 136-174). Hillsdale, NJ: Erlbaum.

Crook, T., & Eliot, J. (1980). Parental death during childhood and adult depression: A critical review of the literature. *Psychological Bulletin, 87*(2), 252-259.

Crook, T., Raskin, A., & Davis, D. (1975). Factors associated with attempted suicide among hospital depressed patients. *Psychological Medicine, 5,* 381-388.

Crumley, F. E. (1979). Adolescent suicide attempts. *Journal of the American Medical Association, 241,* 2404-2407.

de Wilde, E. J., Kienhorst, I., Diekstra, R., & Wolters, W. (1992). The relationship between adolescent suicidal behavior and life events in childhood and adolescence. *American Journal of Psychiatry, 149,* 45-51.

Eagle, M. N. (1987). *Recent developments in psychoanalysis: A critical evaluation.* Cambridge, MA: Harvard University Press.

Farmer, R., & Creed, F. (1986). Hostility and deliberate self-poisoning. *British Journal of Medical Psychology, 59,* 311-316.

Frances, A., Fyer, M., & Clarkin, J. (1986). Personality and suicide. *Annals of the New York Academy of Sciences, 487,* 281-293.

Freud, S. (1957). Mourning and melancholia. In J. Strachey (Ed. and Trans.), *The complete psychological works of Sigmund Freud* (Vol. 14, pp. 237-260). London: Hogarth Press. (Original work published 1917)

Freud, S. (1963). Introductory lectures on psycho-analysis. In J. Strachey (Ed. and Trans.), *The standard edition of the complete psychological works of Sigmund Freud* (Vol. 15, pp. 1-240; Vol. 26, pp. 241-496). London: Hogarth Press. (Original work published 1916-1917)

Friedlander, K. (1940). On the longing to die. *International Journal of Psycho-Analysis, 21,* 416-426.

Friedman, R. C., Corn, R., & Hurt, S. (1984). Family history of illness in the seriously suicidal adolescent: A life-cycle approach. *American Journal of Orthopsychiatry, 54,* 390-397.

Garfinkel, B. O., Froese, A., & Hood, J. (1982). Suicide attempts in children and adolescents. *American Journal of Psychiatry, 139,* 1257-1261.

George, C., Kaplan, N., & Main, M. (1985). *The Berkeley Adult Attachment Interview.* Unpublished protocol, University of California at Berkeley.

George, C., & Main, M. (1979). Social interactions of young abused children: Approach, avoidance and aggression. *Child Development, 50,* 306-318.

Goldberg, S. (1991). Recent developments in attachment theory and research. *Canadian Journal of Psychiatry, 36,* 393-400.

Goldney, R. (1985). Parental representation in young women who attempt suicide. *Acta Psychiatrica Scandinavica, 72,* 230-232.

Goldsmith, S. J., Fyer, M., & Frances, A. (1990). Personality and suicide. In S. J. Blumenthal & D. J. Kupfer (Eds.), *Suicide over the life cycle: Risk factors, assessment and treatment of suicidal patients* (pp. 155-176). Washington, DC: American Psychiatric Press.

Greenberg, J. R., & Mitchell, S. A. (1983). *Object relations in psychoanalytic theory.* Cambridge, MA: Harvard University Press.

Guntrip, H. (1968). *Schizoid phenomena, object-relations and the self.* London: Hogarth Press.

Hale, R. (1985). Suicide and the violent act. *Bulletin of the British Association of Psychotherapists, 16,* 13-24.

Hawton, K., Osborn, M, O'Grady, J., & Cole, D. (1982). Classification of adolescents who take overdoses. *British Journal of Psychiatry, 140,* 124-131.

Hendin, H. (1963). Psychodynamics of suicide. *Journal of Nervous and Mental Disease, 136,* 236-244.

Hendricks, I. (1940). Suicide as wish fulfilment. *Psychiatric Quarterly, 14,* 30-42.

Hill, A. B. (1965). The environment and disease: Association and causation? *Proceedings of the Royal Society of Medicine* (London), *58,* 295-300.

Hill, O. W. (1972). Child bereavement and adult psychiatric disturbance. *Journal of Psychosomatic Research, 16,* 357-360.

Jones, I. H., & Barraclough, B. M. (1978). Auto-mutilation in animals and its relevance to self-injury in man. *Acta Psychiatrica Scandinavica, 58,* 40-47.

Jones, I. M., Congiu, L., & Stevenson, J. (1979). A biological approach to two forms of human self-injury. *Journal of Nervous and Mental Disease, 167*(2), 74-78.

Klein, M. (1935). A contribution to the psychogenesis of manic depressive states. *International Journal of Psycho-Analysis, 16,* 145-174.

Kobak, R., Sandler, N., & Gamble, W. (1991). Attachment and depressive symptoms during adolescence: A developmental pathways analysis. *Development and Psychopathology, 3,* 461-474.

Kobak, R., & Sceery, A. (1988). Attachment in late adolescence: Working models, affect regulation, and representations of self and others. *Child Development, 59,* 135-146.

Lewontin, R. C. (1992, May 28). The dream of the human genome. *New York Review of Books,* pp. 31-40.

Lloyd, C. (1980). Life events and depressive disorder reviewed: I. Life events as predisposing factors. *Archives of General Psychiatry, 37,* 529-535.

Lyons-Ruth, K., Repacholi, B., McLeod, S., & Silva, E. (1991). Disorganized attachment behaviour in infancy: Short-term stability, maternal and infant correlates, and risk-related subtypes. *Development and Psychopathology, 3,* 377-396.

Main, M., & Goldwyn, R. (1984). Predicting rejection of her infant from mother's representation of her own experience: Implications for the abused-abusing intergenerational cycle. *Child Abuse and Neglect, 8,* 203-217.

Main, M., Kaplan, N., & Cassidy, I. (1985). Security in infancy, childhood and adulthood: A move to the level of representation. In I. Bretherton & E. Waters (Eds.), Growing points of attachment theory and research. *Monographs of the Society for Research in Child Development, 50*(1-2, Serial No. 209), 66-104.

Main, M., & Stadtman, I. (1981). Infant response to rejection of physical contact by the mother: Aggression, avoidance and conflict. *Journal of the American Academy of Child Psychiatry, 20,* 292-307.

Maltsberger, J. T. (1986). *Suicide risk: The formulation of clinical judgment.* New York: New York University Press.

Masterson, J. F. (1976). *Psychotherapy of the borderline adult: A developmental approach.* New York: Brunner/Mazel.

Masterson, J. F. (1983). Abandonment depression in borderline adolescents. In H. Golombek & B. Garfinkel (Eds.), *The adolescent and mood disturbance* (pp. 135-144). New York: International Universities Press.

Menninger, K. A. (1933). Psychoanalytic aspects of suicide. *International Journal of Psycho-Analysis, 14,* 376-390.

Menninger, K. A. (1938). *Man against himself.* New York: Harcourt, Brace & World.

Miller, A. (1981). *The drama of the gifted child* (R. Ward, Trans.). New York: Basic Books. (Original work published 1979 as *Prisoners of childhood*)

Mitchell, S. A. (1988). *Relational concepts in psychoanalysis.* Cambridge, MA: Harvard University Press.

Munro, A. (1969). Parent-child separation: Is it really a cause of psychiatric illness in adult life? *Archives of General Psychiatry, 20,* 598-604.

Munro, A., & Griffiths, A. B. (1969). Some psychiatric non-sequelae of childhood bereavement. *British Journal of Psychiatry, 115,* 305-311.

Newcombe, N., & Lerner, J. C. (1982). Britain between the wars: The historical context of Bowlby's theory of attachment. *Psychiatry, 45,* 1-12.

Parker, G., Tupling, H., & Brown, L. B. (1979). A parental bonding instrument. *British Journal of Medical Psychology, 52,* 1-10.

Pellegrini, D. S. (1990). Psychosocial risk and protective factors in childhood. *Journal of Developmental and Behavioral Pediatrics, 11,* 201-209.

Pfeffer, C. (1981). Suicidal behavior of children: A review with implications for research and practice. *American Journal of Psychiatry, 138*(2), 154-159.

Rosenthal, P. A., & Rosenthal, S. (1984). Suicidal behavior in preschool children. *American Journal of Psychiatry, 141,* 520-525.

Ross, M. W., Clayer, J. R., & Campbell, R. L. (1983). Parental rearing patterns and suicidal thoughts. *Acta Psychiatrica Scandinavica, 67,* 429-433.

Rutter, M. (1985). Resilience in the face of adversity: Protective fators and resistance to psychiatric disorders. *British Journal of Psychiatry, 147,* 598-611.

Rutter, M. (1987). Psychosocial resilience and protective mechanisms. *American Journal of Orthopsychiatry, 57,* 316-331.

Schlesselman, J. J. (1987). "Proof" of cause and effect in epidemiological studies: Criteria for judgement. *Preventive Medicine, 16,* 195-210.

Schneider-Rosen, K., Braunwald, K., Carlson, V., & Cicchetti, D. (1985). Current perspectives in attachment theory: Illustration from the study of maltreated infants. In I. Bretherton & E. Waters (Eds.), Growing points in attachment theory and research. *Monographs of the Society for Research in Child Development, 50*(1-2, Serial No. 209), 194-210.

Schrut, A. (1964). Suicidal adolescents and children. *Journal of the American Medical Association, 188,* 1103-1107.

Silove, D., George, G., & Bhavani-Sankaram, V. (1987). Parasuicide: Interaction between inadequate parenting and recent interpersonal stress. *Australian and New Zealand Journal of Psychiatry, 21,* 221-230.

Sroufe, L. A. (1983). Infant-caregiver attachment and patterns of adaptation in preschool: The roots of competence and maladaptation. In M. Perlmutter (Ed.), *Minnesota Symposia in Child Psychology* (Vol. 16, pp. 41-83). Hillsdale, NJ: Erlbaum.

Sroufe, L. A. (1988). The role of infant-caregiver attachment in development. In J. Belsky & T. Nezworski (Eds.), *Clinical implications of attachment* (pp. 18-38). Hillsdale, NJ.: Erlbaum.

Sroufe, L. A., & Fleeson, J. (1986). Attachment and the construction of relationships. In W. Hartnap & Z. Rubin (Eds.), *Relationships and development* (pp. 51-71). Hillsdale, NJ: Erlbaum.

Sroufe, L. A., & Rutter, M. (1984). The domain of developmental psychopathology. *Child Development, 55,* 17-29.

Stanley, E. J., & Barter, J. T. (1970). Adolescent suicidal behavior. *American Journal of Orthopsychiatry, 40,* 87-96.

Stern, D. N. (1985). *The interpersonal world of the infant.* New York: Basic Books.

Suomi, S. J. (1977). Development of attachment and social behaviors in rhesus monkeys. In T. Alloway, P. Pliner, & L. Krames (Eds.), *Attachment behavior: Advances in the study of communication and affect* (pp. 197-224). New York: Plenum.

Suomi, S. J. (1985). Ethology: Animal models. In H. I. Kaplan & B. J. Sadock (Eds.), *Comprehensive textbook of psychiatry* (4th ed., pp. 226-236). Baltimore: Williams & Wilkins.

Tennant, C., Bebbington, P., & Hurry, J. (1980). Parental death in childhood and risk of adult depressive disorder: A review. *Psychological Medicine, 10,* 289-299.

Tennant, C., Bebbington P., & Hurry, J. (1981). The role of life events in depressive illness: Is there a substantial causal relation? *Psychological Medicine, 11,* 379-389.

van der Kolk, B. A., Perry, J. C., & Herman, J. L. (1991). Childhood origins of self-destructive behavior. *American Journal of Psychiatry, 148,* 1665-1671.

Weissman, M. M., Fox, K., & Klerman, G. L. (1973). Hostility and depression associated with suicide attempts, 1960-1971. *American Journal of Psychiatry, 130,* 450-455.

West, M., Keller, A., Links, P., & Patrick, J. (1993). Borderline personality disorder and attachment pathology. *Canadian Journal of Psychiatry, 38*(Suppl. 1), 516-522.

West, M., & Sheldon, A. E. R. (1988). The classification of pathological attachment patterns in adults. *Journal of Personality Disorders, 2,* 153-160.

Zilboorg, G. (1936). Suicide among primitive and civilized races. *American Journal of Psychiatry, 92,* 1346-1369.

CHAPTER 12

Parental Bonding and Depressive Disorders

GORDON PARKER

In this chapter, I consider the general hypothesis that disturbances in the parent-child bond establish a predisposition or diathesis in the child to develop depression subsequently in adulthood. The chapter focuses on the parental contribution to the parent-child relationship, largely ignoring the extent to which both characteristics of the child (e.g., temperament and personality) and characteristics of the parent-child interaction contribute to establishing any such diathesis, as the latter (though conceded in general terms) have resisted empirical delineation.

ATTACHMENT AND BONDING

There is an immediate need to distinguish between parent-child "attachment" and "bonding." I argue that "attachment" is a more appropriate term to describe instinctively determined behaviors, whereas the term "bonding" includes or focuses on how the parent and the child each perceive, experience, and judge the interaction with the other. Thus, this discussion focuses on aspects of the parent-child bond, after a few introductory comments about attachment and its assumed contribution to bonding.

The ethological/evolutionary view of attachment holds that most animal species are born with instinctive mechanisms that promote the development of attachment to a primary adult caretaker, and hence the development of the interactive relationship (Osofsky & Connors, 1979). Bowlby (1969) argued that the development and maintenance of attachment between the child and its mother are consequences of a number of behavioral systems within the child that are designed to ensure proximity to the mother and thus increase the chances of the child's survival. Such behavioral systems are products of both genetic action and environmental influences, with certain stimuli (perhaps internal ones, such as hormones, as well as external factors) acting to elicit, initiate, orient, or terminate behavior. Bowlby detailed a whole series of repertoires with which an infant is equipped that serve to promote attachment to a care-giver. He also described the ontogeny of such attachment behaviors, suggesting that initially such behaviors are entirely instinctual, but that subsequently they are modified by environmental and other factors. Thus, as the infant develops, initially highly instinctive attachment behaviors (e.g., following with the eyes, grasping, clinging, smiling, and babbling) are followed by repertoires that are seemingly less instinctive (i.e., no longer specific and stereotyped) and more suggestive of a "goal-corrected part-nership," being responsive to and modified by the care-giver and other environmental factors. Such variations from "wired-in" behaviors demonstrate, define, and reflect aspects of the parent–child "bond."

It has been argued that adults are also equipped with complementary behavioral caregiving systems that are, at least initially, instinctive. Trause, Klaus, and Kennell (1982) have summarized stereotyped maternal behaviors in mammals, arguing that certain biological mechanisms are responsible for the mother's receptivity to an infant at the time of birth. Such processes are also time-limited; nonhormonal and other mechanisms (whether biologically or socially mediated) are able to override and determine maternal behaviors, again building to and defining the parental contribution to the bond.

DISRUPTION OF THE PARENTAL BOND

It has long been held that "parental deprivation" predisposes a child to develop depression as an adult, with the essential hypothesis conceding that deprivation may occur as a consequence of separation and/or distortions in the parental contribution. Both components have generated considerable empirical research. For an extended period it was held that parental loss, particularly in the first 16 years of the child's life, was a distinct risk factor for subsequent depression. A number of the key studies and reviews have recently been summarized (Parker, 1992), demonstrating that clear and consistent evidence is lacking. Several theoretical problems are likely to have contributed to the inconsistent findings. For instance, "parental loss" is a term used to describe a wide variety of circumstances, ranging from the sudden death of a much-loved parent whose loss is not met by any restitutive social support, to trivial loss (e.g., parent–child separation because of holiday or school boarding arrangements). Again, the "loss" of a destructive and brutalizing parent (perhaps by divorce or other circumstances) may theoretically be beneficial to many children, particularly if the residual parental support is of some worth; thus "parental loss" is hard to evaluate as a categorical issue, and evaluating it without consideration of qualitative issues and restitutive factors is unwise. In addition, because parental death and divorce are likely to be overrepresented in families where the parental contribution to the parent–child bond is dysfunctional, it is likely that the dysfunctional parental style (whether before or after the loss) contributes more than ongoing effects of the actual loss to any subsequent depression in the child.

When the numerous parental loss studies are considered (Parker, 1992), they are remarkable for their lack of consistency, whether in failing to demonstrate an increased chance of subsequent depression in a child (apart from the immediate postseparation period) or in defining determinants of any "risk." Maternal and paternal loss have varyingly been held to be more important; varying age periods have been promoted as salient for the child; and little attention has been paid to the nature of the parental and family support systems that are in place before and after any parental separation. Tennant, Bebbington, and Hurry (1980) concluded that when such potential confounding effects are accounted for, there is either a nonexistent or negligible long-term psychopathological effect. Similarly, Richards and Dyson (1982) concluded that if effects exist they must be relatively weak or the studies would have been able to demonstrate them more consistently. The most recent review (Parker, 1992) of some 60 research studies and integrative analyses therefore suggests that although the death of a parent is clearly associated with acute distress in a child, it remains quite unclear whether loss per se disposes the child to depression in adulthood, and any ill effects that follow may be more closely related to inadequate parental care preceding or subsequent to the loss than to the loss itself.

Similar conclusions are reached, whether separation involves parental death or other types of separation experience. Tennant (1988) reviewed a wide range of such experiences, and concluded again that preseparation parenting and postseparation relationships between children and parents are more important determinants of psychological morbidity in a child, both in childhood and in later life. Thus, recent reviews consistently point to the possibility that any determining variable may emerge primarily from parental psychopathology (or bond distortions) before and after the separation, rather than from bond disruption per se.

DISTORTIONS OF THE PARENTAL BOND

We need, then, to examine those components of the parental contribution to the parent–child bond that may establish a diathesis to later depression. Theorists have argued for two important parental characteristics as determinants of psychopathology in the child: care and control (or overprotection). For instance, Bowlby (1977) noted that caregivers have two roles: (1) to be available and responsive (essentially, a caring dimension);

and (2) to know when to intervene judicially, avoiding extremes of over-protection and neglect. Clinicians have also frequently described the relevance of two broad parental styles (i.e., lack of care and overprotective or controlling parenting) as being of key relevance to child psychopathology, with terms such as "schizophrenogenic" and "asthmatogenic" parenting being used to describe such anomalous characteristics.

Factor-analytic studies (e.g., Parker, Tupling, & Brown, 1979; Arrindell et al., 1986) have confirmed the relevance of such constructs as reflecting key dimensions underlying parental attitudes and behaviors. Such multivariate studies have consistently generated a first dimension of "care," with parents ranging from highly caring to indifferent and/or rejecting. The next most commonly generated dimension has variably been defined as "overprotection" or "control," with parents ranging from over-protecting, controlling, encouraging dependency, and infantilizing the child to encouraging the child's socialization, autonomy, and progressive independence. Such dimesions are not unique to parenting; Hinde (1974) has suggested that they underpin all important interpersonal relationships, be they parent–child, husband–wife, teacher–pupil, or therapist–patient.

Measuring such parental characteristics is clearly problematic. Attempts to measure current parenting run the risk that responses will be biased toward "social desirability" by parents aware that their attributes are under examination. Even if current characteristics can be validly measured, they may not represent any more formative parental attitudes and behaviors expressed in earlier years. Most measures of parental style are retrospective ones, relying on the child to rate his or her earlier memories of parenting. Gerlsma, Emmelkamp, and Arrindell (1990) have recently reviewed 14 such measures and concluded that only three meet basic psychometric criteria—one, the Children's Reports of Parental Behavior Inventory (CRPBI; Schaefer, 1965), which is completed by children; and two, the Parental Bonding Instrument (PBI; Parker et al., 1979) and the Egna Minnen Betraffande Uppfostran ["Own Memories of Child-Rearing Experiences"] (EMBU; Perris, Jacobson, Lindstrom, Von Knorring, & Perris, 1980), which are completed retrospectively by adults. The majority of studies assessing the relevance of parental style to subsequent depressive experience have involved the PBI, and this measure is now described in some detail.

THE PARENTAL BONDING INSTRUMENT: PSYCHOMETRIC AND APPLIED STUDIES

The PBI (Parker et al., 1979) was designed to be a refined measure of parental care and protection, with subjects being requested to score their parents as remembered from their own first 16 years. Such an extended period was set deliberately to obtain a "product moment" of innumerable parental interactions, and not merely recent or stage-specific attitudes and behaviors. It was assumed that in the main, any parent's general level of caring and overprotection would be relatively consistent over time, so that an overprotective parent (for instance) would remain overprotective over the child's early years and adolescence, although the actual manifestations of the overprotection might vary over different stages in the child. The PBI has 12 items on its Care scale and 13 items on its Protection scale. Each item requires the respondent to judge whether the descriptor was "very" or "moderately" like or unlike that parent over the extended period of the respondent's childhood and early adolescence, with forms being completed for the mother and father separately. Although biological parents have been scored in most studies, a few studies have allowed respondents to rate the "most influential" parent figures, to allow for the possibility that any restriction to biological parents may have some obvious limitations (especially if a respondent has no memory of such a parent).

The test-retest reliability of the PBI was initially assessed over a brief interval and shown to be impressive (Parker et al., 1979). More recently, the long-term reliability in scoring parents on the PBI was assessed over a 10-year period (Wilhelm & Parker, 1990), with the overall levels of agreement for Care (.68) and Protection (.62) scale scores being impressive when comparisons were made against a number of other measures, including trait personality ones. In addition to allowing levels of parental Care and Protection to be rated by use of the raw scores, the PBI allows contrasting parental styles to be examined. On *a priori* grounds, a combination of high Care-low Protection is held to represent "optimal parenting"; low Care-low Protection, "neglectful parenting"; high Care-high Protection, "affectionate constraint"; and low Care-high Protection, "affectionless control."

By design, the PBI is an experiential measure, weighting the recipient's memories and experiences of the parent, which of course may or may not correspond with the parent's actual "parental style." This orientation was deliberate; our argument was that if children are influenced by the interpersonal characteristics of parents, they are more likely to be influenced by the way in which they perceive the parent than any "actual" reality (assuming some dissonance between each "reality"). Although this argument has intuitive and logical appeal to the clinician, it risks misinterpretation if applied blindly to the formulation of causal hypotheses. For instance, even if it were to be demonstrated that adult depressives were more likely to remember their parents as "uncaring," such a finding does not establish a causal process linking uncaring parenting with subsequent depression in a child. A number of noncausal postulates must be considered, including the possibility that depressives (as a consequence of their mood state or personality) might misperceive interpersonal interactions and so misinterpret caring parents as uncaring, or even that a future depressive adult has certain early interpersonal characteristics as a child that act so as to elicit uncaring parenting from a parent. (These postulates and others are discussed in more detail later.) Thus, any argument that depressives are more likely to perceive their parents as demonstrating anomalous interpersonal characteristics is limited by reliance on the use of any self-report measures, unless it can be demonstrated that the measure also provides an accurate rating of the "actual" parenting.

The validity of the PBI, both as an experiential measure and as a measure of "actual" parenting, has therefore been examined in a number of studies. The first set of studies can be briefly summarized, as an overview has been provided previously (Parker, 1983a). In the first one, subgroups of nonclinical and clinical subjects were asked to score their parents on the PBI; each subject was then required to pretend to be a nominated sibling and complete another set of PBIs as he or she judged that the parents had related to that sibling. In addition, the nominated sibling was similarly required to complete sets of PBIs on his or her own behalf and that of the respondent. Examination of the multitrait–multimethod matrix suggested high levels of agreement when the relevant validity diagonals were examined, but an important caveat emerged: It became clear that subjects tended to score parents in a rather similar way, regardless of whether they were asked to complete the PBI for themselves or in relation to their siblings, suggesting an experientially driven set.

The second study had a group of young adults complete the PBI. Their mothers were then approached and interviewed by a rater who was blind to the PBI scores; as this study focused on determinants of overprotection, the interviewer assessed only whether a mother gave evidence of overprotective behaviors during an open-ended interview assessing the child's developmental years. Those mothers who were rated as high on Protection by their children on the PBI were significantly more likely to be rated at interview as having earlier been more controlling, as having prevented independent behavior, and as having infantilized the respondent children. These two studies are important in suggesting that PBI scores are likely to reflect actual parenting and not distorted self-perceptions. Several as yet unpublished North American studies have used quite complicated genetic modeling approaches in twin study paradigms, and again suggest support for the PBI as a valid measure of actual parenting.

A large number of studies have been undertaken using the PBI in relation to depression, and these have recently been summarized (Parker, 1992). There have been seven studies of nonclinical groups, with relatively consistent associations linking higher depression levels with low parental Care scores and, less distinctly, with high parental Protection scores. Studies of clinical depressive groups have suggested the specificity of anomalous parenting to the nonmelancholic or nonendogenous depressive disorders, but have failed to find any clear relationship to melancholia/endogenous depression. For instance, I (Parker, 1979) studied some 50 bipolar depressed patients and found no differences in the way they scored their parents, compared to age- and sex-matched routine attenders of a general practice; a replication New Zealand study (Joyce, 1984) returned similar findings. A subsequent study (Parker, Kiloh, & Hayward, 1987), involving endogenous depressives whose diagnoses had been allocated nearly two decades earlier by Kiloh, Andrews, Neilson, and Bianchi (1972), again failed to find any differences in PBI scores between those depressives and age- and sex-matched controls.

By contrast, all case–control studies of nonmelancholic (essentially "neurotic" or "dysthymic") depressives have established those depressives as more likely to rate their parents low on Care and/or high on Protection on the PBI (Parker, 1979, 1983a; Parker et al., 1987; Hickie, Wilhelm, & Parker, 1990). In most studies, nonmelancholic depressives have distinguished themselves from controls in being most likely to report exposure to "affectionless control" (low Care–high Protection scores) from one or both parents, with odds ratios ranging from 3 to 7 across the several studies, suggesting a significantly increased risk factor. A possible interaction between sex of parent and sex of subject was suggested in one study (Parker, 1983b), with male depressives being more likely to report anomalous parenting from their fathers, while the female depressives were more likely to report anomalous parenting from their mothers. The specificity phenomenon (i.e., the finding that anomalous parenting is relevant only to nonmelancholic depression) has been recently confirmed in an additional study of 150 depressed patients (Parker & Hazdi-Pavlovic, 1992). In that study, 65 melancholic patients returned PBI scores similar to those of controls, whereas the nonmelancholic patients were much more likely to provide low parental Care and/or parental high Protection ratings. The suggestion of specificity is consistent with the view that melancholia/endogenous depression is essentially a genetic disorder with an imputed biological etiology, whereas nonmelancholic depressive disorders reflect an interaction of a vulnerable personality (perhaps determined in part by parental interactive attitudes and behaviors) with life event stressors.

The question of how low parental care or parental overprotection may contribute to the "vulnerable personality" is considered later. The last study cited (Parker & Hazdi-Pavlovic, 1992) considered an important issue—the extent to which the style of one parent that puts a child at risk for depression may be modified or added to by characteristics of the other parent. Clear evidence of additive effects were demonstrated for the nonmelancholic depressives, with low Care scores (for instance) from both parents raising the risk of depression some 4-7 times in one sample and

13-27 times in the other sample (when compared against low Care scores for one parent only). Further analyses in that sample suggested that the highest risk for adult depression was associated with exposure to one of two broad types of parenting—"affectionless control" (the combination of low Care and high Protection) and "neglectful parenting" (the combination of low Care and low Protection).

EXAMINING NONCAUSAL EXPLANATIONS

A number of noncausal explanations are possible for links between anomalous parenting (as defined by the PBI) and nonmelancholic depression, and several of these have been assessed in considerable depth. For instance, it is frequently suggested that a depressed mood will cause subjects to perceive themselves, their interpersonal relationships, and their futures in a negative way; thus, depressives may merely (as a consequence of mood state) rate their parents in a negative way, resulting in associations between anomalous PBI scores and depression levels. The specificity findings suggest, however, that if this explanation were valid, the phenomenon would be restricted to nonmelancholics. Several studies (e.g., Parker, 1981; Plantes, Prusoff, Brennan, Anderson, & Parker, 1988) have examined this possibility by having clinical depressives (nonmelancholic, in the main) score their parents on the PBI when depressed and subsequently when recovered or improved. These studies have shown that reports of anomalous parenting persist in nonmelancholic depressives, both when depressed and upon recovery; such an explanation can thus be rejected.

A second possibility is a variant of the first—that nonmelancholic depressives may, as a consequence of a distinct personality style, be more likely to perceive their parenting in a negative light. Various descriptors have been used to describe the at-risk personality style of such depressives, and characteristics such as "interpersonal sensitivity," "neuroticism," "internal locus of control," "dependency," and "low self-efficacy" have been nominated. Although definitive studies have not been undertaken to exclude this possibility, some preliminary studies (see Parker, 1983a) have shown that when "neuroticism" and "dependency" levels are controlled for, links between anomalous PBI scores and higher depression levels remain. Support for this noncausal hypothesis would be demonstrated if nonmelancholic depressives were demonstrated to score all significant interpersonal relationships in a negative light. Several studies (e.g., Hickie, Wilhelm, & Parker, 1990; Hickie, Parker, Wilhelm, & Tennant, 1990) have examined this issue by intercorrelating scores on a marital measure (rating Care and Control) with PBI scores returned by nonmelancholic depressives; this research failed to show links on either the Care or Control/ Protection scales, which would be anticipated if there were a general tendency to judge all such interpersonal relationships under the influence of a negative (e.g., plaintive set) or positive (e.g., social desirability) response bias.

A third noncausal explanation concedes a genetic influence. Thus, it could be that a genetically determined factor (e.g., "neuroticism") might both cause a parent to demonstrate anomalous parenting (i.e., to be uncaring and overprotective) *and* also cause depression in the child, so creating a spurious link between those two outcomes. This hypothesis was investigated (Parker, 1982) in a study of adoptees, who were required to score their adoptive parents on the PBI and themselves on measures of anxiety and depression. Associations between PBI scores and mood levels were found to be as high as those demonstrated in other nonclinical samples, in which subjects had scored their biological parents. If a genetic factor had been operant, clearly associations would not have been expected.

EXPLORING THE CAUSAL PROPOSITION

Although a causal hypothesis can never be proved conclusively, and can only be progressively supported and refined by rejection of alternative hypotheses, the view that uncaring and/or overprotective parenting is a risk factor for nonmelancholic depression has been consistently confirmed in empirical studies, and the level of risk to adult depression has been shown to be considerable. The PBI approach respects the dimensions (of care and protection) held by clinicians and theoreticians to be important, has refined and allowed quantification of their relevance, and has allowed estimates of the magnitude of the risk. How that risk is brought about remains speculative, but the question has been considered previously (Parker, 1983a). In essence, the argument is that low parental care and overprotective parenting act in somewhat differing ways to establish a diathesis to depression in the recipient.

Parental care is an important determinant of the child's self-esteem. A child exposed to uncaring parenting (whether by neglect or by active rejection) will be more likely to have low self-esteem, or self-esteem that has lacunae and therefore allows the individual to be "spooked" by particular life events. Thus, exposure to an actively rejecting parent may lay the foundation for the recipient subsequently to be susceptible to sharp, demeaning, and rejecting comments in an adult interpersonal relationship, and even to perceive such interactions when such a stimulus is slight or nonexistent.

Parental overprotection is likely to act in a differing way. The hypothesis here is that there is a normal process of separation-individuation in the child and that its socialisation should proceed with respect for stage-specific nuances. An overprotective parent tends to "hold back" the child's development so that social competence is limited or restricted. A child may function quite well while under the protective umbrella of the parent or parental home, but may reveal social and interpersonal limitations in a wider arena, either in childhood or adulthood. Thus, the child may appear self-confident within the family (even at times inappropriately so, when the overprotective parent invests the child with false values and expectations), but the child's self-esteem may be revealed as having lacunae in nonfamily interactions; any failure to have achieved genuine independence also places the recipient at risk in social situations.

Although many would regard "overprotection" as a surfeit of care, my colleagues and I favor a differing interpretation, supported by negative correlations between PBI Care and Protection scores. In essence, we argue that overprotective parents are *less* likely to be able to care effectively for a child, because their anxiety levels, intrusiveness, and vigilance tend to cause them to have difficulty in sustaining an interactive partnership with a child and in relaxing sufficiently to allow care to be expressed directly. Thus, the combination of low care and overprotection is not uncommon, and its particularly malignant effects on the later development of depression in adulthood can be seen to emerge from these two differing mechanisms.

CONTINUITY IN BONDING STYLE

One final issue is addressed here; although it is not central to this chapter, it is an issue addressed in several other chapters. As an extension to our research, my colleagues and I have focused on the issue of continuity versus discontinuity in interpersonal relationships. In particular, we have been interested in whether early parent–child socialization experiences establish a diathesis to repeat those experiences in subsequent significant interpersonal relationships. Bowlby (1977) held that "attachment behavior is held to characterise human beings from the cradle to the grave" (p. 203). He suggested that "mental models" are constructed by the child on the basis of experiences of significant others, and that these expectations tend to persist relatively unchanged throughout the rest of life, determining aspects of adult attachments. A number of studies (e.g., Main, Kaplan, & Cassidy, 1985) have suggested that secure attachments in childhood dispose the recipients to have secure attachments with their own children subsequently. Hazan and Shaver (1987) have reported that adults with unfavorable descriptions of their childhood relationships with their parents had "insecure" attachments in their most important adult romantic relationships. This hypothesis has encouraged us to examine whether we might find links between PBI scores and measures of adult social attachments (Parker, Barrett, & Hickie, 1992). We have reviewed some 20 studies intercorrelating PBI scores with scores on differing measures of adult social networks. Most studies have found links between PBI Care scores and measures of general social support. Three broad explanations of those links can be suggested:

1. Some studies have incorporated parents into both the PBI and social support measures, leading to a spurious link.

2. Links may be determined by general response biases to score all interpersonal relationships either positively or negatively, reflecting personality sets.

3. There is a causal link: Levels of parental care affect the extent and, more strongly, the satisfaction with adult support levels.

When the hypothesis is refined, and restricted to adult intimate (usually marital) relationships, a differing finding emerges. Several studies (e.g., Hickie, Wilhelm, & Parker, 1990; Hickie, Parker, et al., 1990) have looked for links between PBI scores and a similar measure of adult intimate relationships, the Intimate Bond Measure (IBM; Wilhelm & Parker, 1988), with its Care and Control scales. All such studies have failed to show significant correlations between PBI and IBM scores, except that when an individual returns an extremely low PBI Care score, there is an increased chance of the individual's also rating his or her current intimate partner as uncaring. Rejection of the continuity hypothesis (at least in relation to links between parenting and subsequent intimate relationships) does not necessarily mean rejection of the view that there can be links between the past and present in interpersonal relationships, but it does suggest a need to acknowledge that early developmental trajectories are capable of significant modification. The revelant PBI studies suggest that exposure to harshly uncaring parenting does result in a diathesis, or perhaps conditions the recipients to seek and expect similar characteristics in ongoing relationships, so that they select or associate with adult intimates who provide little nurturance. But, apart from this group of those exposed to gross parental deprivation, the general proposition of continuity is hard to demonstrate—perhaps because there is a continuum in development, with any early diathesis being modified by later relational experiences with both intimates and significant others.

This last point requires some clarification. A number of studies have shown that close affectional bonds in adulthood may be instrumental in modifying and undoing the effects of earlier parental deprivation (Parker & Hazdi-Pavlovic, 1984; Brown & Harris, 1978). In the former study, exposure to an uncaring parent (as measured on the PBI) and to an un-caring partner resulted in a high risk of adult depression; conversely, high caring from both resulted in a low rate. For those who were initially exposed to uncaring parenting, but who "made up" for this by having caring intimates, the earlier parental risk was "undone" to the extent of reducing the chance of adult depression by four-fifths. For those who started with caring parenting but who were currently in relationships with uncaring partners, the risk of adult depression was almost as high as for those who reported lack of care from all support figures. Thus, although our research has focused on the parental characteristics that act as risk factors for a depressive disorder in the recipient in adulthood, I must emphasize an important caveat: Distortions in parent–child bonding are unlikely to establish an immutable diathesis to adult depression. This finding should encourage clarification of those interventions and adult social interactions that may modify exposure to any such early risk.

REFERENCES

Arrindell, W. A., Perris, C., Perris, H., Eisenman, N., Van Der Ende, J., & Von Knorring, L. (1986). Cross-national invariance of dimensions of parental rearing behavior: Comparisons of psychometric data of Swedish depressives and healthy subjects with Dutch target ratings on the EMBU. *British Journal of Psychiatry, 148,* 305–309.

Bowlby, J. (1969). *Attachment and loss: Vol. 1. Attachment.* London: Hogarth Press.

Bowlby, J. (1977). The making and breaking of affectional bonds. *British Journal of Psychiatry, 130,* 201–210.

Brown, G. W., & Harris, T. O. (1978). *The social origins of depression.* London: Tavistock.

Gerlsma, C., Emmelkamp, P. M. G., & Arrindell, W. A. (1990). Anxiety, depression and deception of early parenting: A meta-analysis. *Clinical Psychology Review, 10,* 251–277.

Hazan, C., & Shaver, P. (1987). Romantic love conceptualized as an attachment process. *Journal of Personality and Social Psychology, 52,* 511–524.

Hickie, I., Parker, G., Wilhelm, K., & Tennant, C. (1990). Perceived interpersonal risk factors of non-endogenous depression. *Psychological Medicine, 21,* 399–412.

Hickie, I., Wilhelm, K., & Parker, G. (1990). Perceived dysfunctional intimate relationships: A specific association with the non-melancholic depressive type. *Journal of Affective Disorders, 19,* 99–107.

Hinde, R. A. (1974). *Biological basis of human social behavior.* New York: McGraw-Hill.

Joyce, P. R. (1984). Parental bonding in bipolar affective disorder. *Journal of Affective Disorders, 7,* 319–324.

Kiloh, L. G., Andrews, G., Neilson, M., & Bianchi, G. N. (1972). The relationship of the syndromes called endogenous and neurotic depression. *British Journal of Psychiatry, 121*, 183-196.

Main, M., Kaplan, N., & Cassidy, J. (1985). Security in infancy, childhood and adulthood: A move to the level of representation. In I. Bretherton & E. Waters (Eds.), Growing points of attachment theory and research. *Monographs of the Society for Research in Child Development, 50*(1-2, Serial No. 209), 66-104.

Osofsky, J. D., & Connors, K. (1979). Mother-infant interaction: An integrative view of a complex system. In J. D. Osofsky (Ed.), *Handbook of infant development* (pp. 519-548). New York: Wiley.

Parker, G. (1979). Parental characteristics in relation to depressive disorders. *British Journal of Psychiatry, 134*, 138-147.

Parker, G. (1981). Parental reports of depressives: An investigation of several explanations. *Journal of Affective Disorders, 3*, 131-140.

Parker, G. (1982). Parental representations and affective disorder: Examination for an hereditary link. *British Journal of Medical Psychology, 55*, 57-61.

Parker, G. (1983a). *Parental overprotection: A risk factor in psychosocial development.* New York: Grune & Stratton.

Parker, G. (1983b). Parental "affectionless control" as an antecedent to adult depression. *Archives of General Psychiatry, 48*, 956-960.

Parker, G. (1992). Early environment. In E. S. Paykel (Ed.), *Handbook of affective disorders* (Vol. 2, pp. 171-183). London: Churchill Livingstone.

Parker, G., Barrett, E., & Hickie, I. (1992). From nurture to network: Examining for links between earlier parenting experiences and social bonds in adulthood. *American Journal of Psychiatry, 149*, 877-885.

Parker, G., & Hadzi-Pavlovic, D. (1984). Modification of levels of depression in mother-bereaved women by parental and marital relationships. *Psychological Medicine, 14*, 125-135.

Parker, G., & Hadzi-Pavlovic, D. (1992). Parental representations of melancholic and non-melancholic depressives: Examining for specificity to depressive type and for evidence of additive effects. *Psychological Medicine, 22*, 657-665.

Parker, G., Kiloh, L., & Hayward, L. (1987). Parental representations of neurotic and endogenous depressives. *Journal of Affective Disorders, 13*, 75-82.

Parker, G., Tupling, H., & Brown, L. B. (1979). A parental bonding instrument. *British Journal of Medical Psychology, 52*, 1-10.

Perris, C., Jacobson, L., Lindstrom, H., Von Norring, L., & Perris, H. (1980). Development of a new inventory for assessing memories of parental rearing behavior. *Acta Psychiatrica Scandinavica, 61*, 265-274.

Plantes, M. M., Prusof, B. A., Brennan, J., Anderson, G., & Parker, G. (1988). Parental representations of depressed outpatients from a US sample. *Journal of Affective Disorders, 15*, 149-155.

Richards, M. P. M., & Dyson, M. (1982). *Separation, divorce and the development of children: A review.* London: Department of Health and Social Security.

Schaefer, E. S. (1965). A configurational analysis of children's reports of parental behavior. *Journal of Consulting Psychology, 29*, 552-557.

Tennant, C. (1988). Parental loss in childhood: Its effect in adult life. *Archives of General Psychiatry, 45*, 1045-1050.

Tennant, C., Bebbington, P., & Hurry, J. (1980). Parental death in childhood and risk of adult depressive disorders. *Psychological Medicine, 10,* 289-299.

Trause, M. A., Klaus, M. H., & Kennell, J. H. (1982). Maternal behavior in mammals. In M. H. Klaus & J. H. Kennell (Eds.), *Parent-infant bonding* (pp. 130-140). St. Louis: Mosby.

Wilhelm, K. & Parker, G. (1988). The development of a measure of intimate bonds. *Psychological Medicine, 18,* 225-234.

Wilhelm, K.., & Parker, G. (1990). Reliability of the Parental Bonding Instrument and Intimate Bond Measure scales. *Australian and New Zealand Journal of Psychiatry, 24,* 199-202.

CHAPTER 13

Psychotherapy Strategies for Insecure Attachment in Personality Disorders

MALCOLM WEST
ADRIENNE KELLER

In one of his last publications, Bowlby questioned whether the field of attachment had retained the clinical promise of its early years. In *A Secure Base* (1988), Bowlby stated (concerning the clinical relevance of attachment) that

> whereas attachment was formulated by a clinician for use in the diagnosis and treatment of emotionally disturbed patients and families, its usage hitherto has been mainly to promote research in developmental psychology. Whilst I welcome the findings of this research as enormously extending our understanding of personality development and psychopathology, and thus as of the greatest clinical relevance, it has none the less been disappointing that clinicians have been so slow to test the theory's uses. (pp. ix-x)

Bowlby was clearly appreciative of the abundant research literature that the study of attachment has generated. In suggesting that this work has not somehow found its place in the clinic, Bowlby implied that we ought to examine more thoroughly the clinical usefulness of the attachment concept.

The fact remains, however, that of the many aspects of attachment theory, Bowlby paid the least attention to a theory of psychotherapy. He made only one reference to the therapeutic implications of attachment theory in the second part of "The Making and Breaking of Affectional Bonds" (Bowlby, 1977). If Bowlby himself did not leave to us a complete theory of an attachment-based psychotherapy, he did, however, provide the core concept around which such a theory could be organized. In "Pathological Mourning and Childhood Mourning," Bowlby (1963) demonstrated convincingly that yearning for an experience that never happened or that happened only inconsistently (a close, loving relationship with a parental figure) is the basic problem in neurotic difficulties and personality disorders. In addition, Bowlby did elaborate in a most lucid manner the consequences of the individual's failure to master this "lost" relationship in terms of patterns of insecure attachment. Taken together, these two ideas are highly relevant to the description of an attachment theory of psychotherapy.

In the recent literature on personality disorder research, the concept of attachment has attained considerable currency for depicting the interpersonal difficulties that are a predominant feature of personality disorders. We thus begin this discussion of the clinical implications of attachment theory by starting with a brief account of some representative studies from this literature. Our consideration of the relations of personality disorders and attachment problems necessarily introduces the following topics: the different kinds of patterns of insecure attachment, and the broader question of the nature of insecure attachment. We argue that the dynamic of feared loss of the security invested by individuals in their attachment relationships is the pivotal concept in clinical and theoretical understandings of insecure adult attachment. In the light of this discussion, we formulate in attachment terms how patterns of relating may change through psychotherapy, and in this connection we develop the idea that the principal aim of therapy is to help individuals mourn the loss of that which they never fully experienced but yearned for deeply.

PERSONALITY DISORDERS AND ATTACHMENT PATHOLOGY

It is easy to demonstrate that disturbed or impoverished interpersonal relationships are the hallmark of most personality disorders. The language of personality disorders is replete with terms referring to types of relationships—"close friends," "confidants," "social relationships," "close relationships." According to Widiger and Frances (1985, p. 620),

> An interpersonal nosology is particularly relevant to personality disorders. Each personality disorder has a characteristic and dysfunctional interpersonal style that is often the central feature of the disorder. There is also some empirical support for the hypothesis that a personality disorder is essentially a disorder of interpersonal relatedness.

The central question is how to specify the meaning of interpersonal relationships within the context of personality disorders.

Like many terms in common use, the term "close interpersonal relationships" appears to have an obvious meaning or referent. Approaching the task of classifying such relationships intuitively, we could designate three types: (1) spousal relationships; (2) best friend/closest confidant relationships; (3) relationships with other close friends. Unfortunately, people resolutely fail to confine one relationship to one category (Ainsworth, 1982; Hinde, 1982). For example, one common pattern is for individuals to identify their spouses or partners as their best friends. Alternatively, relationships may look similar in most circumstances, but may prove to be dissimilar in certain crucial ways. This is what George Brown and his colleagues found in the study of Camberwell women (Brown & Harris, 1978). Close affiliative relationships were classed as type a, type b, or type c. Type a and type b were both confidant relationships. In type a relationships, the subject lived with the identified confidant; in type b relationships, the subject did not live with the confidant, but saw him or her frequently and regularly. Type a and type b relationships appeared to be equivalent, except that type a relationships provided "almost complete protection" against psychiatric sequelae to stressful life events. Type b relationships, on the other hand, failed to provide "even relative protection" (Brown & Harris, 1978, p. 234).

In these circumstances, we may be tempted to conceive of attachment relationships as a subset of an individual's affiliative network. Hence the *Diagnostic and Statistical Manual of Mental Disorders*, third edition, revised (DSM-III-R) tends to regard "attachment" as simply a name for the closest affiliative relationship. But this assumption of an intensity continuum between affiliation and attachment is inadequate for differentiating relationships; the function(s) of the relationship must also be taken into account. In this regard, we have demonstrated that the general dimension of interpersonal relationships can be meaningfully differentiated into functionally distinct components: the attachment component, based on the expectation of finding security and safety in an enduring relationship; and the affiliative component, serving to meet intimacy needs and to promote exploration and expansion of interests from the secure base provided by attachment (Sheldon & West, 1989).

This excursion into the conceptual discrimination of two types of interpersonal relationships should not obscure the necessity of demonstrating the usefulness and relevance of attachment to clinicians faced with the practical problem of treating personality-disordered individuals. Happily, there is a growing body of empirical research directed to the examination of attachment problems in personality disorders. To date, the findings of this research are as follows:

1. The criterion of desire for, but fear of, an attachment relationship is more characteristic of those individuals without an attachment figure and diagnosed as having avoidant personality disorder than of those with the same diagnosis who simply have a low level of social skills (see Sheldon & West, 1990).

2. Insecure attachment is central to the style of relating of individ-

uals with dependent personality disorder (see Livesley, Schroeder, & Jackson, 1990).

3. Insecure attachment is as characteristic of avoidant personality disorder as it is of dependent personality disorder (see Sheldon, 1991; Trull, Widiger, & Frances, 1987).

4. Individuals with borderline personality disorder, in response to anticipatory anxiety over being able to meet their needs for security, direct both care-seeking and angry behaviors toward their attachment figures (see Melges & Swartz, 1989; Livesley & Schroeder, 1991; West, Keller, Links, & Patrick, 1993; Sperling, Sharp, & Fishler, 1991).

Taken together, these studies underscore the clinical value of attachment problems to the understanding of personality disorders, which, as Vaillant and Perry (1980, p. 1563) observe, "continually demonstrate to mental health professionals the limits of their expertise." The attachment point of view has many immediate implications. The notion of a person's seeking to find security in a special other, and constructing a representational world of self in relation to others through successive relationship experiences, is fundamental in explaining the personality-disordered individual's inability to feel secure within an attachment relationship. In this case, psychotherapists are allied with developmental psychologists in their concern with the antecedents and consequences of the failure to experience secure attachment.

THE DYNAMIC OF FEARED LOSS IN INSECURE ATTACHMENT

Freud (1926/1959) noted that among the basic anxiety situations, the most significant, and the prototype of all later anxiety, is separation protest: Anxiety "can be reduced to a single condition, namely, that of missing someone who is loved and longed for . . . *anxiety appears as a reaction to the felt loss of the object* (p. 136; emphasis added). Since 1926, when Freud made his reinterpretation of anxiety, later theorists such as Sullivan (1953), Fairbairn (1954), and Winnicott (1965) have considered that no particular attribute of personality, such as motives or affects, can be meaningfully understood apart from the interpersonal context of the person.

Following this accent on relatedness as a motive in its own right, Bowlby, as summarized by Sroufe (1986, p. 845), amassed evidence to show that "the quality of any attachment relationship depends on the quality of care experienced with that partner and the quality of primary attachment relationships strongly influences early personality organization, specifically the child's concept of self and others." Thus one theme in Bowlby's (1969, 1973) organizing theory or story line comes through strongly: The developing child is more or less hurt by a lack of empathic care, or, to use Stern's (1985) term, by the lack of the caregiver's "affect attunement" to the child. Things do not go well, either in childhood or in later life, when this basic parental provision is lacking. Subsequent relational efforts are hampered by the individual's glum and pessimistic beliefs, which predict that attachment needs will be unmet, current attachment figures will be unresponsive, and security will be lost and not restored. Instead of having a sustained confidence in the future of the relationship, the insecurely attached person lives "in constant anxiety lest he lose his attachment figure" (Bowlby, 1977, p. 207). The cast of characters in such an individual's attachment story share the remembered and predicted traits of unresponsiveness and unavailability. Consider, for example, the following clinical vignette in which the pervasive and persistent nature of feared loss is demonstrated:

> Joan, in her late 40s, has experienced symptoms of chronic anxiety for over 10 years, and has been diagnosed according to DSM-III-R criteria as having dependent personality disorder. Her primary attachment figure is her husband. She indicates that she feels very close to him and states, "I need him to always be there," such that when he is away she worries about "falling apart" and has to force herself to keep going. Although she states that her husband is very supportive and understanding, she reports fearing that nobody will be there "to catch me if I fall." In this vein, she is also fearful of losing him. Although he is in good health, she frequently mentions that she worries about his dying, and hardly a day goes by without these thoughts passing through her mind. She also worries when he is away. During his absence, she feels convinced that something terrible will happen to him, and she usually needs to arrange for additional support on these occasions. Joan also becomes very concerned if he is a little late in returning from work or any other trip outside the home, fearing that "something might have happened to him and I'd be totally alone."
>
> Most events that lead to an exacerbation of Joan's symptoms are ones that resonate with underlying expectations about the potential inaccessibility of her attachment figure. Any loss or death causes a crisis. Even the death of someone vaguely known, such as a distant relative or a friend of a friend, precipitates a crisis. Visiting someone who has been hospitalized for a non-life-threatening condition causes intense anxiety that can last for weeks. Under these stressful conditions, Joan responds with intensified care seeking and clings desperately to her husband.

The intensity of these affectively charged beliefs brought about by the feared loss of the current attachment relationship is prefigured by the individual's representational world. Specific expectations embedded in this world that have been carried forward to adulthood are *not* solely the result of early childhood working models. Rather, those beliefs that endure until adulthood have been given special pressure for continuity through having been confirmed by subsequent attachment experiences. This view is consistent with Khan's (1963) notion of cumulative trauma—that is, the idea that chronic failures in caregiver responsiveness summate and can have as great an organizing effect as an acute, sudden trauma such as the death of a parent. Thus successive experiences within relationships (i.e., the degree of success in having needs met) interact with early experiences, through the representational world, to determine the person's current state of mind with regard to attachment. The *validation* of the person's early working model in the form of continued lack of success in achieving felt security contributes significantly to its persistence.

In the instance of insecure attachment, then, we are concerned with a set of beliefs and feelings (typically anger, sadness, yearning, and guilt) that are carried forward as potentials awaiting to be expressed in current relationships. Because, as Guntrip (1969) has observed, the representational world has a life of its own independent of external reality, an insecurely attached individual can experience constant fear of the loss of the present attachment relationship. This fear often becomes obvious when the individual is confronted with the need to take a new and larger step toward relational intimacy. For example, the clinician is likely to see avoidant/schizoid individuals after their usual style of relating has been threatened or demolished by a quantitative or qualitative increase in close relationships. Consider a man's behavior that is consistent with what would be described as "schizoid personality" (Guntrip, 1969; Fairbairn, 1954), as "false self" (Winnicott, 1965), or as avoidant personality disorder (DSM-III-R):

> In his psychotherapy, David's withdrawal from personal relationships was developed around the childhood loss of a loving parental relationship. As discussed above, Khan's (1963) concept of cumulative trauma broadens the idea of loss to include the effects of long-lasting situations such as the lack of empathetic parental care. Eventually, this work led him to an attempt at intimacy. He met and dated a woman from a small liberal arts college where both of them taught. Although this opportunity for closeness resurrected the old danger of feared loss, which had first of all led to David's compensatory self-sufficiency, it was also evident that the almost overwhelming anxiety he experienced derived from the reality of the woman's emotional availability. For someone who had turned away from others, and who lacked a belief in himself as worthy of caring, the hope or expectation of attaining a meaningful attachment was indeed a fright-

ening feeling. As Main, Kaplan, and Cassidy (1985) point out in another context, the development of defensive attachment patterns enables many children to compensate for serious caregiver responsiveness failures. Yet, as noted above, the clinician may well see such people as adults after the attachment patterns of their lives have been threatened or undermined. Clearly, the possibility of an intimate relationship had repercussions for David's defensive attachment pattern. We can recognize here a conflict: retrenchment expressed in terms of further withdrawal and denial of his attachment emotions, or a commitment to a leadership role in order to meet and enrich the woman's offer of emotional availability.

The stress of threatened loss in their attachment relationships leaves insecurely attached individuals vulnerable to intense affective distress (Kobak & Sceery, 1988). Often because of their intensity, feelings such as passionate yearning, fearsome possessiveness, aggressiveness, or despair are always just around the corner, awaiting activation, in the current attachment relationship. And once these feelings are expressed toward the attachment figure, they have the very great likelihood of evoking corresponding feelings in that person, creating in this way a representational identity between past and present attachment experiences. Repetitive affect patterns therefore lead to further disappointing and frustrating experiences in achieving felt security. In this manner, what happens in the present attachment relationship and the individual's glum beliefs about attachment reciprocally reinforce each other to maintain the representational world as an impermeable fortress.

The representational world is synonymous with a pattern of attachment. From the discussion that follows, it will be apparent that the patterns of insecure attachment, although variously named, move from the distant and detached (Bowlby's [1977] "compulsive self-reliance" and Main's [1985] "dismissing" classification) to the close and enmeshed (Bowlby's "anxious attachment" and Main's "preoccupied" classification). Such clearly defensive attachment patterns are always connected ultimately with an unbearable threat: anticipation of the loss of the attachment figure and the attachment relationship.

ADULT PATTERNS OF INSECURE ATTACHMENT AND DEFENSIVE EXCLUSION

In the study of patterns of insecure attachment, we are concerned with a faithful adherence to a maladaptive style of relating that cannot be wholly described in terms of the attachment concept of "defensive exclusion." Defensive exclusion operates by persistently excluding from complete internal processing certain types of attachment information; that is, what should be treated as "signal" is ignored as "noise." Defensive exclusion is easily translated into behavioral consequences in the case of compulsive self-reliant/dismissing patterns of attachment. For these patterns, the activation of the attachment system itself is defensively excluded. The connection is less straightforward for the anxious/preoccupied patterns. In fact, we have failed to find, either in Bowlby's own writings or in related works, a coherent explication of the defensive exclusion underlying these patterns. It may well be that the anxious/preoccupied patterns prevent the establishment of satisfactory defensive exclusion. Thus, individuals who have always been anxiously attached to their attachment figures may not have developed adequate defenses against separation anxiety, leaving them prey to overreactions to anticipated or actual separations from their attachment figures. For example, we (West et al., 1993) and Livesley and Schroeder (1991) use hypersensitivity to the continuity of the attachment relationship to characterize the borderline individual's intense and unstable relationships. Perhaps, then, in the context of the anxious/preoccupied patterns, the individual is relatively defenseless.

Defensive exclusion is conceptually problematic, in that it is defined exclusively from an intrapsychic standpoint. In this important respect, Bowlby (1980), like Freud, borrowed a theory for attachment from a popular theory within another branch of scientific inquiry. Thus, Freud's concept of defense is based on an analogy to the mechanics of energy as understood by 19th-century physics; Bowlby's formulation of defensive processes is based on an analogy to the mechanics of information processing as understood by 20th-century cognitive research. Although the language and imagery of the two models are clearly different, both models are primarily mechanistic. Both, as noted above, locate the defensive process in the individual's intrapsychic machinery: One is conceived to operate according to the inexorable laws of 19th-century physics, the other according to a computerized version of attachment that de-emphasizes the role of affects in determining patterns of attachment.

When we speak of "defensive attachment patterns," we are referring essentially to an inauthentic style of relating. The forming and sustaining of meaningful attachments have a good deal to do with affective authenticity, in the sense of an openness to one's own feelings and a readiness to respond to another person's feelings. Inauthentic affective communication is a significant form of defense because it creates relational distance. This is seen most clearly in the case of the compulsive self-reliant/dismissing patterns. The detachment from, and loss of recognition of, one's true feelings result in the inability to endure intimate relationships. In the case of the anxious/preoccupied patterns, the unmodulated and exaggerated expression of a narrow range of feelings (typically, angry yearning and fearsome expectations about being left) permit only a shallow concern with and sharing of the other person's feelings or point of view. In either case, "defensiveness" means an allegiance to a constricted pattern of gaining security, in order to protect the person from re-experiencing a situation of helplessness that caused anxiety or sadness.

The qualities of these defensive attachment patterns can be related to variations of an incomplete mourning reaction. From the point of view of pathological mourning, the single most important cause of insecure attachment lies in the person's inability to master the loss of a longed-for but never fully experienced tender relationship to the caretaker. Unresolved mourning is always associated with the giving up of authentic relatedness to others and a relative detachment from one's attachment emotions. In the compulsive self-reliant/dismissing pattern, the detachment and withdrawal are of a much greater magnitude than in the case of the anxious/preoccupied pattern. The turning away from intimate personal relationships is often massive. As Bowlby (1977, p. 207) observed of the compulsive self-reliant individual, "So far from seeking the love and care of others, a person who exhibits this pattern insists on keeping a stiff upper lip and doing everything for himself whatever the conditions." The self-sufficiency is in many ways a pseudo-self-sufficiency that covers a soft-hearted center full of perpetual feelings of loneliness and "unexpressed yearning for love and support."

Main et al.'s (1985) characterization of dismissing individuals provides the best and most obvious explanation of their withdrawal from meaningful contacts with other persons. Specifically, the idealized versions given by these individuals of their childhood attachment experiences bespeak repressed feelings and denial of loss. The inability of dismissing individuals to face feelings of anger and sadness that accompany disappointments in the relationship with their parents suggests that grief has only been experienced in part, loss only partially admitted. As has often been observed, this inability to recognize and express anger and sadness leads to the inability to feel and express attachment emotions. A dismissing individual's detachment from any kind of deep feeling is general and pervasive.

In the case of the anxious/preoccupied pattern, the individual seems not to believe that it is obligatory to say goodbye to a lost attachment relationship. Rather, there is a persistent effort to recover this lost relationship, accompanied by intense anger and reproach expressed toward the parent. The inability to break free from an enmeshed dependency on an ambivalently regarded parent necessarily compromises the individual's ability to form authentic ties to new attachment figures.

It is our contention that insecure attachment in the adult stems from the person's inability to master the consequences of parental responsiveness failures in childhood. The results of this inability, as we have seen, are disavowed feelings of grief, anger, and sorrowful yearning, and a distrust or lack of confidence in others' availability and responsiveness. In the final section of this chapter, we characterize an attachment-based psychotherapy in terms of the creation of a safe environment that enables the individual to recapture and assimilate disavowed feelings associated with the memory of painful attachment experiences.

THE THERAPEUTIC YIELD: FOCUSING ISSUES OF THERAPY[1]

With every kind of psychotherapy, there is implicit agreement that the therapeutic relationship is a decisive component of the curative process. What Ainsworth (1989) described as the secure base provided by the childhood caregiver becomes a compelling metaphor for the therapeutic relationship. In ordinary situations of bereavement, Bowlby (1980, p. 232) also compared the role of a companion to a caregiver whose presence has the following salutary effects: "the bereaved's anxiety is reduced, his morale fortified, his evaluations made less harsh, and the actions necessary to meet a new situation selected and planned more judiciously." Similarly, the therapist becomes a companion with whom the person can re-experience grief and acknowledge loss.

Although the essence of psychotherapy is that it establishes the therapist as a protective figure, this should not obscure the fact that the person's active use of this secure base is required to achieve change; that is, change needs exploration as well as attachment. Rapport on its own runs the particular risk of leading to either an enmeshed dependency on the therapist or withdrawal and escape from the therapist. Rather, the use of the therapist as an auxiliary secure base creates a "background of safety," to use Sandler's (1960) term, which permits the individual to begin to uncover the secrets and landmarks of his or her past attachment experiences. As noted by Bowlby (1988, p. 138), reliance upon the therapist as a protective figure establishes "a secure base from which he can explore the various unhappy and painful aspects of his life, past and present, many of which he finds it difficult or perhaps impossible to think about and reconsider without a trusted companion to provide support, encouragement, sympathy, and, on occasion, guidance."

Before discussing the nature of the therapeutic process, let us consider one additional aspect of the therapist as a protective figure. The therapeutic relationship, in the minds of most object relations theorists—such as Balint (1968), and Winnicott (1958)—is literally akin to the child's relationship with a maternal caregiver. In any of these theories, the therapist is portrayed as a reparative parental figure who provides relational experiences that were missing during the individual's childhood. At the same time, the individual's attachment to the therapist is conceived as a regressive infantile longing or as a symbolization of the earliest mother-child relationship. As Mitchell (1988, p. 156) points out, adult attachment desires in this approach "are depicted as regressive symbiotic yearnings, unresolved residues from earliest childhood."

There is, however, a dilemma implicit in this type of therapeutic relationship: If the therapist is primarily understood as a reparative parental figure, can the individual's desire to form an adult attachment to the therapist (in terms other than as a vestige of infantile needs) be adequately attended to? Perhaps a resolution lies in understanding adult attachment needs in such a way that they can be seen in the context of a relational conflict. Could we not understand what the individual experiences as an intense longing for closeness as reflecting one polar element of an inner attachment drama? Within this internal drama, we can recognize the concurrence of two aspects of a conflictual situation—desire and fear. The desire component, as mentioned above, is essentially a longing for meaningful relatedness. The fear component of the drama arises when expression of the attachment desire is suffused with anxiety about the individual's own vulnerability and anxiety about the other person's responsiveness. Our therapeutic approach to this desire-fear attachment drama is to separate the desire from the fear, leaving the desire component as an uninterpreted background against which the fear component may be examined as figure. This approach is fully consistent with Malan's (1979) precept that only negative transference reactions require interpretation; thus the positive transference is left as an uninterpreted and essentially ambiguous backdrop in therapy.

THE SIGNIFICANCE OF ENACTMENT

At this point we wish to introduce a new thought about the unfolding of events in the therapeutic process. From the beginning in Freud's cathartic method, the uncovering of the individual's inner drama has almost always been conceived to proceed in this stepwise sequence: Interpretation provides insight, and insight is later translated into both actions and changes in behavior. A somewhat modified sequence of events is suggested by Weiss and Sampson's (Weiss, Sampson, & the Mount Zion Psychotherapy Research Group, 1986; Weiss, 1993) theory of therapy. They hold that the achievement of a sense of safety within the therapeutic setting depends upon the individual's recreating danger situations. The individual's effort to disconfirm his or her pessimistic beliefs about the therapist's empathic reliability is chiefly accomplished through the medium of experience. Eagle (1984) has hailed Weiss and Sampson's attention to the therapeutic value of *action* as an important antidote to the classical view of the curative pathway, in which change is depicted as a linear movement from insight to subsequent behavioral change, uninterrupted by creative experience.

Just as Bowlby was careful to show that an individual's representational world evolves from the specific and accurate perception of past experience (from the outside), so we have to allow that modification of this world may similarly begin with behavioral change. The term "enactment," first introduced by Eagle (1984), nicely captures this sequence of events in therapy. Early in therapy, the individual, perhaps buttressed by the secure base provided by the therapist, undertakes a new mode of action. These actions take many different forms, such as enrolling in a university course, asserting oneself a bit more in social situations, and so on. The actual behavioral initiative is not as important as the place it assumes in the person's inner attachment drama. Although not extensively explored at this early stage of therapy, the significance of this new mode of action is that it represents an externalization of the person's attachment drama, or at least reflects an element of it. For example, disavowed attachment wishes may be brought out into the open as an aspect of the enactment. However, subsequent therapeutic work is more often organized around the fears aroused by the initiative than around the wish component of the inner drama.

Let us turn again to a clinical example to illustrate how a behavioral initiative reflects both a core element of the person's inner attachment drama and the therapist's inevitable enmeshment as a coactor in that drama. The woman's problems discussed below are consistent with the DSM-III-R's description of self-defeating personality disorder or Bowlby's (1977) "compulsive caregiving" attachment pattern. The details of the account are derived from a previous discussion of the deviant pattern of attachment behaviors of compulsive caregiving (West & Keller, 1991).

> Mary, a woman in her late 20s, had been so dominated by her mother's neediness that she felt that pursuing her own life meant turning her back on her mother. An episode recalled from childhood dramatically captures the responsibility Mary felt for her mother's welfare. In this scene, her father sent her into the garden to speak with her mother. There, she found her mother frantically running around pulling her hair out and screaming, "It's my nerves—I can't go on!" In recalling other similar incidents, Mary said, "She didn't try to control herself." She feared that her mother would commit suicide or desert her. In response, Mary appeased her mother, catering to and serving her in many ways in the hope of making her happy.

To use Winnicott's (1965) term, the problem was "impinge-ment"; that is, the parent's relationship to the child ignored the child's attachment needs. Mary had fashioned herself to comply with her mother's definition of relatedness. She became bound to her mother by the need to meet her mother's neediness with her own caregiving. Among the psychological sequelae of this premature caregiving responsibility was her inability to assert genuine aspects of her indi-viduality ("I felt like a bud that wants to bloom but can't").

Early in therapy, Mary enrolled in a university program. This initiative arose from her having assumed increasing responsibility in her secretarial role without the accompanying authority—a disparity clearly reminiscent of her childhood situation. In terms of the enact-ment of Mary's inner drama, her enrollment in a university program represented the desire component of the drama—that is, the asser-tion of her right to do something that was of value to her. Although she wanted the therapist's approval for this effort to change her life, the transference was predominantly organized around Mary's fear that the therapist would intrude into this act of self-assertion. In par-ticular, she was very apprehensive that the therapist would interpret this act of personal assertion as defiance and compel her to renounce it. Mary believed, in other words, that therapy was a reductionistic process in which she would have to submit to the therapist's inter-pretations, and that when she did so, the legitimacy of her desire to change her life would be undermined.

In psychotherapy, much of the work, often intensely affect-laden, centers around an effort to understand and work through the effects that the individual's inner attachment drama has on the therapeutic relationship. In Mary's case, many sessions revolved around her transference reaction of fearing the therapist's intrusive-ness. This situation ended when she came to the realization that de-cisions she made independently of the therapist would not threaten the relationship. This work led to the recognition of the possibility of a new type of relationship that would enhance rather than threaten security, and would be based upon reciprocity rather than unsatis-factory complementarity.

The notion of an inner attachment drama is close to the heart of the concept of transference. Almost all accounts of transference mention or imply the rekindling of an old relational gestalt and the imposition of it onto the therapist. The pressure to weave the therapist into this gestalt derives principally, of course, from the unmourned "trauma" of chronic failures in caregiver responsiveness. Disavowed feelings of anger, yearn-ing, guilt, and anxiety, and cynical distrust of others, appear in response to the therapist. In Piagetian terms, individuals assimilate the therapist into their internal "relational templates" by distorting what they perceive to suit their needs. But, paradoxically, they are changed in doing so.

When the therapist declines the gambit—that is, through interpretative efforts, the therapist does *not* act the role assigned to him or her in the person's inner attachment drama—a discontinuity of experience results. Such a refusal to be cast into playing a role in this drama can precipitate the best kind of corrective emotional experience. Over time, this experiential discontinuity favors accommodation of the therapist as a new and different coactor in a manner, to use Weiss et al.'s (1986) formulation, that allows for the disconfirmation of the individual's pathogenic beliefs.

Inevitably, the process of both consciously and unconsciously comparing past attachment experiences and current experiences with the therapist arouses painful and depressive feelings. This is so because, prior to the therapist's engaging in a different and broadened way of relating, the individual has been unable in one sense, and unwilling in another sense, to conduct relationships differently. The wasting of attachment possibilities and the missed opportunities for giving and receiving love are now deeply felt. Implicitly, such feelings and mourning are inextricably conjoined.

LOSS, MOURNING, AND INTEGRATION

We have suggested earlier that the most important cause of insecure attachment lies in the inability of the person to master the loss of an empathic relationship with the childhood caregiver. Chronic experiences of caregiver insensitivity or rebuff summate and become for the individual miniexperiences of loss. These experiences create relational distance and perpetual feelings of not being understood, the results of which are loneliness and the despair of alienation. The typical response to loss is an amalgam of sorrowful yearning, anger, guilt, and partial or complete withdrawal from meaningful relationships. Such pathological mourning, as Bowlby (1963) demonstrated, is marked by denial of loss and repression of feelings.

Pathological mourning is indeed a challenge to those psychotherapists who assume that a person's relational difficulties are exclusively the results of the effects of the cumulative and unassimilated trauma inflicted by caregiver empathic failures. According to Green (1986, p. 142), "If one had to choose a single characteristic to differentiate between present-day analyses and analyses as one imagines them to have been in the past, it would surely be found among the problems of mourning." Green suggests here that individuals have been unable to master not only their actual losses, but also the loss of that which they have deeply desired but never fully experienced. It is certainly true that many people who come for therapy are still searching for an experience that never happened. As suggested above, a basic problem of insecurely attached individuals is that they have been unable to say goodbye to "lost" attachment figures; that is, they have been unable to forgive, forget, and reconcile themselves to the reality of unsuccessful past attachments.

In an essential way, then, attachment-based psychotherapy strives to complete a delayed mourning process. It is principally concerned with the undoing of a denied loss (a longed-for but never fully experienced loving relationship with the childhood caregiver) so that connected feelings are expressed and then followed into the childhood past. The mourning process thus provides a direct pathway to the reality and consequences of caregiver empathic failures. In another sense, it simplifies and organizes the relationship between these prior attachment experiences and present affectively charged beliefs about attachment.

If the work of mourning is to lead to forgiveness and reconciliation with past attachment figures, feelings of disappointment, anger, and sadness need to appear, as in the case of Mary (see above):

> As Mary began to acknowledge her losses, she often fell into a sad mood. In some sessions, she remained silent and simply wept after she had untangled the impact of the missing tender relationship with her mother. In other sessions, as she became able "to be what you think you really are," Mary railed against her mother's failure to be an attachment figure (someone stronger and/or wiser) for her. By making these feelings conscious, Mary was able to acknowledge and reconcile herself to her apparent failure to elicit her mother's tender attentions.

Finally, the account of early attachment events and situations as remembered by the individual needs to be integrated into the representational world if it is to have therapeutic value beyond a cathartic effect. This involves a turning back on oneself by directing reflection upon one's own representational world, so that the influence of past attachment experiences on present relationships can be examined. By recalling neglected or forgotten details of these past events, and becoming aware of the meaning they have assumed in the representation of attachment, the person increases the "permeability" of his or her representational world and enhances the integration of present and past, perception and memory, ideas and affects. The individual begins to see the subtle but often painfully obvious effects of caregiver responsiveness failures upon his or her current attitudes toward and expectations about attachment. Once connectedness between these areas is recognized, an enlarged and more open concept of attachment reality results. Insight, then, is based on understanding this connectedness coupled with a conviction of its reality.

The development of insight is akin to a creative process, in that it consists of the putting together of two previously unconnected frames of reference. But, as Koestler (1966) points out, this act of discovery operates in a "Janusian" fashion. Any new awareness derives first from the individual's escaping from blind representational alleys and disrupting cognitive biases that distort the affective appraisal of attachment experiences. Only then can new frames of perception be constructed and coded in such a way that the person may "feel free to imagine alternatives better fitted to his current life" (Bowlby, 1988, p.139).

NOTE

1. In this section, we describe the therapeutic effects of organizing an attachment-based psychotherapy around the completion of a mourning reaction. Within the domain of personality disorders, there is an important element of incomplete mourning in most of these disorders. Two common variations of incomplete mourning in personality-disordered individuals are (1) withdrawal from meaningful attachments, and (2) the persistent search for a relationship experience that never happened, eventuating in an anxious enmeshment with the current attachment figure. We do not believe that there are basic differences in approach in the psychotherapy of the "withdrawn" personality disorders (schizoid, avoidant) as compared to the "enmeshed" disorders (borderline, dependent).

REFERENCES

Ainsworth, M. D. S. (1982). Attachment: Retrospect and prospect. In C. M. Parkes & J. Stevenson-Hinde (Eds.), *The place of attachment in human behavior* (pp. 3-30). New York: Basic Books.

Ainsworth, M. D. S. (1989). Attachments beyond infancy. *American Psychologist, 44,* 709-716.

Balint, M. (1968). *The basic fault: Therapeutic aspects of regression.* London: Tavistock.

Bowlby, J. (1963). Pathological mourning and childhood mourning. *Journal of the American Psychoanalytic Association, 11,* 500-541.

Bowlby, J. (1969). *Attachment and loss: Vol. 1. Attachment.* New York: Basic Books.

Bowlby, J. (1973). *Attachment and loss: Vol. 2. Separation: Anxiety and anger.* New York: Basic Books.

Bowlby, J. (1977). The making and breaking of affectional bonds. *British Journal of Psychiatry, 130,* 201-210.

Bowlby, J. (1980). *Attachment and loss: Vol. 3. Loss: Sadness and depression.* New York: Basic Books.

Bowlby, J. (1988). *A secure base: Clinical applications of attachment theory.* London: Routledge.

Brown, G., & Harris, T. (1978). *Social origins of depression: A study of psychiatric disorder in women*. London: Tavistock.

Eagle, M. (1984). *Recent developments in psychoanalysis*. New York: McGraw-Hill.

Fairbairn, W. R. D. (1952). *An object-relations theory of the personality*. New York: Basic Books.

Freud S. (1959). Inhibitions, symptoms and anxiety. In J. Strachey (Ed. and Trans.), *The standard edition of the complete works of Sigmund Freud* (Vol. 20, pp. 77-175). London: Hogarth Press. (Original work published 1926)

Green, A. (1986). *On private madness*. Madison, CT: International Universities Press.

Guntrip, H. (1969). *Schizoid phenomena, object-relations and the self*. New York: International Universities Press.

Hinde, R. A. (1982). Attachment: Some conceptual and biological issues. In C. M. Parkes & J. Stevenson-Hinde (Eds.), *The place of attachment in human behavior* (pp. 60-76). New York: Basic Books.

Khan, M. (1963). The concept of cumulative trauma. *Psychoanalytic Study of the Child, 18*, 286-306.

Kobak, R. R., & Sceery, A. (1988). Attachment in late adolescence: Working models, affect regulation, and perceptions of self and others. *Child Development, 59*, 135-146.

Koestler, A. (1966). *The act of creation*. London: Pan Books.

Livesley, W. J., & Schroeder, M. (1991). Dimensions of personality disorder: The DSM-III-R cluster B diagnoses. *Journal of Nervous and Mental Disease, 179*, 320-328.

Livesley W. J., Schroeder M., & Jackson, D. N. (1990). Dependent personality disorder and attachment problems. *Journal of Personality Disorders, 4*, 131-140.

Main, M. (1985). *An adult attachment classification system: Its relation to infant-parent attachment*. Paper presented at the bennial meeting of the Society for Research in Child Development, Toronto.

Main, M., Kaplan, N., & Cassidy, J. (1985). Security in infancy, childhood and adulthood: A move to the level of representation. In I. Bretherton & E. Waters (Eds.), Growing points of attachment theory and research. *Monographs of the Society for Research in Child Development, 50*(1-2, Serial No. 209), 66-104.

Malan, D. H. (1979). *Individual psychotherapy and the science of psychodynamics*. London: Butterworths.

Melges, F., & Swartz, M. (1989). Oscillations of attachment in borderline personality disorder. *American Journal of Psychiatry, 146*, 1116-1120.

Mitchell, S. A. (1988). *Relational concepts in psychoanalysis: An integration*. Cambridge, MA: Harvard University Press.

Sandler, J. (1960). The background of safety. *International Journal of Psycho-Analysis, 41*, 325-356.

Sheldon, A. E. R. (1991). *The discrimination of attachment and affiliation: Theoretical propositions and application to specific personality disorders*. Unpublished doctoral dissertation, University of Calgary.

Sheldon, A. E. R., & West, M. L. (1989). The functional discrimination of affiliation and attachment: Theory and empirical demonstration. *British Journal of Psychiatry, 155*, 18-23.

Sheldon, A. E. R., & West, M. L. (1990). Attachment pathology versus low social skills in avoidant personality disorder: An exploratory study. *Canadian Journal of Psychiatry, 35,* 596-599.

Sperling, M. B., Sharp, J. L., & Fishler, P. H. (1991). On the nature of attachment in a borderline population: A preliminary report. *Psychological Reports, 68,* 54-546.

Sroufe, L. A. (1986). Appraisal: Bowlby's contribution to psychoanalytic theory and developmental psychology. *Journal of Child Psychology and Psychiatry, 27,* 841-849.

Stern, D. (1985). *The interpersonal world of the infant.* New York: Basic Books.

Sullivan, H .S. (1953). *The interpersonal theory of psychiatry.* New York: Norton.

Trull, T. J., Widiger, T. A., & Frances, A. (1987). Covariation of criteria sets for avoidant, schizoid, and dependent personality disorders. *American Journal of Psychiatry, 144,* 767-771.

Vaillant, G. E., & Perry, J. C. (1980). Personality disorders. In H. I. Kaplan, A. M. Freedman, & B. J. Sadock (Eds.), *Comprehensive textbook of psychiatry* (3rd ed., pp. 1562-1590). Baltimore: Williams & Wilkins.

Weiss, J. (1993). *How psychotherapy works.* New York: Guilford Press.

Weiss, J., Sampson, H., & the Mount Zion Psychotherapy Research Group. (1986). *The psychoanalytic process: Theory, clinical observation, and empirical research.* New York: Guilford Press.

West, M. L., & Keller, A. E. R. (1991). Parentification of the child: A case study of Bowlby's compulsive care-giving attachment pattern. *American Journal of Psychotherapy, 14,* 425-431.

West, M. L., Keller, A. E. R., Links, P., & Patrick, J. (1993). Borderline personality disorder and attachment pathology. *Canadian Journal of Psychiatry, 38*(Suppl. 1), 516-522.

Widiger, T. A., & Frances, A. (1985). The DSM-III personality disorders: Perspectives from psychology. *Archives of General Psychiatry, 42,* 615-623.

Winnicott, D. W. (1958). *Through paediatrics to psychoanalysis.* London: Hogarth Press.

Winnicott, D. W. (1965). *The maturational processes and the facilitating environment.* New York: International Universities Press.

CHAPTER 14

Representations of Attachment and Psychotherapeutic Change

MICHAEL B. SPERLING
LISA SANDOW LYONS

THEORIES OF MENTAL REPRESENTATIONS

The construct of "mental representations" suggests that within each of us there are enduring matrices of memories, expectations, and affects associated with significant interpersonal (usually attachment) relationships. These integrated representations are formed through actual interpersonal experience, yet evolve into internal constructions that do not usually retain isomorphic properties of these experiences. Furthermore, these internal representations are reified through the generation of internal and external relational narratives, which then recursively influence the assimilation and organization of new interpersonal experience. This synergistic representational process is one of the fundamental mechanisms governing mental functioning; it has generated interest principally within attachment, psychoanalytic, and cognitive theories, and secondarily within systems and social-constructionist theories. There have, however, been too few attempts at explicitly integrating this breadth of work on mental representations within the clinical sphere of psychodynamic psychotherapy. The intent here is to do so in the service of examining the possibilities for a dynamically informed psychotherapy within a nonenactive transferential mode that focuses directly on facilitating change in mental representations, particularly representations of attachment.

We have chosen to address this topic because the literature within psychoanalysis and psychodynamic psychotherapy (as opposed to psychoanalytic theory) that covers representational notions usually does so indirectly. The more common direct focus on the dynamics of transference enactments within the therapeutic relationship often treats representational considerations as either implicit or secondary. This secondary role, however, disguises the important convergences and divergences between the notions of representation and transference. Part of the heuristic dilemma may be mnemonic, in that the construct of mental representations is invoked using many different but associated terms: "self-representation," "object representation," "internal working model," "introjected object," "internal object," "representational world," "psychical representation," "schema," "self schema," "personal-construct system," "life history narrative," "core conflictual relationship theme," and "evocative memory."

Each of the theoretical domains addressing representational process describes the concept using somewhat different language, although with remarkable conceptual overlap. Within attachment theory, which has given mental representations much attention, the term "internal working model" is used to connote the dynamic process through which environmental and intraorganismic information about attachment experiences is selected, processed, reified, and encoded into representational models (Bowlby, 1969). Drawing on Bowlby's work, Main, Kaplan, and Cassidy (1985) provide a succinct definition of working models in reference to attachment as "a set of conscious and/or unconscious rules for the organization of information relevant to attachment and for obtaining or limiting access to that information, that is, to information regarding attachment-related experiences, feelings, and ideations" (pp. 66-67). Thus, a model can be regarded as analogous to an "average" accumulation of associated representations, which are themselves accumulations of associated (and internally processed) interpersonal experiences (Stern, 1985).

Important to psychoanalytic applications of transference theory to the concept of working models is the notion that these models must apply to real *and* imagined interpersonal situations, and must be able to "evoke in consciousness representation of an absent object" (Beres & Joseph, 1970, p. 8). These points constitute a major aspect of the related concept of "object representations," developed initially by Freud and expanded by developmental psychoanalytic and object relations theorists. For example, Sandler and Rosenblatt (1962) and Jacobson (1964) postulated that interpersonal experience lays the foundation for an internal representational world constructed from self- and object representations. These cathected representations are then differentiated and activated by what Kernberg (1976) refers to as the "emotional valences" of internal objects. The eventual developmental goal is that of attaining temporal and affective stability within one's representational world—that is, "libidinal object constancy" (Fraiberg, 1969; Mahler, Pine, & Bergman, 1975).

Related concepts are found in cognitively focused theory and therapy, especially in the work of personal-construct and cognitive-developmental theorists. George Kelly (1955) based his theory of "personal constructs" on the philosophical position of constructive alternatism, which holds that there are many alternative ways of viewing the same events. He postulated that each individual perceives events through a filter of highly personal and idiosyncratic constructs about the world. The fundamental postulate of Kelly's theory is that "a person's processes are psychologically channelized by the ways in which he anticipates events" (1955, p. 46).

Originally the sole domain of cognitive-developmental science (e.g., Bartlett, 1932; Piaget, 1955), the term "schema" has recently come to denote more broadly the mental structures through which individuals of any age filter and give meaning to both internal and external events. It connotes a "top-down" way of processing conscious and unconscious information, as opposed to a "bottom-up" or data-driven method (Singer & Salovey, 1991). The term is now used, with differing but related definitions, by researchers and clinicians working in a range of theoretical domains on a range of clinical and theoretical problems (e.g., Beck, Rush, Shaw, & Emery, 1979; Greenberg & Beck, 1990; Singer & Salovey, 1991; Slap & Slap-Shelton, 1991). Schemata are used, for example, to track and describe perceptions of reality in transference responses during therapy (Luborsky, Crits-Christoph, Friedman, Mark, & Schaffler, 1991), to diagram complex patterns in interpersonal relationships (Horowitz, 1991), and to study and redefine diagnostic classifications (Horowitz, 1991). Of particular integrative significance are the systematic research efforts of Horowitz (e.g., Horowitz, 1991) on the cognitive notion of person schemata, and his attempts to reconcile this notion with similar psychoanalytic constructs (Horowitz, 1988). He suggests that person schemata "are structures of meaning that integrate knowledge about self and others. These mental structures may operate consciously and unconsciously to organize thought, complex mood states, self appraisal, and interpersonal actions" (Horowitz, 1991, p. 1). Schemata thus are mental representations, both conscious and unconscious, of intrapsychic and interpersonal events.

Attachment, psychoanalytic, and cognitive theories appear to be the primary areas to offer specific and precise definitions of mental representations or their equivalents; yet there certainly has been interest in related disciplines. For example, systems theory has only recently developed a distinct interest in representations, and incorporates these terms definitionally from attachment and psychoanalytic theories (Heard, 1982). The incorporation into systems theory of the influence of mental representations on individual functioning is understandable, given the attention within this theory to the dimensions and differentiation of the "self within systems" (e.g., Fogarty, 1976), and the effect of collective self-representations on the treatment of the system as a whole (Byng-Hall, 1991). The application of representational constructs to families then necessarily involves examining the array of legends or scripts that each family member brings to the system (Byng-Hall, 1988).

It is noteworthy that all of the differing theoretical applications of representational constructs (e.g., "internal working model," "object representation," "personal construct," "schema") are organized largely around representations of meaningful attachment relationships, although this is not explicitly stated in most cases. A relationship need not conform to the characteristics of attachment (i.e., perceived security when distressed, proximity seeking, discomfort when separated) to bear a strong affective-cognitive meaningfulness—but most seem to. Similarly, interpersonal relationships, especially those early in life, that are formative for the development of representations need not be attachment relationships—but most are. Although this point is not always stated when the term "representation" is invoked, it is understood that the notions of representation (in a relational context) and attachment are themselves developmentally linked.

CLINICAL PROCESS IN REPRESENTATIONAL CHANGE

In discussing the representational dialectic between the interpersonal and the intrapsychic, Stern (1988) suggests that representations are conservative historical structures, in which "past experience will have enormous weight in the construction of present subjective experience. People will repeat the same behaviors, selective inattentions, interpretations, etc." (p. 510). In short, interpersonally we do what we know, and what we know is in large part a product of our formative representations of attachment experiences. This simply stated argument gets right to the heart of the matter when it comes to psychotherapeutic means of effecting either character change or realignment of defenses within a given character structure. Schafer (1968/1990) expressed this point a different way by writing that

> whether they do so unconsciously or otherwise, people marshal those details ("representations") that provide the narrative content that they expect to be most useful both in pursuing the aims they have set for themselves and in giving subsequent accounts of their pursuits and accomplishments. They tell the lives they enact and they enact the lives they tell. (p. xxii)

The narrative representational formulations voiced by Stern and Schafer are most commonly attributed to a psychoanalytic sensibility, although a representational focus demands a constructivist perspective that serves as a point of integration between psychoanalytic and other theoretical domains.

The question remains of how therapeutic change in this multiply determined representational process can be brought about. Our extensive review of the literature (Sperling & Lyons, 1994) indicates that those modes of therapy that have attempted to focus somewhat directly, albeit not exclusively, on correcting dysfunctional mental representations appear to fall into four fundamental but not mutually exclusive categories: (1) therapies that work to provide alternative representations of interpersonal functioning through relational modeling within the therapist–patient attachment bond; (2) a more specific application of relational modeling that attempts to reparent through establishing a corrective emotional attachment with the therapist, or between a child and his or her primary caretaker, that competes with and substantially alters dysfunctional representations; (3) therapy that aims to cognitively and emotionally analyze, reassess, and thereby change mental representations and the defenses that maintain them; and (4) a variant of the reassessment technique that focuses specifically on reconstruction of representational narratives. Few of these therapies address representations explicitly, but the first two categories generally incorporate more traditional though useful applications of psychoanalytic or developmental theory, along with an emphasis on use of the therapist–patient attachment relationship; the latter two categories offer some relatively novel approaches that integrate cognitive with psychoanalytic and developmental theory, and generally de-emphasize therapist–patient attachment per se as a critical therapeutic tool, although they may nonetheless operate from an interpersonal stance.

The scope of this chapter prohibits a fuller elaboration of these categories of therapeutic work that are *implicitly* associated with mental representations. Of immediate interest are therapeutic models that focus *explicitly* on effecting change in representations through an interpersonally (either attachment-enactive or attachment-nonenactive) oriented therapy. Among the few models that give such attention to representations are the systematic work of Kelly (1955) and subsequent cognitive approaches to personal-construct change, as well as the attachment, psychoanalytic, and cognitive theories that pay attention to representational process as a interpersonal and empirical variable (e.g., Blatt, Wiseman, Prince-Gibson, & Gatt, 1991; Horowitz, 1988; Luborsky & Crits-Christoph, 1990). Notwithstanding the work cited above, specific discussions of dynamic psychotherapies that use mental representations as a *central* element in defining pathology, and that in addition focus therapy on correcting dysfunctional representations of attachment, appear only sporadically in the literature.

Bowlby (1988) is one of the few theorists or clinicians who has addressed the clinical implications of mental representations quite explicitly. With regard to representations of attachment, his perspective is quite compatible with a transference-based, insight-oriented therapy, while also including a cognitive component:

> A therapist applying attachment theory sees his role as being one of providing the conditions in which his patient can explore his representational models of himself and his attachment figures with a view to reappraising and restructuring them in the light of the new understanding he acquires and the new experiences he has in the therapeutic relationship. (p. 138)

Consistent with this, Bowlby described five main roles the therapist adopts toward the patient: providing a secure base; encouraging exploration of relationships and expectations with significant figures; encouraging examination of the relationship with the therapist; fostering consideration of how relational perceptions, expectations, feelings, and actions (i.e., working models) may be the products of parental experiences and expectations; and, finally, enabling the patient to recognize that these models may or may not be appropriate to present and future circumstances. This perspective is particularly consistent with psychoanalytic investigators who advocate a similar transferential–cognitive stance, particularly those presenting short-term dynamic models (e.g., Malan, 1963/1975; Strupp & Binder, 1984), although they do lack an explicit representational focus.

A formative recent contribution in the area of reassessing and reanalyzing representational constructions is that of West, Sheldon, and Reiffer (1989), who propose a model for brief psychotherapy that specifically integrates attachment and psychoanalytic theories. Their model uses cognitive and affective (principally transferential) means both to understand patients' mental representations of attachment figures and to modify them. Awareness of representations is conceptualized as coming first through analysis of the ways they are reflected in the relationship with the therapist (essentially, analyzing the transference), and then later through exploration of the relationship between the attachment to the therapist and early caretaking experiences. As described to this point, the West, et al. approach is quite consistent with other transference-based models of short-term dynamic psychotherapy; however, their representational focus, albeit through the transference, remains paramount and increasingly becomes a focus of intervention as the therapy progresses.

As a first step in revising mental representations, West et al. (1989) recommend examining the defensive operations that maintain them. Drawing upon Bowlby (1980), they consider the exclusion of attachment-relevant information to be the defensive operation most significant to the maintenance of dysfunctional representations of attachment, and thus to attachment-related interpersonal problems. According to their model, information gets excluded during the representational process because it causes pain; similar information continues to be excluded as the individual evaluates and internalizes subsequent experiences. For instance, they suggest that if attachment figures were consistently unavailable when needed, awareness of the need for attachment would be shut off, because the ongoing experience of not having the need met is too painful. Thus the principal transformative element in therapy becomes the recognition and acceptance of representations characterized by denied and dissociated feelings of anger, yearning, and loss relevant to attachment.

In the service of reassessing and adjusting representational models, it cannot escape notice that, as Bowlby (1969) asserted, "a special and unique feature of man's behavioural equipment is language. An obvious benefit it confers is that, instead of each one of us having to build his environmental and organismic models entirely for himself, he can draw on models built by others" (p. 83). Language in general, and narratives (both oral and written) in particular, provide a complex and uniquely human tool in the construction and reconstruction of relational representations, particularly those enduring representations that are formed subsequent to the onset of autobiographical memory at about age 4 (Nelson, 1991). Language also allows for representational models to be reified within an individual, and shared between individuals and over time (e.g., Schafer, 1983; Spence, 1982).

Although hermeneutic application of narrative construction has received much attention within nontherapeutic areas of psychology and related disciplines, the bridge between hermeneutic and therapeutic uses of narrative constructions about representations has received little direct attention. However, one such recent effort to apply narrative construction psychotherapeutically within a systems theory frame is a work by White and Epston (1990). Their discussion focuses on the interrelated triad of story (or narrative), knowledge (or known "truths"), and power (or interpersonal cybernetics), and its influence on representations. They view therapy from the assumption that

> persons experience problems, for which they frequently seek therapy, when the narratives in which they are "storying" their experience, and/ or in which they are having their experience "storied" by others, do not sufficiently represent their lived experience, and that, in these circumstances, there will be significant aspects of their lived experience that contradict these dominant narratives. (pp. 14-15)

So in their view, the discrepancy between lived experience and self- and/ or other-constructed storied experience (i.e., problematic assimilation in a Piagetian sense) is what creates the conflict that often leads a person to seek therapy. What they do not appear to account for is the fact that representations are not isomorphic summative conglomerations of lived experience, but are themselves metabolized constructions. White and Epston's (1990) suggestions for a psychotherapy organized around narrative/representational change are more paradigmatic than technical. They emphasize the sense of authorship and reauthorship in the retelling of one's lived experience, and invite "a reflexive posture and an appreciation of one's participation in interpretive acts" (p. 83).

A NONENACTIVE TRANSFERENTIAL CONSTRUCTION OF REPRESENTATIONAL CHANGE

To some extent, any psychotherapy model informed by psychoanalytic theory, and especially those informed by object relations, self psychology, and interpersonal orientations, attempts to effect some change in mental representations of significant attachments. For example, many object relations models target integration of part-object representations into internalized whole-object representations. Yet (as noted already), rarely is the emphasis on representations explicit, and even more rarely are technical considerations aimed specifically at this issue. The little extant discussion addressing representational or schematic change in an attachment/ interpersonal sphere operates within a transferential frame (e.g., Bowlby, 1988; Slap & Slap-Shelton, 1991; West et al., 1989). In other words, within psychoanalytic theory, analysis of the patient's transference toward the therapist is seen as the primary means of gaining access to representational models and of changing them. Although interpersonal theories sometimes make less explicit use of transference in clinical interventions in favor of the vicissitudes of the here-and-now therapeutic relationship, they are nonetheless usually organized around formulations about the patient from a transferential perspective. Within some cognitively based therapies (e.g., Greenberg & Beck, 1990; Kelly, 1955), there is more direct focus on changing representations or personal constructs; however, the adherence is principally to here-and-now understandings and behavioral– cognitive analysis, and there is very little direct focus on the complex interactions between past and present. Horowitz (1988) does suggest a theoretical integration of cognitive and psychoanalytic conceptualizations of representations with transferential considerations, labeling this resulting matrix "recurrent interpersonal relationship patterns" or "schemata," but he barely addresses psychotherapy strategies. Our clinical experience suggests that a useful area for further examination, and one that has not been adequately explored in the literature, is a dynamic psychotherapy organized directly around understanding and modifying representations, using an interpersonal but nonenactive transferential mode with regard to the therapeutic relationship.

In exploring such an approach, it is important to distinguish between applications of the concepts of "transference" and "representation." Many nuances of meaning have evolved for each term. Although when loosely defined and broadly applied they seem almost identical, and there certainly is much overlap between them, significant differences do emerge.

"Transference" is often used as a catchall phrase to refer to any transfer of memories, expectations, or affects about relationships from one situation to another; however, this loose understanding of the term does not accurately describe its theoretical and clinical significance. Within psychoanalytic theory, "transference" refers specifically to the re-enactment *within the therapeutic relationship* of derivatives of unconscious impulses that engendered early intrapsychic conflict as a result of their problematic external enactments (Dewald, 1971). The term is closely intertwined with theoretical and technical considerations concerning resistance to treatment, interpretation, and the development of a therapeutic alliance. A "representation" of attachment, in some contrast, is a summative construction of relational experiences and expectations, usually derived from several attachment sources. "Representations" develop and change over time as the interaction of ongoing intrapsychic and interpersonal experience gets processed through the "stereotype plates" (Freud, 1912/1958) concerning relationships that each person constructs from a combination of inborn characteristics and early relational experiences.

There are two important distinctions to be made between "transference" and "representation": (1) "Transference" usually refers to the enactment of a relational paradigm within the therapeutic relationship, whereas "representations" may be identified without their enactment in the therapy relationship; and (2) "transference" is used more often to link current relationships to early dyadic and triadic attachment models and experiences, whereas "representation" is used additionally to refer to both the conscious and unconscious anticipation of future outcomes, and the recursive effect that such anticipation has on the interpretation of past and present events. "Transference," then, except when used in the broadest sense to refer to any transposition of expectations from one situation or relationship to another, is a subcategory of representation that is "rooted in the building blocks of a script theory or a life-narrative theory of personality" (Singer & Singer, 1992, p. 533). Given this understanding, it becomes a plausible (though formidable) task to distinguish the patient's enactment of transference responses within the therapeutic relationship from his or her extratherapeutic representational responses.

Why might a nontransferential yet representational approach with regard to the therapeutic relationship be useful to examine? A compelling theoretical argument is that if (as suggested by the discussion above) transference is an enactive subset of a wider array of active representations, a therapist–patient transferential mode is often not necessary to achieve the therapeutic goals, and may divert attention away from or impede the examination and development of the capacity for change in representations (Singer & Singer, 1992). Pragmatically, it seems that dynamic psychotherapies are more often supportive than insight-oriented in nature, and therefore do not normally use the therapist–patient transference as a therapeutic tool. This may be attributable to constraints on session frequency, motivation, or patients' ability to tolerate the emotional intensity of the experience and the systematic analysis of transference and transference resistance.

The mode of dynamic psychotherapy being discussed in this chapter is ego-supportive with regard to the therapist–patient transference, and insight-oriented (or expressive) with regard to interpretation of extratherapeutic representations. As many have argued (e.g., Dewald, 1971; Rockland, 1989), an obvious caveat that needs to be made explicit is that inattention to therapist–patient transference does not mean that it is nonexistent; rather, it is not the focal point of intervention in working toward the goal of structural change. In fact, when a therapist works within an ego-supportive frame, although still within a technically neutral (i.e., insight-oriented) stance with regard to interpretation of representational enactments, transference responses toward the therapist are more likely to be diminished. However, a nontransferential mode with regard to the therapeutic relationship does not necessitate a dogmatically nonrepresentational mode within the therapeutic relation, in that the therapist interprets transferential responses when they arise as specific cases of larger representational patterns, rather than encouraging the transference to expand and become a target of intervention.

As with, for example, family therapies that operate from a general systems theory understanding, so too therapy operating from a representational stance is often less a matter of technique than of theoretical perspective. To put it another way, within this mode of psychotherapy theory *must* guide technique. The therapist of course makes use of psychoanalytic technical principles, which are the fundamental tools of any dynamic psychotherapy, but what the therapist does to be helpful with a patient is primarily a function of the theoretical sensibility he or she brings to the clinical situation. Therefore, a psychotherapy organized around an attachment-representational stance would vigilantly attend to the patient's report of current and past attachment experiences, attempting always to discern emergent representational patterns and the ways in which these patterns are used by the patient to give meaning to current events and the anticipation of future events; the overall goal, then, is the creation and reworking of a shared "story" for further examination.

In this therapeutic process, the therapist tries to guide the patient in constructing defining relational narratives that serve to clarify particularly meaningful and/or conflictual aspects of attachment experiences. This clarity comes in large part from allowing the patient to develop a more conscious awareness of the idiosyncratic rules and expectations that govern his or her representations, and to learn to use them as anticipatory markers against which new experiences can be compared and evaluated. The interpretive process thus takes on a somewhat psychoeducational quality, similar to that in many brief dynamic psychotherapies or cognitive therapies, as the therapist "narrates" interpretations in a full and recursive way that allows the patient increasingly to integrate and share this understanding of his or her representational patterns. The eventual therapeutic aim, synergistic in nature, is the modification of representations, which in turn affects the experience and processing of current interpersonal behavior, which then further modify representations. Ultimately, it is expected that this approach will make available to the patient an increased ability to engage in and consciously process new interpersonal experiences, along with a wider range of affects.

This emphasis on modifying representations directly, rather than indirectly through the medium of the transference, constitutes a clear and perhaps somewhat controversial departure from standard psychoanalytic technique. We discuss it not to be iconoclastic, but because of our experience of its clinical utility, as in this case example:

A 30-year-old married female, in twice-weekly psychotherapy for 11 months, had a long history of dependency in attachment relationships; enormous sensitivity to and reliance on tracking of interpersonal cues for self-definition; and difficulty in maintaining a job because of seemingly inevitable interpersonal difficulties. She presented as an individual for whom interpersonal reactions were rich and complicated, and as one who would very readily experience both positive and negative transference responses. It seemed to her therapist that analysis of these responses might iatrogenically consume the better part of a therapy; instead, her ongoing interpersonal distress might be more effectively ameliorated through a representational mode that maintained a focus on her broader extratherapeutic expectations and experiences of her attachment world.

Doing this involved critical choice points. For instance, many sessions were dominated by the patient's discussion of her sense of agitated hopelessness at getting the recognition she so wanted in close relationships, particularly with men. This content was understandable, given her abandonment by her father at a very young age, and her ongoing (fruitless) search for unconditional paternal affection. After having ended one of these sessions by discussing her discomfort with not being able to easily track the therapist's feelings toward her, she began the next session by invoking the metaphor of keeping the closet door closed on her "monsters" (i.e., conflictual internal attachment objects) rather than letting them out and wrestling with them. At this point, the therapist might have productively interpreted a current "monster" as himself, focusing on the struggle to trust and engage with such an enigmatic figure. Instead, he commented that for the patient to allow herself to reconnect with these already too familiar monsters might be a frightening and confusing experience. In pursuing this interpretation, the therapist explicitly began to narrate her active efforts at delimiting access to the monsters (i.e., disallowing examination of her troubling early family attachments) as reflecting a defensive representational pattern. It was also acknowledged that this pattern had been so overlearned and internalized that it would seem overwhelming now to contemplate letting the monsters out, thereby allowing full access to the affective context of the attachments. This narrative interpretation of the defense against experiencing conflictual early attachments was then restated and reworked several times in the ensuing discussion until the patient understood and began to narrate it herself, as well as apply it to other current interpersonal experiences.

The following session, the patient reported having had variations on two recurrent dreams, both apparently reflecting the "monster control" representational issue: In the first, she suddenly found herself unclothed in a shopping mall and frantically running for cover; in the second, she was being chased and physically threatened by a large man. In this second dream, however, in contrast to her usual passive approach to resolving interpersonal conflict, at one point she turned and began to attack back, only then to shrink down and pass through a small window to escape. Again, these dreams could potentially be used in the service of transference analysis, perhaps around the image of the therapist as a pursuing aggressor and her vulnerability to him. Such an approach might lead eventually to larger representational issues. The dreams were immediately discussed instead with an explicit representational focus organized around her extratherapeutic experience of close male figures as offering wished-for yet threatening contact, and her ongoing regulation of "exposing" herself to this threat.

A marker of positive response to such a representationally focused treatment is the ability to narrate and independently invoke reconstructed representations. This process should promote both increased interpersonal comfort and functional gains, allowing for representational analysis to be consciously applied to new interpersonal experiences. For this patient, the approach has proved useful in both her marital and work relationships: She has begun to experience more adult-like gratifications, rather than largely reifying earlier representations and their associated fears and attributions.

Another case, of relatively short-term dynamic psychotherapy, illustrates a situation where a transferential focus would have been too stressful for the patient:

A 40-year-old single woman presented with a childhood history of an alternately caring and physically abusive alcoholic father, and an emotionally rejecting and often physically unavailable mother. Up until the time she presented for treatment, the patient's adult life had been characterized by avoidance and fear of emotionally intimate relationships. This manifested itself both in extreme social isolation and in an inability to take committed action that would lead to a stable and satisfying career. She came to treatment because of her perceived inability to make changes in her rigid and unsatisfying personal and professional lives.

It quickly became clear in treatment that although many transferential issues emerged, working directly with them was intolerable to this patient. She consistently refused to consider transferential implications of relational events, and denied any but the most warm and affectionate feelings for the therapist. Any attempts at further examining some of the feelings that arose toward the therapist were rejected. Thus, for example, transferential interpretation of anger expressed not with words but with tone of voice, or analysis of projections such as immediately assuming that the therapist was very angry when a misunderstanding led the patient to show up 20 minutes late for the first session, were rejected. The patient steadfastly denied that any of her projections onto the therapist reflected anything but a consensual view of reality, apparent to all the world. In addition, the patient initially expressed great relief in knowing of the time limitations on treatment, and thanked the therapist profusely for telling her.

Given what was known of this patient's past history and current functioning, events such as the ones described were taken as indications that for her it was important to maintain a perception of control over the setting and to set clear limits on the dose of intimacy to be experienced with the therapist. The question became how to work within these restrictions in a way that would lay the groundwork for their eventual modification, while also facilitating a useful treatment outcome within the time period allotted for this treatment. It was clear that the therapist could easily have spent much of the 7 months of treatment working with the patient's resistance to examining transferential elements within the therapeutic relationship, particularly those elements relating to the patient's representations of attachment. However, it also seemed clear that given the patient's resistance to that kind of work, as well as the time limitations on treatment, this might accomplish very little. Therefore, the therapist decided early to put transference issues on a back burner. They were not ignored, however. The therapist tracked transference manifestations carefully, and used them for herself as markers of change and indicators of problematic representations. Transferential issues were occasionally introduced in sessions, in an attempt to test whether the patient could tolerate and work with them. However, they were not the prime focus of sessions; the focus with the patient became her functioning outside of the treatment situation.

Notwithstanding her vigilant defenses against awareness of the apparently considerable transference responses she experienced, the patient brought in rich material concerning her extratherapeutic interpersonal and intrapsychic experiences. In examining these experiences, she was able both to acknowledge patterns of relating to others and to see them as manifestations of enduring representations of attachment; she also gained some understanding of the genetic origins of these representations, as well as of the ongoing and self-perpetuating influence they exerted on her processing of experience. In gradually understanding the origins and function of her need to control the dosage of intimacy in relationships, she came to recognize her characteristic style of nonaction, the self-protective function it served, and the way in which it was maintained by the anticipation of negative outcomes in both interpersonal and professional situations. She was then able to see how taking any steps whose probable outcome was not easily expectable and controllable led her to quickly reject opportunities for intimacy and change. This process led eventually to understanding of how her need to control intimacy often resulted in her seeking intimacy with unavailable partners, and to connect these patterns with the recursive influence of enduring representations formed through her early attachment experiences. By the end of the 7-month treatment period, the patient was beginning to seek out and form more adaptive relationships; she was also beginning to plan some changes in her professional life, the mere contemplation of which at the start of therapy had created unbearable levels of anxiety.

Part of the process of change for this patient also involved a shift in the ways that she narrated her life history. At the beginning of treatment, she found it difficult to give a coherent account of either who she was or how she got that way. As she began in therapy to integrate the experiential parts of her life and personality, she also began to narrate a more coherent biographical story. With that ability, she became more able to see herself as the author of the yet-to-be-lived part of her biography. Furthermore, she was increasingly able to see herself as having options in the enactment of her story.

In the two clinical examples presented, the positive response to working within a representational but nonenactive transferential mode was apparent from the eventual symptomatic relief and functional changes initiated by the patients. As we have attempted to discuss conceptually and clinically, such an approach has proven very useful under certain conditions with certain patients. Our current research within this area aims to expand upon this initial work in addressing some important technical and outcome questions. For example, are the changes effected in working nontransferentially toward representational change as potentially comprehensive and enduring as might be accomplished by working within the transference enactments? At what level does change occur—characterological, defensive realignment, symptom masking, or other nonspecific factors not directly attributable to this mode of work? What adjustments in psychodynamic technique, in addition to the narrative interpretive focus away from transference enactments, need to be made? What are the differential indicators that would allow a therapist to decide during early treatment sessions which mode is likely to be most effective? We have suggested some responses to these questions; we hope to be able to answer them more systematically as our efforts, and those of other investigators in integrating attachment-representational theory and dynamic psychotherapy, continue.

ACKNOWLEDGMENTS

Preparation of this chapter was supported in part by a Grant-in-Aid from Fairleigh Dickinson University. An earlier version of this work was presented at the 100th Annual Convention of the American Psychological Association, Washington, DC, August 1992.

REFERENCES

Bartlett, F. C. (1932). *Remembering: A study in experimental and social psychology.* Cambridge, England: Cambridge University Press.

Beck, A. T., Rush, A. J., Shaw, B. F., & Emery, G. (1979). *Cognitive therapy of depression.* New York: Guilford Press.

Beres, D., & Joseph, E. D. (1970). The concept of mental representation in psychoanalysis. *International Journal of Psycho-Analysis, 51,* 1-9.

Blatt, S. J., Wiseman, H., Prince-Gibson, E., & Gatt, C. (1991). Object representations and change in clinical functioning. *Psychotherapy, 28,* 273-283.

Bowlby, J. (1969). *Attachment and loss: Vol. 1. Attachment.* New York: Basic Books.

Bowlby, J. (1980). *Attachment and loss: Vol. 3. Loss: Sadness and depression.* New York: Basic Books.

Bowlby, J. (1988). *A secure base: Parent–child attachment and healthy human development.* New York: Basic Books.

Byng-Hall, J. (1988). Scripts and legends in families and family therapy. *Family Process, 27,* 167-179.

Byng-Hall, J. (1991). The application of attachment theory to understanding and treatment in family therapy. In C. M. Parkes, J. Stevenson-Hinde, & P. Marris (Eds.), *Attachment across the life cycle* (pp. 199-215). London: Routledge & Kegan Paul.

Dewald, P. A. (1971). *Psychotherapy: A dynamic approach* (2nd ed.). New York: Basic Books.

Freud, S. (1958). The dynamics of transference. In J. Strachey (Ed. and Trans.), *The standard edition of the complete psychological works of Sigmund Freud* (Vol. 12, pp. 97-108). London: Hogarth Press. (Original work published 1912)

Fogarty, T. F. (1976). Systems concepts and the dimensions of self. In P. J. Guerin (Ed.), *Family therapy: Theory and practice* (pp. 144-153). New York: Gardner Press.

Fraiberg, S. (1969). Object constancy and mental representation. *Psychoanalytic Study of the Child, 24,* 9-47.

Greenberg, M. S., & Beck, A. T. (1990). Cognitive approaches to psychotherapy: Theory and therapy. In R. Plutchik & H. Kellerman (Eds.), *Emotion: Theory, research, and experience. Vol. 5: Emotion, psychopathology, and psychotherapy* (pp. 177-194). San Diego: Academic Press.

Heard, D. (1982). Family systems and the attachment dynamic. *Journal of Family Therapy, 4,* 99-116.

Horowitz, M. J. (1988). *Introduction to psychodynamics: A new synthesis.* New York: Basic Books.

Horowitz, M. J. (Ed.). (1991). *Person schemas and maladaptive interpersonal patterns.* Chicago: University of Chicago Press.

Jacobson, E. (1964). *The self and the object world.* New York: International Universities Press.

Kelly, G. A. (1955). *The psychology of personal constructs* (Vols. 1 and 2). New York: Norton.

Kernberg, O. (1976). *Object relations theory and clinical psychoanalysis.* New York: Jason Aronson.

Luborsky, L., & Crits-Christoph, P. (1990). *Understanding transference: The CCRT method.* New York: Basic Books.

Luborsky, L., Crits-Christoph, P., Friedman, S. H., Mark, D., & Schaffler, P. (1991). Freud's transference template compared with the core conflictual relationship theme (CCRT): Illustrated by the two specimen cases. In M. J. Horowitz (Ed.), *Person schemas and maladaptive interpersonal patterns* (pp. 167-195). Chicago: University of Chicago Press.

Mahler, M., Pine, F., & Bergman, A. (1975). *The psychological birth of the human infant.* New York: Basic Books.

Main, M., Kaplan, N., & Cassidy, J. (1985). Security in infancy, childhood, and adulthood: A move to the level of representation. In I. Bretherton & E. Waters (Eds.), Growing points of attachment theory and research. *Monographs of the Society for Research in Child Development, 50*(1-2, Serial No. 209), 66-104.

Malan, D. H. (1975). *A study of brief psychotherapy.* New York: Plenum. (Original work published 1963)

Nelson, K. (1991, April). *Emergence of autobiographical memory at age 4.* Paper presented at the biennial meeting of the Society for Research in Child Development, Seattle.

Piaget, J. (1955). *The language and thought of the child.* New York: Harcourt, Brace.

Rockland, L. H. (1989). *Supportive therapy: A psychodynamic approach.* New York: Basic Books.

Sandler, J., & Rosenblatt, B. (1962). The concept of the representational world. *Psychoanalytic Study of the Child, 17,* 128-145.

Schafer, R. (1983). *The analytic attitude.* New York: Basic Books.

Schafer, R. (1990). *Aspects of internalization.* Madison, CT: International Universities Press. (Original work published 1968)

Singer, J. L., & Salovey, P. (1991). Organized knowledge structures and personality: Person schemas, self schemas, prototypes, and scripts. In M. Horowitz (Ed.), *Person schemas and maladaptive interpersonal patterns* (pp. 33-79). Chicago: University of Chicago Press.

Singer, J. A., & Singer, J. L. (1992). Transference in psychotherapy and daily life: Implications of current memory and social cognition research. In J. W. Barron, M. N. Eagle, & D. L. Wolitzky (Eds.), *Interface of psychoanalysis and psychology* (pp. 516-538). Washington, DC: American Psychological Association.

Slap, J., & Slap-Shelton, L. (1991). *The schema in clinical psychoanalysis.* Hillsdale, NJ: Analytic Press.

Spence, D. P. (1982). *Narrative truth and historical truth: Meaning and interpretation in psychoanalysis.* New York: Norton.

Sperling, M. B., & Lyons, L. (1994). *Mental representations and psychotherapeutic change: An integrative review of clinical process strategies.* Unpublished manuscript, Fairleigh Dickinson University.

Stern, D. N. (1985). *The interpersonal world of the infant.* New York: Basic Books.

Stern, D. N. (1988). The dialectic between the "interpersonal" and the "intrapsychic": With particular emphasis on the role of memory and representation. *Psychoanalytic Inquiry, 8,* 503-512.

Strupp, H. H., & Binder, J. L. (1984). *Psychotherapy in a new key: A guide to time-limited dynamic psychotherapy.* New York: Basic Books.

West, M., Sheldon, A., & Reiffer, L. (1989). Attachment theory and brief psychotherapy: Applying current research to clinical interventions. *Canadian Journal of Psychiatry, 34,* 369-374.

White, M., & Epston, D. (1990). *Narrative means to therapeutic ends.* New York: Norton.

Index